J. Chermet J. M. Bigot

Venography of the Inferior Vena Cava and Its Branches

Translated by M.-T. Wackenheim

With 243 Figures in 323 Separate Illustrations

Springer-Verlag
Berlin Heidelberg New York 1980

Jacques Chermet
Professeur Agrégé, Radiologiste des Hôpitaux
Service de Radiologie (Professeur J. Chalut), Hôpital Saint-Antoine
184, rue du Faubourg St-Antoine, F-75012 Paris

Jean-Michel Bigot
Professeur Agrégé, Radiologiste des Hôpitaux
Chef du Service de Radiologie, Hôpital Tenon
4, rue de la Chine, F-75020 Paris

Translator Marie-Therese Wackenheim
Institut de Radiologie, Université de Strasbourg
11, rue Humann, F-67085 Strasbourg Cedex

The cover design shows Fig. 4.36b, page 76

ISBN-13: 978-3-642-67581-2   e-ISBN-13: 978-3-642-67579-9
DOI: 10.1007/978-3-642-67579-9

Library of Congress Cataloging in Publication Data. Chermet, J. 1941– Venography of the inferior vena cava and its branches. Includes bibliographical references and index 1 Vena cava – Radiography. 2 Veins – Radiography. I. Bigot, Jean-Michel, 1935–. joint author. II Title. [DNLM: 1. Vena cava, Inferior – Radiography 2 Phlebography WG625 V3 C521v] RC695 C46 616 1'4'07572 80-132

Softcover reprint of the hardcover 1st edition 1980

Contents

Chapter 8. Inferior Vena Cavography in Hepatic and Intraperitoneal Diseases

Chapter 9. Renal Venography

List of Contributors

A. Chatel
Chef de Clinique Assistant, Service de Radiologie
Hôpital Tenon, 4, rue de la Chine, F-75020 Paris

F. Joffre
Professeur Agrégé, Radiologiste des Hôpitaux
Service central de Radiologie, Hôpital Rangueil, chemin du Vallon, F-31054 Toulouse

E. Kieffer
Professeur Agrégé, Chirurgien des Hôpitaux
Service de Chirurgie Vasculaire, Hôpital de la Salpétrière, 47, Bd de l'Hôpital
F-75634 Paris Cedex 13

J.P. Monnier
Professeur Agrégé, Radiologiste des Hôpitaux
Service de Radiologie, Hôpital St-Antoine 184, rue du Faubourg St-Antoine
F-75012 Paris

J. Théron
Professeur Agrégé, Radiologiste des Hôpitaux
Chef du Service de Neuroradiologie, Centre Hospitalier Clémenceau, F-14000 Caen

J.M. Tubiana
Chef de Clinique Assistant, Service de Radiologie
Hôpital St-Antoine, 184, rue du Faubourg St-Antoine, F-75012 Paris

Chapter 1. Techniques of Angiographic Investigation of the Inferior Vena Cava

Opacification of the inferior vena cava may be obtained by approach either from below, the bifemoral route being best, or from above through a vein of the upper limb. Isotopic angiography is not dealt with here.

1.1 Cavography by Percutaneous Bifemoral Approach

This is the method of choice and allows an excellent opacification of the inferior vena cava, quickly and easily obtained by bilateral catheterization of the common femoral veins. It is thus an iliocavography.

The patient is placed supine. Scarpa's triangle is disinfected and the femoral vein is located: it is usually midway between the pubic symphysis and the anterosuperior iliac spine, 1 cm medial to the artery. The vein is punctured 2 to 3 cm below the inguinal ligament.

Usually gauge 16 or 18 needles are employed, either metal ones with a shelf (Seldinger type), or with a Teflon catheter. After removal of the stylet, gradual withdrawal of the needle produces a slight dripping of venous blood when its tip is situated in the venous lumen. The dripping may be more or less copious and will be clearly increased while the patient is instructed to perform Valsalva's maneuver. When the dripping is poor, aspiration with a syringe is performed in order to determine when accurate intraluminal placement of the needle is attained. Then the femoral vein is catheterized over a few centimeters with the aid of a flexible guide wire. The correct placement of the needle is always checked fluoroscopically: a rapid injection of contrast medium allows one to check the patency of the vein and the correct position of the catheter, i.e., intraluminal and in the iliofemoral axis. Then the needles are firmly fixed onto the skin. The contrast medium delivery is adapted to the patency or nonpatency of the iliac veins. The needles are connected via a Y-connector to the syringe. Before injecting, it is necessary to verify if reflux occurs in the tubing. The commonly used contrast medium contains 38 mg iodine/ml.

In adults 70 to 80 ml is injected, at 35 ml/s. When only one femoral vein is punctured, only half the amount of contrast medium is used. Some employ an opaque embolus pulsated by the serum.

X-ray pictures are taken from the very beginning of injection; their timing must take into account the extreme rapidity with which the contrast medium passes up the inferior vena cava when the latter is patent, and its marked slowing down as soon as the vein is compressed. Thus, when the vena cava seems fluoroscopically normal, X-ray pictures are taken at 2 to 3 per second for 6 s. When the aorta is to be demonstrated, a pause of 6 to 7 s is followed by additional films at 1 per second for another 3 s. The investigation is always terminated with a roentgenogram of the urinary tract.

Two small transparent polyethylene catheters, most often gauge 7 F with side holes, may be used in a bilateral iliocavography. The catheters are placed according to the Seldinger technique into the external iliac veins, 2 to 3 cm above the inguinal ligament. This technique has the advantage of allowing cavography in both the supine and the prone position, with almost no risk of extravasation during injection in the prone position. Besides, use of a small catheter with side holes prevents the Venturi effect, which produces, at the beginning of the injection, the appearance of a stenosis of the external iliac vein, an artifact dealt with in more detail later. The only drawback of this technique employing catheterization is the risk of venous catheterism, i.e., phlebitis, although this is rather rare.

Transtrochanteral iliocavography is dealt with in Chapter 13.

Roentgenograms are taken in frontal, lateral, and sometimes left anterior oblique projections. Two projections are essential for study of the sometimes quite complex displacements. The diagnostic accuracy of cavography is directly dependent on this technique using two projections together. When equipment allowing projections in two planes is available, the films are taken in one phase during the injection; when there is only one seriograph, however, a frontal projection is first taken and then a lateral projection.

The left anterior oblique projection makes it possible to distinguish the posterior aspect of the inferior vena cava from the spine. The lateral projection, with horizontal beam, may be of interest in some cases to demonstrate invasion and/or compression of the anterior aspect of the inferior vena cava in its retroduodenopancreatic portion by a possible neoplasm. The supine position may be responsible for a layering phenomenon when the injection is too slow. The image may then resemble an extrinsic compression of the anterior aspect of the vena cava (Fig. 1.1a and b).

The centering of the X-ray pictures depends on the area to be studied: When the disease is thought to involve the origin of the inferior vena cava, the roentgenogram is centered on L5. On the other hand, when the disease is suspected to affect its termination, the roentgenogram must include the right atrium – 4 cm above the diaphragm (Fig. 1.2). In a medium-sized subject the usual 35 × 35 cm seriographs allow visualization from the cavosuprahepatic confluence to the external iliac veins. Valsalva's maneuver produces a reflux into the large collateral branches (Fig. 1.3).

1.2 Cavography by Percutaneous Unifemoral Approach

Opacification of the inferior vena cava may be achieved by catheterization of one femoral vein, but the opacification will be poor owing to the flow of nonopaque blood from the contralateral common iliac vein. A venous tourniquet may avert this phenomenon. Unifemoral percutaneous cavography is usually performed, however, when the other side is occluded and there is consequently no diluting flow entering at the bifurcation. For this technique 40 to 50 ml contrast medium is injected at 18 ml/s.

1.3 Retrograde Iliac Venography

Rather than being a specific technique for study of the inferior vena cava, retrograde iliac venography is complementary to phlebography of the lower extremity. It can be used to demonstrate the upper level of an iliofemoral thrombus. The homolateral iliac vein is opacified from above by contralateral venous catheterization using the Seldinger method. The rapidly injected contrast medium outlines the head of the thrombus. Further developments of this technique are studied in Chapter 4.

1.4 Cavography with Intracaval Catheter – Retrograde Femoral Approach

The catheter is inserted into the supra- or infrarenal inferior vena cava through one of the femoral veins according to the Seldinger technique. Usually a catheter with side holes is used which allows rapid injection: 25 to 30 ml/s. The side holes permit uniform opacification of the inferior vena cava. This technique may be helpful as a complementary method in demonstrating obstruction or nonobstruction of the suprarenal inferior vena cava, for example, in cases of apparent or pseudo-obstruction caused by extrinsic compression (Fig. 1.1c and d).

This technique is not, however, to be employed as a routine method, since it could fail to demonstrate congenital anomalies of the inferior vena cava. Bifemoral percutaneous iliocavography remains the basic technique. Retrograde femoral catheterization (Seldinger technique) carries the risk of iatrogenic thromboses; these seem seldom to occur, except in some cavographies in patients with retroperitoneal ganglionic sarcomas.

1.5 Cavography with Intracaval Catheter – Anterograde Approach

Descending retrograde cavography may be additionally performed when a femoral approach either is impossible or has provided insufficient morphologic data (Fig. 1.4). A catheter with side holes is inserted into a vein in the bend of the elbow with the help of an introducer (Desilets). Much less frequently the subclavian or even the internal jugular vein is catheterized. The technique is often used to determine the upper level of obstruction in iliocaval phlebitis, in which case the catheter is positioned in the interrenal portion of the inferior vena cava. The use of this technique in cases of obstruction is dealt with in detail in Chapter 4. The anterograde approach also makes it fairly easy to catheterize some collaterals of the vena cava, such as the suprahepatic veins, which often enter the inferior vena cava obliquely from below.

1.6 Occlusive Cavography

Occlusive cavography is rather rarely employed in investigation of the inferior vena cava, but more often in the study of its collateral branches. It is at present mostly performed for selective catheterization of the inferior vena cava collaterals. It gained new interest with the introduction of the catheters with small balloons.

1.6.1 Uniocclusive Cavography

A catheter with a single balloon is used, the balloon being large enough in diameter to obstruct the trunk of the inferior vena cava. The balloon is inflated with saline solution and a small amount of contrast medium so as to render it radiopaque. The catheter is positioned at the desired level either in the retrohepatic or in the infrarenal vena cava. This is achieved either via the upper descending route or via the retrograde femoral route, depending on the level to be opacified.

The upper approach allows one to obtain excellent reflux into the subjacent branches of the inferior vena cava and thus to demonstrate the iliac and hypogastric axes (up to the first valve). This method provides complementary data for study of iliocaval phlebitis and visualization of the upper level of the thrombus. Ascending occlusive cavography by the femoral route has rare indications. Some use a balloon distal to the farthest hole of the catheter, so as to produce subjacent, instead of suprajacent, opacification.

1.6.2 Biocclusive Cavography

This technique has been described by Gillot; it necessitates general anesthesia, aseptic precautions, and denudation of the arch of the saphenous vein. A catheter with two small balloons 8 cm apart is inserted into the venous lumen up to the desired level. Both balloons are inflated with saline solution, and 10 ml contrast material is injected between the balloons in about 10 s. The technique consists in opacification of the vena cava collaterals located between the occlusions produced by the two balloons, and it is used for study of the renal veins. It has also been proposed for studying the suprahepatic veins, by inflating the upper balloon in the right atrium, and for the follow-up of therapeutic portocaval shunts. Actually, this technique is hardly ever used, since it is far from harmless and enough data are provided by the previously mentioned techniques for therapeutic indications to be decided.

1.7 Carboxyangiography

Carboxyangiography is a vascular exploration method using carbon dioxide gas injected into a peripheral vein as contrast medium. It was used in man for the first time in 1956. It permits exploration of the right atrial wall, and, with a larger amount of gas contrast medium, of the suprahepatic veins and portocaval, truncal, and radicular anastomoses. This method is performed, then, for study of the right side of the heart, but as concerns the inferior vena cava, it is also used in investigating the pathology of the suprahepatic veins and for postsurgical angiography of portocaval shunts. We have no personal experience with this technique.

1.8 Contraindications for Bifemoral Cavography

There are scarcely any contraindications for bifemoral cavography. Hypersensitivity to iodinated contrast material is very rarely encountered in angiography with premedication. If need be, premedication with corticoids or even epsilon-aminocaproic acid could be given the day before and just prior to the examination.

1.9 Complications of Bifemoral Cavography

When the usual aseptic precautions have been taken, complications are rare. It may happen that the artery is punctured while the femoral vein is being located, in which case a few minutes' compression will suffice. Extravasation of contrast material may occur (Fig. 1.5). If the tip of the needle or of the catheter becomes wedged into the wall of the vessel, intraparietal extravasation may occur at that point. Fluoroscopic control of the correct intraluminal position of the catheter helps to avoid this complication. However, it usually has no consequence beyond the pain experienced by the patient for about 10 min. Rupture of the vessel during injection is quite exceptional and should never occur. Air embolism can only be due to a mistake during the filling of the syringe. Phlebitis is not an uncommon phenomenon. Some diseases that produce vena cava compression predispose to phlebothrombosis. The contrast medium is thought to irritate the venous walls; thus, when there exists partial thrombosis or marked compression of the inferior vena cava, with resulting contrast stasis on the last films, it is recommended to inject physiologic saline solution with heparin rapidly into both femoral veins.

References

Bendib M, Toumi M, Boudjellab A (1975) La carboxyangiographie élargie. Traité de radiodiagnostic. Masson, Paris, pp 431–445

Bigot JM, Monnier J-P, Chermet J (1973) Techniques d'exploration radiologique de la veine cave inférieure. Encycl Méd Chir Paris (Radiodiagnostic) 4:1–10

Crummy AB, Jr, Hipona FA (1964) Aortic impression in inferior vena cavography. Clin Radiology 15:130–132

Doppmann J, Foley HT, Hammond W (1967) Inferior vena caval compression: The pseudo-obstruction syndrome. AJR 100:411–413

Farinas PL (1947) Abdominal venography. Roentgenology 58/599–601

Ferris EJ, Hipona FA, Kahn PC, Philipps E, Shapiro JH (1969) Venography of the inferior vena cava and its branches, Williams & Wilkins, Baltimore, pp 33–52

Gabriele OF, Bell D, Martineau R (1967) Pitfalls in inferior vena cavography. AJR 100:417–420

Hayt DB (1966) Upright inferior vena cavography. Radiology 86:865–870

Helander CG, Lindbom A (1959) Venography of the inferior vena cava. Acta Radiol 52:257–259

Kaufman JJ, Burke DE (1956) Abdominal venography; technique of roentgen visualization of the inferior vena cava. AJR 76:807–809

Monnier J-P, Chermet J (1978) Guide pratique de radiologie vasculaire, Masson, Paris

Paupy F, Viallet JF (1976) Iliocavographie rétrograde. Phlébographie 29: 251–256

Ranniger K, Siortz DM (1965) Local obstruction of the inferior vena cava by massive ascites. AJR 93:935–937

Wexler L, Bergel DH, Gabe IT, Makin GS, Miles C (1968) Velocity of blood flow in normal human venae cavae. Circ Res 23:349–350

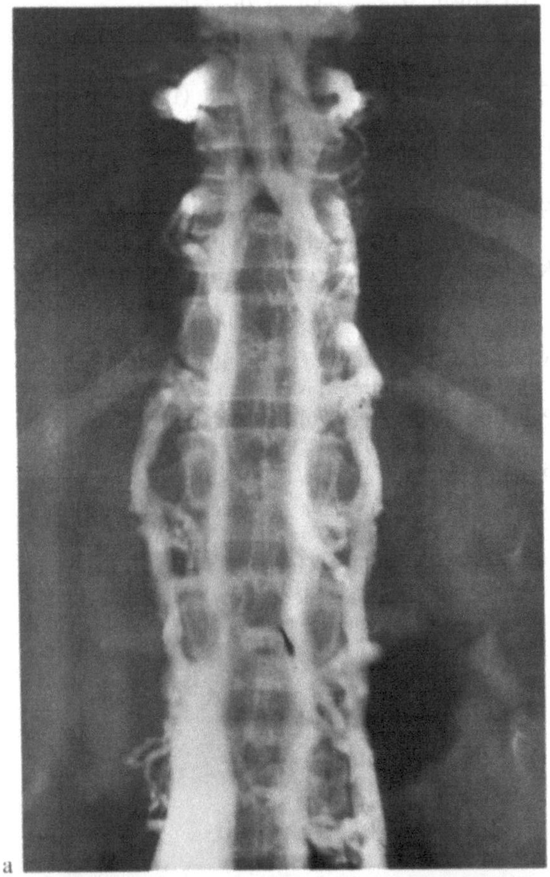

1.1a

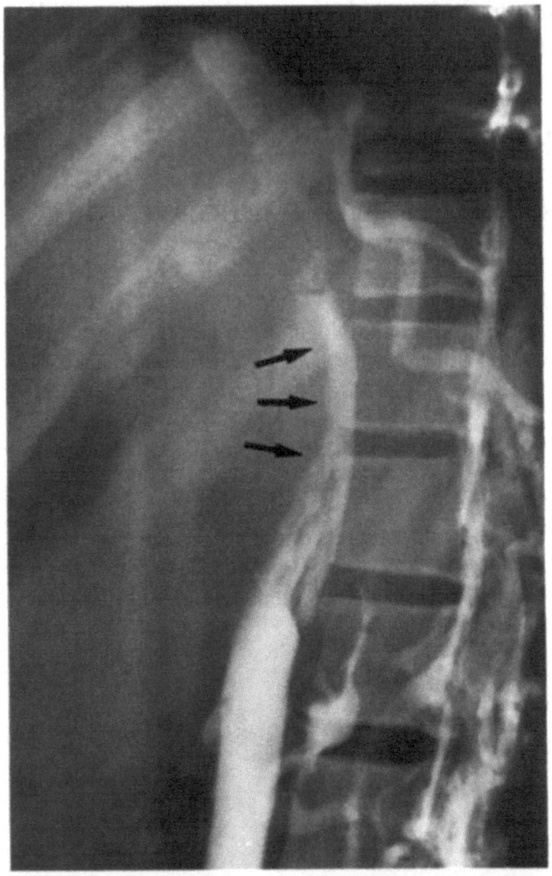

1.1b

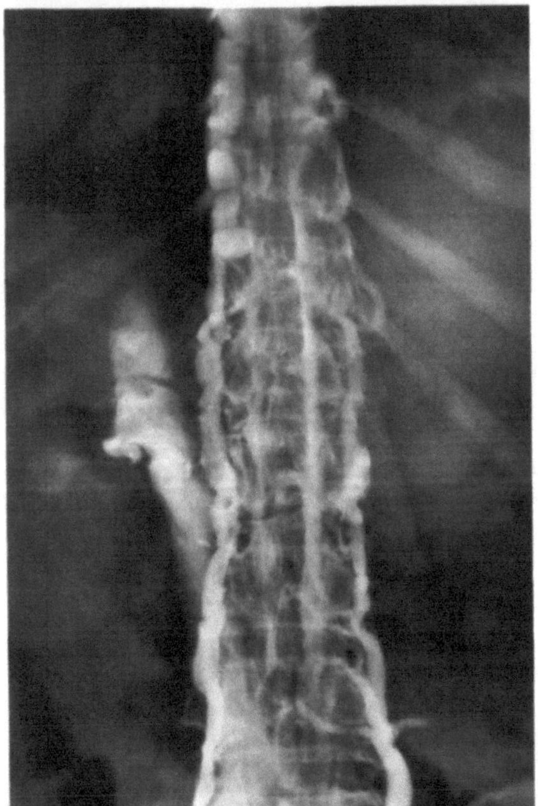

1.1c

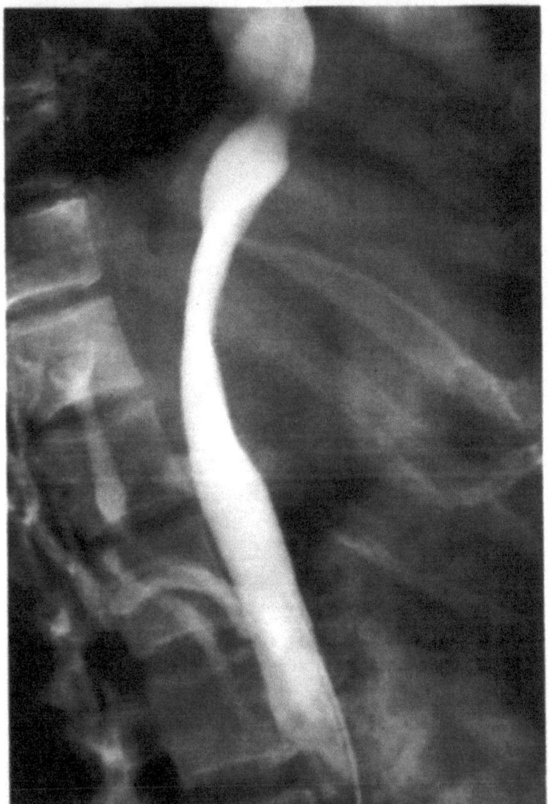

1.1d

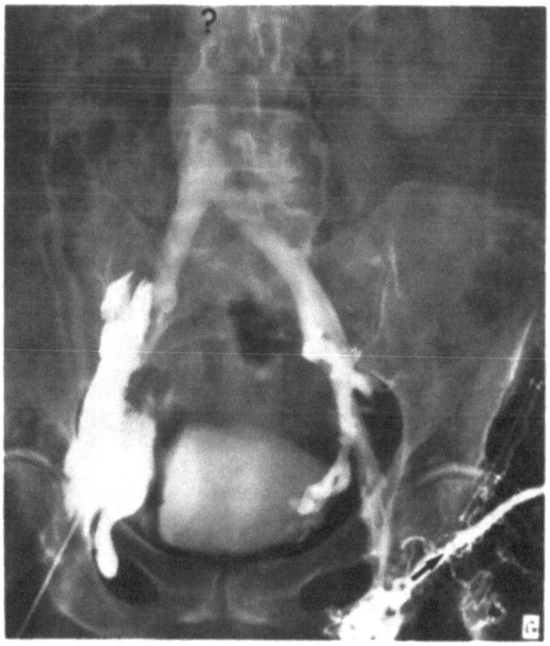

a

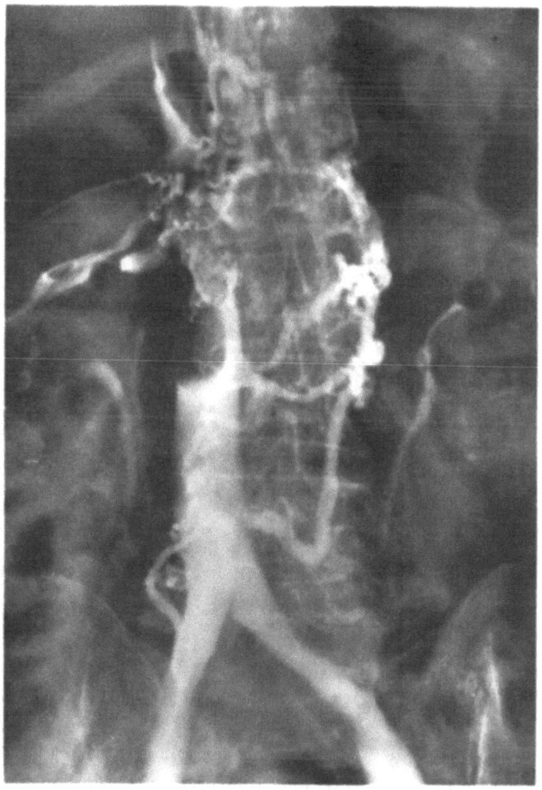

b

Fig. 1.2. a Bilateral percutaneous cavography. Injection into a superficial branch on the left with slight left iliac opacification (↗). Extravasation of the contrast medium on the right. The opacification of the inferior vena cava is not sufficient for conclusive diagnosis. The inter- and suprarenal segments of the inferior vena cava are not displayed (?). b Cavography centered higher up. Carcinoma of the right kidney with intracaval thrombus extending up to the right atrium. Postmortem confirmed the presence of thrombosis of the inter- and suprarenal segments of the vena cava, extending up to the right atrium. These two films prove the absolute necessity of obtaining a picture centered on the entire iliocaval axis, from the iliofemoral system up to the inferior aspect of the right atrium

---

◁ Fig. 1.1. a Bifemoral percutaneous cavography, frontal projection. Thrombosis of the inter- and suprarenal segment of the inferior vena cava. Drainage through the azygos system. b The usefulness of a lateral projection with horizontal beam is here apparent: the suprarenal segment of the inferior vena cava is not obstructed but markedly compressed by a hepatic mass (↗). c Other patient: The retrohepatic segment of the vena cava fails to opacify. Drainage through the azygos system. d Same patient as c, injection with intra-caval catheter in the retrohepatic segment of the inferior vena cava: no obstruction, it was only compression

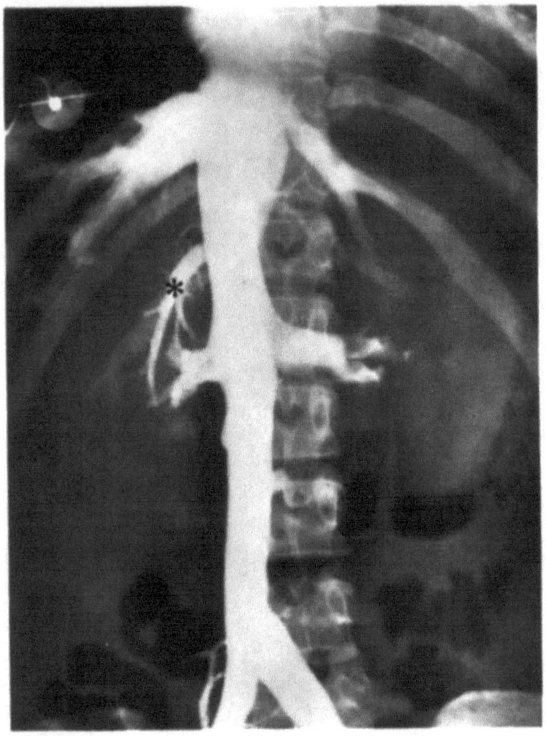

Fig. 1.3. Bifemoral percutaneous cavography. The examination is performed after Valsalva's maneuver has been correctly carried out. Normal aspect of the trunk of the inferior vena cava up to the right atrium. Right and left suprahepatic reflux. Accessory suprahepatic reflux (*). Right and left renal reflux

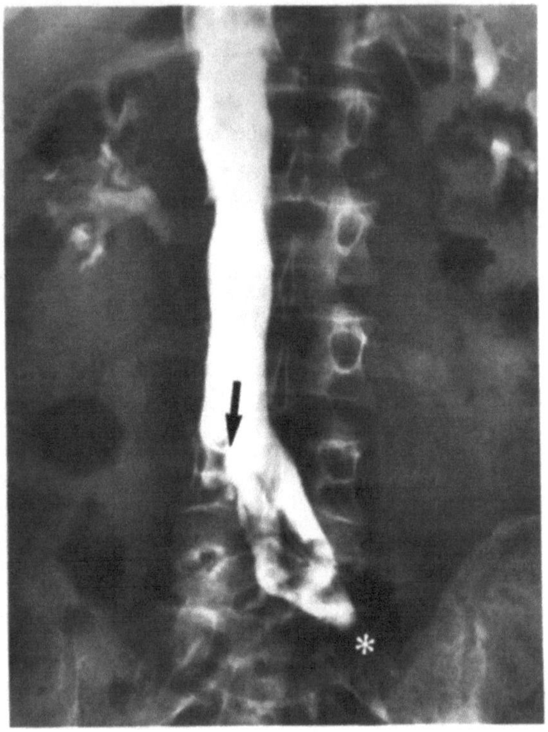

Fig. 1.4. Descending cavography with intracaval catheter (↓). The catheter is of the "pigtail" type. The suprarenal segment of the inferior vena cava is patent. Obstruction of the right iliac vein. Duplication of the left primary iliac system with obstruction of the left external iliac vein (*). Additional investigations are necessary to ascertain precisely the upper level of the thrombus in bilateral iliac phlebitis

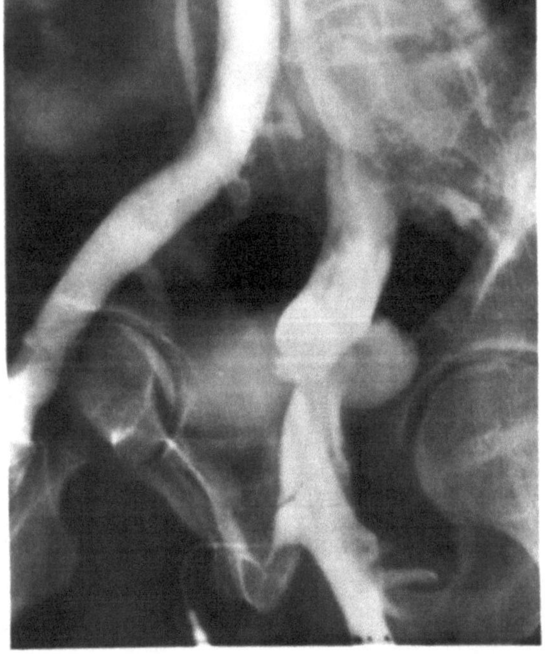

Fig. 1.5. Bifemoral percutaneous cavography. A left anterior oblique view shows extravasation of the contrast medium at the level of the femoral vein. The injection was both intra- and extraparietal

Chapter 2. Radioanatomy of the Inferior Vena Cava Pitfalls in Interpretation

2.1 Anatomy

A thorough knowledge of the course and anatomic relations of the inferior vena cava is essential if one is to understand the effect on it of neighboring pathologic conditions.

2.1.1 Course (Fig. 2.1 and 2.2a)

At the level of the inguinal ligament, the femoral vein becomes the external iliac vein. The latter joins with the internal iliac vein to form the common iliac vein. The two common iliac veins unite at the level of the fifth lumbar vertebra, slightly to the right of the midline. The right common iliac vein has a more vertical course and is shorter than the left. It ascends behind, and then lateral to, its artery. The left common iliac vein usually lies behind its artery at the level of its origin. The inferior vena cava is the largest vein of the body, since it drains the inferior members, the pelvis, the retroperitoneal space, and finally the whole abdominal cavity via the superior hepatic veins.

2.1.2 Anatomic Relations

With the *aorta* (Fig. 2.3a) the relations vary according to the level. At its origin, the inferior vena cava ascends to the right of and slightly behind the aorta. In ascending, the vena cava becomes more and more lateral and eventually anterior to the aorta. Indeed, when it perforates the diaphragm (between the right medial and intermediate crus of the diaphragm), the vena cava is clearly anterior to the aorta.

Lying posterior to the liver, it is enclosed by the pericardium and opens into the lower posterior part of the right atrium (Fig. 2.2b). The valve of the posterior vena cava – the Eustachian valve – is situated at the termination of this vein and is occasionally visible on a lateral projection, as a vertical radiolucent line in front of the atrial orifice.

Posteriorly, the inferior vena cava rests on a muscular plane mainly formed by the psoas muscle. It is thus related to the branches of the retrocaval aorta, i.e., the right lumbar arteries, and especially the right renal artery.

On the left side, it is related to the aorta and to the latero-aortic ganglionic chain.

Anteriorly, (Fig. 2.3b) the inferior vena cava is separated from the intra-abdominal organs by the posterior peritoneum; thus it is crossed by the root of the mesentery, the horizontal and the superior part of the duodenum, and the head of the pancreas. The liver and the portal vein are anterior to it. Just in contact, behind the peritoneum, pass the right testicular artery and branches of the periaortic sympathetic plexus.

On the right side, the inferior vena cava is closely related to the right ureter and right kidney. The proximity of the inferior vena cava to the renal hilus accounts for the importance of venous investigations in tumors of the right kidney. Above this level, it is also related to the liver. The inferior cava is situated behind the liver and often causes an imprint on its posterior surface. This imprint is usually a groove and may become a canal, when a small tongue of liver tissue covers the inferior vena cava from behind. This intrahepatic course is sometimes responsible for changes in the caval caliber.

2.1.3 Tributaries of the Inferior Vena Cava

In the retroperitoneal space the following tributaries join: the renal veins, the right suprarenal vein, the lumbar veins, the inferior phrenic veins, and the right sex vein. After passing through the liver all the venous blood coming from the digestive system is drained by the termination of the inferior vena cava via the hepatic veins.

2.2 Physiology

Several physiologic factors have an effect upon the blood flow in the inferior vena cava. It is essential to be aware of them in order to understand temporary features appearing in certain films of a series. Principal among them are cardiac and respiratory factors.

2.2.1 Cardiac Factors

During ventricular systole the blood flow in the inferior vena cava ranges from 30 to 45 ml/s. It increases during diastole by about 30%–75%. The venous flow is thus pulsatile. This can often be observed at the time of femoral vein puncture. On film recording a very transient systolic reflux may be seen into the hepatic veins; this reflux diminishes clearly during diastole and appears again with the next systole. Cardiac abnormalities, mainly right or global ventricular insufficiency, may cause decreased inferior caval flow. In some long-standing cardiac failures the inferior vena cava may become markedly dilated, with slowed blood flow.

2.2.2 Respiratory Factors

Significant variations in the inferior vena caval caliber occur during respiration. These changes are well visualized by echography. Inspiration increases the blood flow velocity in the inferior vena cava. By producing a blockage in this vein, the Valsalva maneuver causes marked reduction in caval flow and increases the diameter of the vein. Thus, if the patient is instructed to perform the Valsalva maneuver during injection of contrast material, it will ensure significant reduction in blood flow, inferior caval dilatation, and a better, longer-lasting opacification of the tributaries of the inferior vena cava.

2.3 Radioanatomy Pitfalls in Interpretation

A certain number of technical and anatomic factors must be taken into account in the interpretation of an inferior vena cavogram. Let us recall that two perpendicular projections are indispensable.

2.3.1 Technical Factors

The fact of there being tributaries to the inferior vena cava may lead to two types of phenomenon during contrast injection, reflux of contrast material into the collaterals, and conversely, dilution of the contrast material by nonopaque blood entering from the collaterals.

There may be a *physiological reflux* of contrast material into the tributaries of the inferior vena cava, but it will be minimal and transient. It occurs mainly into the hepatic and renal veins, and in the latter case especially into the right.

Dilution phenomena are caused by the inflow of nonopaque blood from these same collaterals. It is often seen at the site of the major collaterals, such as the renal veins (Fig. 2.4) and hepatic veins. Indeed, the amount of blood coming from the hepatic veins and from the kidneys is clearly greater than that coming from the other areas drained by the inferior vena cava. At the point where a major collateral joins the inferior vena cava the nonopaque blood causes a defect in the contrast column. This phenomenon is particularly visible at the end of the passage of the contrast material: the dilution is less and less marked the further downstream from the confluence one looks.

In some cases this dilution phenomenon is visible in the suprarenal, lumbar, or sex veins. With very rapid injections, the phenomenon is visible only at the end of the injection. Conversely, when the contrast material is injected slowly, the phenomenon is clearly enhanced.

A third technical factor is the *Venturi effect*, a hydraulic effect producing the appearance of an extended and regular stenosis at the beginning of an injection at high delivery rate through a catheter without side holes. The iliac vein is incompletely filled and complete opacification of the iliac system is only obtained on late films, i.e., 2 to 3 s after the start of injection (Fig. 2.5a, b). This pseudostenosis should be recognized as an artifact occurring at the beginning of a cavography.

2.3.2 Anatomic Factors

Neighboring anatomic structures, particularly the arteries, may cause impressions on the inferior vena cava, owing to the low tonicity of the venous wall and the low venous pressure (2 to 5 mm Hg).

Arterial Impressions (Fig. 2.6a, b)

The iliac arteries and the right renal artery are mainly responsible for impressions. The common iliac arteries cross the left common iliac vein anteriorly. It is normal for a bifemoral cavography to display an anterior compression of the inferior vena cava in front of the sacrum, at the level of the termination of the left common iliac vein. This compression is usually due to the right common iliac artery, as late aortographic films would show. Sometimes, the impression of the left common iliac artery – especially when there is an arterial siphon – is also visible.

The right renal artery passes behind the inferior vena cava to join the right kidney. It may cause an impression on the posterior caval aspect, which is readily displayed on a cavographic projection with the patient supine (Fig. 2.7). The right renal artery, at the level of the second lumbar vertebra, causes a small, smooth, rounded indentation on the posterior aspect of the cava.

Compressions by the Aorta

Inflexion of the abdominal aorta or severe atheromatosis may be responsible for an S-shaped or tortuous aortic course and may thus result in compression of the inferior vena cava. Aneurysm of the abdominal aorta can also affect the inferior vena cava. All these changes in the relationships between aorta and vena cava are readily detected on delayed roentgenograms (aortography).

Effects of the Liver upon the Inferior Vena Cava

On a frontal view the intrahepatic segment of the inferior vena cava may seem narrower than the segment below. A lateral view shows this anomaly to be merely due to an increased AP diameter where the right-to-left diameter is reduced. This physiological feature emphasizes the importance of orthogonal projections for appreciating the caval caliber. Changes in the volume of the liver will result usually in posterior or lateral displacements of the inferior vena cava, but hypertrophy of the caudate lobe causes a forward displacement of the inferior vena cava at this level.

Changes in the intra-abdominal hydrostatic pressure due to ascites cause alterations in the upper caval segment: there will be smooth and progressive narrowing, commencing above the level of the renal veins. When the ascites is punctured, the inferior vena cava regains its normal volume. This feature must also be recognized and differentiated from narrowing of the inferior vena cava due to cirrhosis.

Compressions of Vertebral Origin

Any modification in the statics of the vertebral column, whether exaggeration of the lumbar lordosis or scoliosis of the spine, may distort the shape or affect the caliber of the inferior vena cava. On a frontal view, lumbarthrosis may cause irregularities on the left lateral margin of the inferior vena cava. The left anterior oblique projection and lateral view show the defects to be localized at the level of the intervertebral disk spaces, facing the osteophytes (Fig. 2.8).

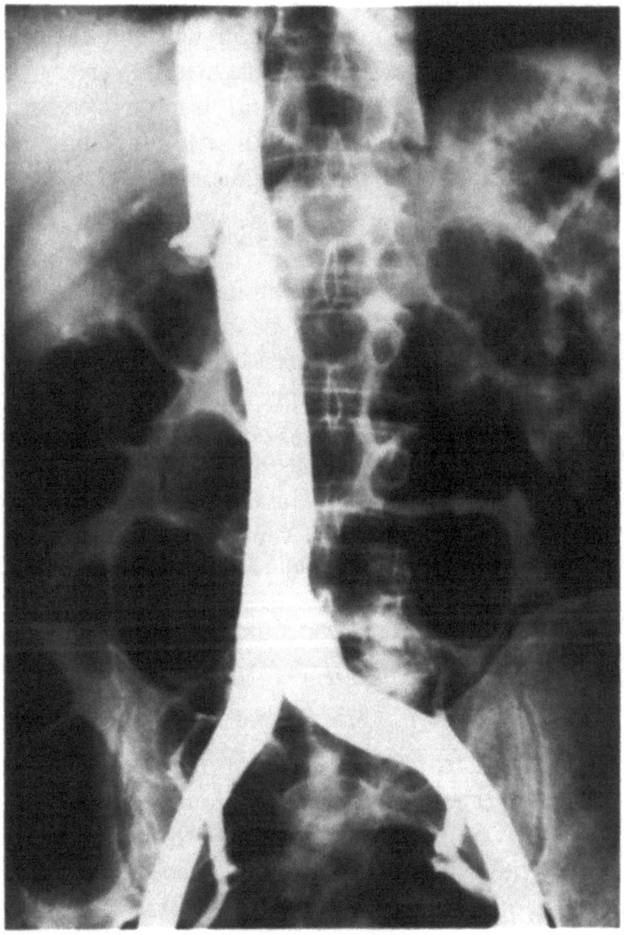

Fig. 2.1. Inferior vena cava trunk on a frontal projection. Note that the inferior vena cava runs along the right margin of the vertebral bodies

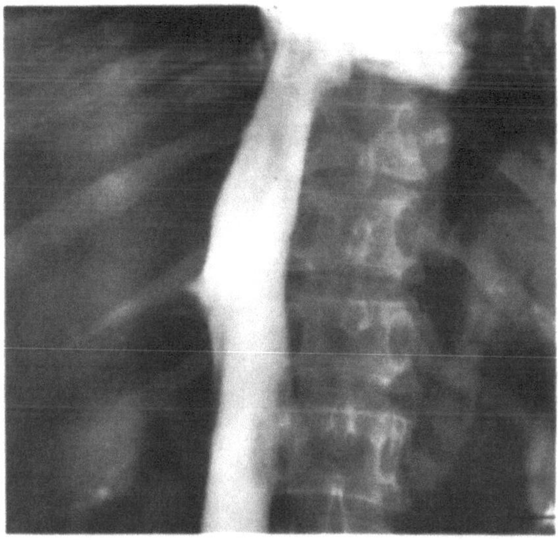

a

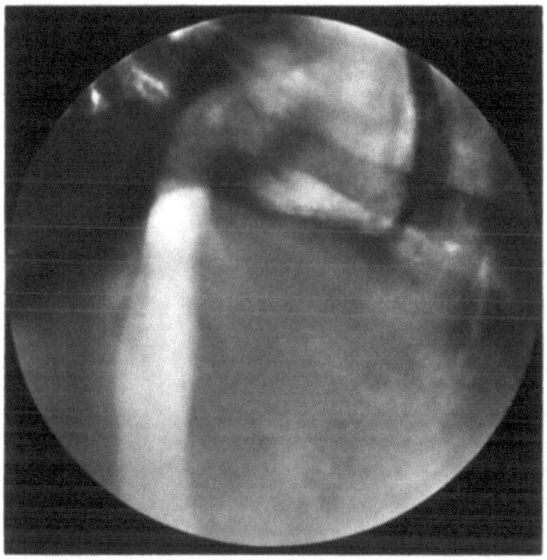

b

Fig. 2.2a, b. Inferior vena cavography. a Frontal view centered on the termination of the inferior vena cava and the inferior aspect of the right atrium. b Lateral view

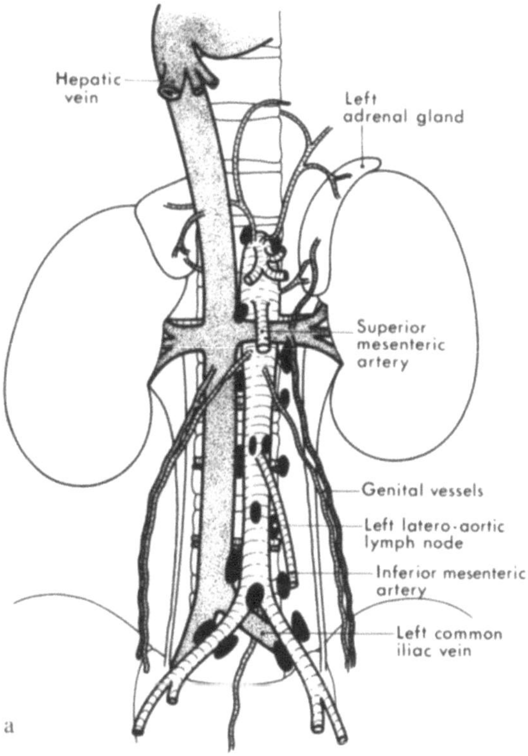

a

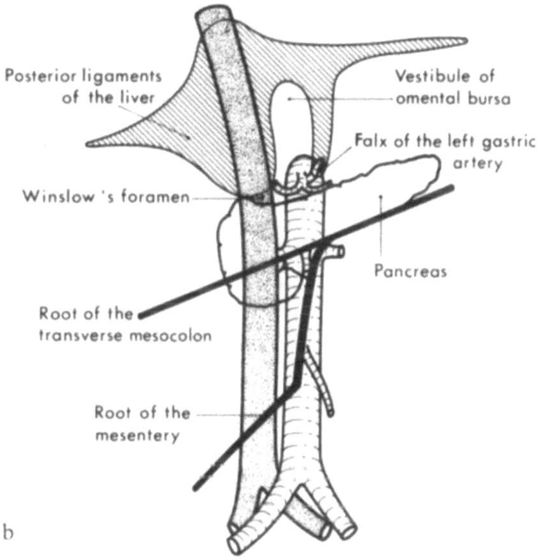

b

Fig. 2.3. a Anatomic relations with aorta and retroperitoneal space. b Anatomic relations with the posterior peritoneum

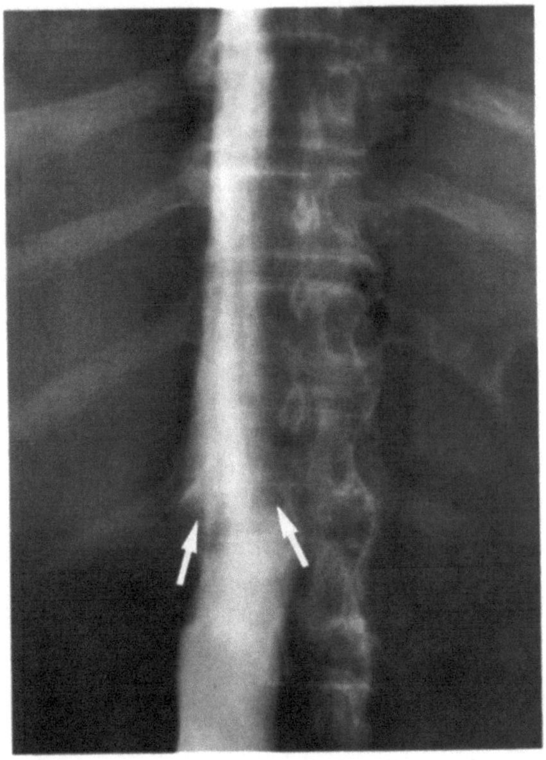

Fig. 2.4. Inferior vena cavography showing the dilution flow at the level of the right and left renal veins (↗)

Fig. 2.5. a Venturi effect with pseudostenosis at the beginning of the injection. b At the end of the injection the pseudostenosis has disappeared and the external iliac vein has a normal caliber

▽

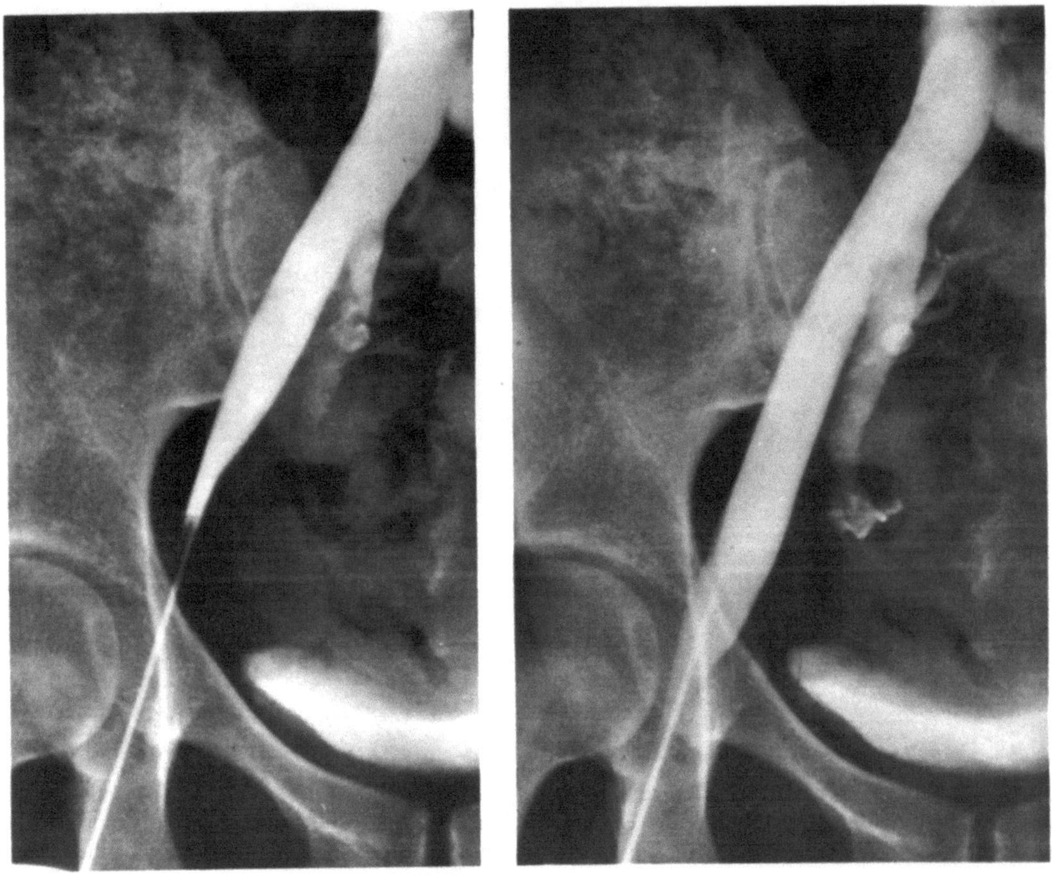

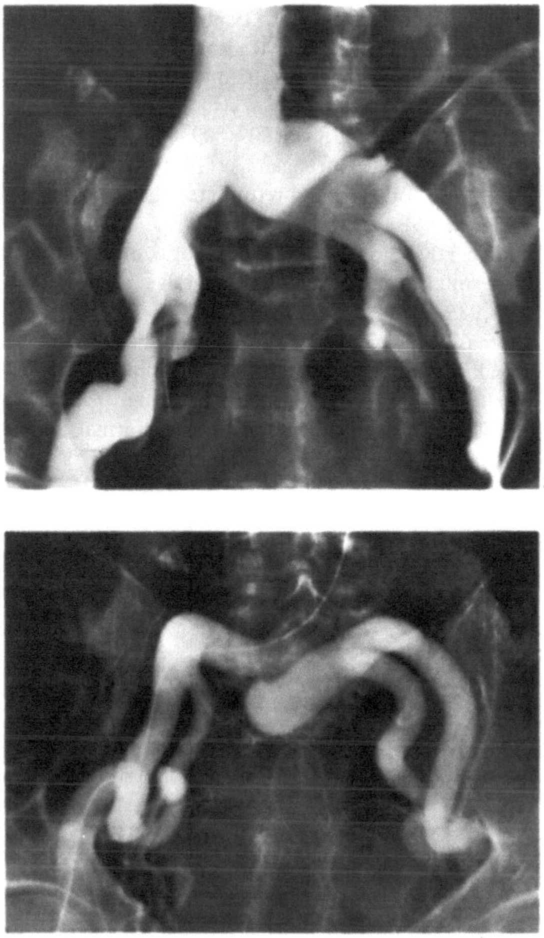

a

b

Fig. 2.6. a Cavography: Multiple compression defects on the left and right iliac vein. b Arteriography: Kinking and buckling of the iliac arteries

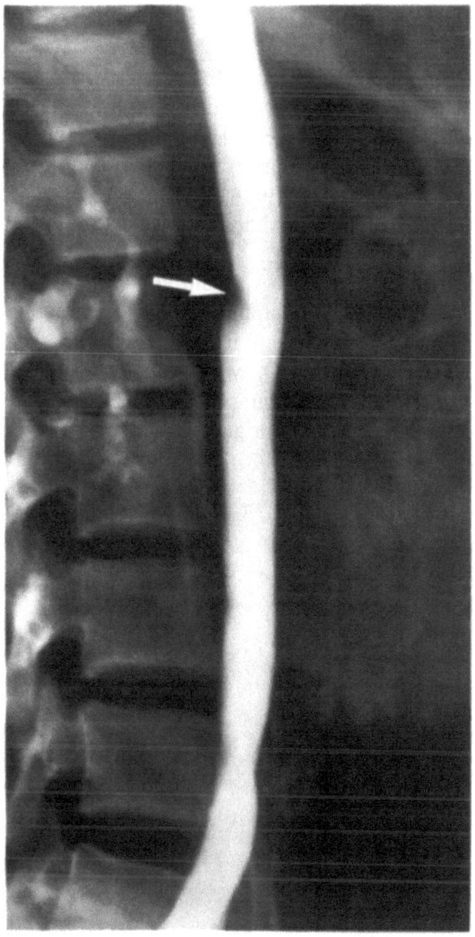

Fig. 2.7. Inferior vena cavography with the patient supine, horizontal beam. Impression of the right renal artery on the posterior aspect of the cava (→)

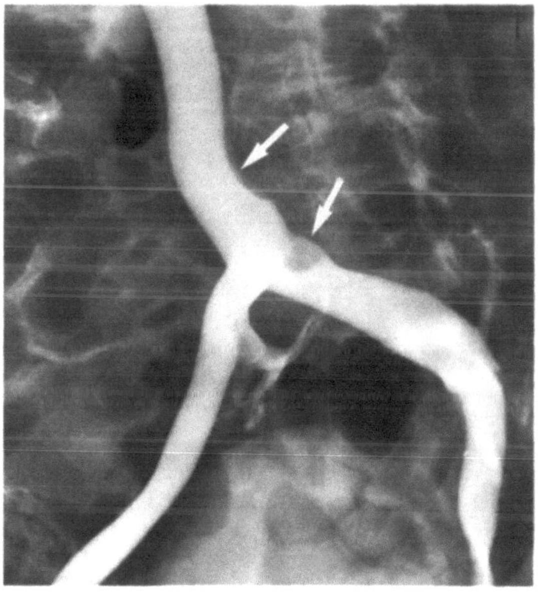

Fig. 2.8. Percutaneous bifemoral inferior cavography. Left anterior oblique projection. Multiple arcuate compression defects (↙) due to arthrosis of the lower lumbar spine

References

Crummy AB Jr, Hipona FA (1964) Aortic impression in inferior vena cavography. Clin Radiol 15:130–131

Doppman J, Foley HT, Hammond W (1967) Inferior vena caval compression: The pseudo-obstruction syndrome. AJR 100:411–413

Farinas PL (1947) Abdominal venography. Roentgenology 58:599

Ferris EJ, Hipona FA, Kahn PC, Philipps E, Shapiro JH (1969) Venography of the inferior vena cava and its branches, Williams & Wilkins, Baltimore,

Gabriele OF, Bell D, Martineau R (1967) Pitfalls in inferior vena cavography. AJR 100:417–420

Hayt DB (1966) Upright inferior vena cavography. Radiology 86:865–870

Helander CG, Lindbom A (1959) Venography of the inferior vena cava. Acta Radiol 52:257–259

Kaufmann JJ, Burke DE (1956) Abdominal venography: Technique of roentgen visualization of the inferior vena cava. AJR 76:807–809

Nordenstrom B, Horhagen A (1965) Effects of respiration on venous return to the heart. AJR 95:655–661

Ranniger K, Siortz DM (1965) Local obstruction in the inferior vena cava by massive ascites. AJR 93:935–937

Thomas L, Carty H (1975) The appearance of artefacts on lower limb phlebograms. Clin Radiol 26:527–533

Wexler L, Bergel DH, Gabe IT, Makin GS, Mills C (1968) Velocity of blood flow in normal human venae cavae. Circ Res 23:349–350

Chapter 3. Congenital Anomalies of the Inferior Vena Cava

Embryology is important for our understanding of the variations of the inferior vena cava. The variations have been known for years; they necessitate particular cavographic techniques and have radiosurgical applications, which are dealt with later on.

Using the diagram of Huntington and McClure, we shall discuss the most frequently occurring anomalies of the inferior vena cava, i.e., the anomalies of its postrenal (infrarenal) segment. Although their diagram is based on the inferior vena cava system of the cat, it does allow one to classify accurately the human anomalies of this segment, since the human and feline systems are similar (Fig. 3.4). It was subsequently utilized by Ferris et al. in 1969 in their book on the inferior vena cava and then simplified by Chuang et al. in 1974.

Then, with the help of Boutelier and Couinaud's anatomic classification we shall study the anomalies of the retrohepatic segment. After that we shall consider the congenital anomalies of the left renal vein with or without persistence of the periaortic venous ring. Finally, we shall study the very rare abnormal terminations of the inferior vena cava itself and of certain venous systems that flow into it.

3.1 Review of the Embryology

The embryogenesis of the inferior vena cava is very complex and comprises the development of certain anastomoses and the regression of three paired and symmetrical venous systems: the posterior cardinal, subcardinal, and supracardinal veins.

3.1.1 Posterior Cardinal Veins

In the embryo most of the venous return from the infradiaphragmatic area is via the posterior cardinal veins (Fig. 3.1). They are paired, symmetrical, and posterior, and situated dorsally to the mesonephric ridge. In their cranial segment they join the anterior cardinal veins to form the duct of Cuvier which opens into the sinus venosus. Dorsally to the aorta, the posterior cardinal veins are connected by anastomoses, including an interrenal and an interiliac anastomosis. During embryogenesis the posterior cardinal veins regress. Only the caudal part persists, giving rise to the common iliac veins.

3.1.2 Subcardinal Veins

The subcardinal veins appear later and are less developed than the posterior cardinals. They are also paired and symmetrical, and are situated anteriorly and medially with regard to the posterior cardinal veins. They are connected via multiple anastomoses to the corresponding posterior cardinal veins, and also to each other. These anastomoses are preaortic, whereas those between the posterior cardinal veins are retroaortic. Each subcardinal vein has a cranial and a caudal portion, respectively above and below the renal vein. As the embryo develops, the following changes are seen:

1) A communication develops between the right vitelline vein and the right subcardinal vein (cranial portion), thus forming the retrohepatic or prerenal segment of the inferior vena cava in the adult.
2) The left subcardinal vein (cranial portion) becomes less important and forms, in the adult, the left suprarenal vein and the part of the left renal vein situated between the sex vein and the inferior vena cava.
3) The caudal portion of the subcardinal veins regresses and gives, in the adult, the sex veins.

The development of the prerenal division of the inferior vena cava, the intersubcardinal anastomoses, and the atrophy of the left subcardinal vein allow the blood flow to be diverted to the retrohepatic segment of the inferior vena cava, and presage the right asymmetrical pattern that exists in the adult (Fig. 3.2).

3.1.3 Supracardinal Veins

The supracardinal veins are situated medially to the posterior cardinals and laterally to the subcardinal veins. They are symmetrically paired and are connected by anastomoses to each other and with the posterior cardinal and subcardinal venous systems.

The cranial end of this venous system forms the azygos system. The caudal end forms the postrenal division of the inferior vena cava. This postrenal segment is initially paired; but progressively only the right part persists and forms the right-sided infrarenal system. In the interrenal area the supracardinal veins anastomose with the subcardinal veins and become part of a venous ring. At this stage of development, a circumaortic venous ring is found which is formed laterally by supracardinal–subcardinal anastomoses, anteriorly by intersubcardinal anastomoses, and posteriorly by intersupracardinal anastomoses. The abdominal aorta passes through this venous ring.

On the right side, the system persists and forms the renal segment of the inferior vena cava. On the left, the venous ring is formed by a dorsal and a ventral part. The retroaortic dorsal segment disappears, and the preaortic, ventral segment persists to form the left renal vein, which drains the left suprarenal and sex veins.

3.1.4 Conclusion

Normally, the inferior vena cava results from the evolution of three symmetrically paired venous systems with a history of anastomoses, developments, and atrophies, leading finally to a right-sided system comprising the following divisions (Fig. 3.3):

Branches of Origin: the Common Iliac Veins

The common iliac veins derive from the posterior cardinal veins. The left common iliac vein, more precisely, derives from the anastomosis between the posterior cardinal veins, which accounts partly for some of the anomalies encountered at this level.

The Inferior Vena Cava at Its Origin

The most caudal part, i.e., the junction of the two common iliac veins, derives from a part of the right posterior cardinal vein and from a part of the caudal anastomosis between the two posterior cardinal veins.

Postrenal Segment

The postrenal segment is formed caudally by the caudal part of the right supracardinal vein and by the anastomosis of the latter with the corresponding subcardinal vein.

Interrenal Segment

The interrenal segment is formed by the intermediate portion of the right subcardinalvein and the right-hand part of the circum-aortic venous ring.

Prerenal Segment

The prerenal segment develops from the anastomosis connecting the right subcardinal vein and the right vitelline vein.

Infra-atrial Portion

This area, situated between the confluence of the hepatic veins and the right atrium, derives very likely from the terminal portion of the right vitelline vein, which also forms the right upper hepatic veins. The left vitelline vein forms the left hepatic veins and presents a transverse anastomosis with its right mate; its connection with the heart disappears, so that the left hepatic flow is drained by the right vitelline vein. Into this anastomosis opens the canal of Arantius which, in the embryo, connects the left umbilical vein with the inferior caval system. As we have seen, the embryologic development of the inferior vena cava is very complex, and this accounts for the relative frequency of its congenital anomalies.

A review of the embryology of the azygos system is also essential, since this system plays a role as collateral route in numerous cases of congenital anomaly of the cava; moreover, it may itself show some congenital variations.

The azygos system derives from the longitudinal venous plexus (internal sympathetic veins). This venous plexus develops at the same time as the supracardinal veins. It communicates at its cranial end with the posterior cardinal veins. It also has multiple anastomoses with the subcardinal veins.

Nevertheless, the supracardinal system is the major constituent of the final azygos system. On the right, the cranial part of the supracardinal vein constitutes the great azygos vein. Its upper end joins the right anterior cardinal vein and forms the arch of the azygos vein. On the left, the supracardinal vein loses its normal communication with the posterior cardinal vein; it forms the hemiazygos vein, which is connected to the great azygos vein through a transverse anastomosis.

The medial root of the inferior hemiazygos vein arises, in 88% of cases, from the renal vein; it often communicates with the first or the second lumbar vein, thus forming a collateral renoazygolumbar route (renoazygolumbar canal). Usually but not always, the inferior phrenic, the main suprarenal, and the lumbar veins open into the caval trunk on the right side. From the caval trunk arises, inconstantly, the internal root of the azygos vein.

3.2 Congenital Anomalies of the Postrenal Segment

Four major embryonic trunks participate in the formation of the postrenal segment of the inferior vena cava (Fig. 3.4):

A. Right posterior cardinal vein
B. Right supracardinal vein
C. Left supracardinal vein
D. Left posterior cardinal vein

The variants of the postrenal segment of the inferior vena cava are constituted by one or more of these four trunks. We shall designate them by the letters of the persistent segments.

Type A: Retrocaval ureter. This variation is due to the persistence of the right posterior cardinal vein and is known as retrocaval ureter (Fig. 3.5). In the embryo, the ureter lies ventral to the supracardinal vein, and dorsal to the posterior cardinals. This location determines the relations of the ureter and inferior vena cava in the adult. In normal development the posterior cardinal vein regresses and the ureter lies anterior to the supracardinal vein, and thus anterior to the postrenal segment of the inferior vena cava in the adult. This explains why the sex veins, which derive from the subcardinal veins, cross in front of the ureter.

Persistence of the posterior cardinal vein as the postrenal segment of the inferior vena cava causes displacement of the ureter toward the midline and caval compression of the ureter as it passes from behind, at the level of the fourth lumbar vertebra, then to the left, and, finally, anterior to the inferior vena cava.

This embryologic review shows why in type A the proximal ureter lies dorsal to the inferior vena cava and why it emerges, lower down, from between this vein and the right aspect of the aorta, before winding around the anterior aspect of the inferior vena cava.

Numerous cases of retrocaval ureter were reported by Bateson and Atkinson in 1969. This condition is always seen on the right side; a single case of left retrocaval ureter has been reported, but since it was in a case of situs inversus, it cannot be considered a true left retrocaval ureter. Gladstone has reported a case with bilateral retrocaval ureter due to the persistence of both posterior cardinal veins (Gladstone's acardiac monster).

This anatomic variation has no specific symptoms. Intravenous pyelography may suggest its presence by showing proximal obstruction in the right collecting system with a very characteristic bayonet-shaped course of the ureter at the level of the third and fourth lumbar vertebrae. Only inferior vena cavography can demonstrate a retrocaval ureter clearly. Involvement of the urinary tract (hydronephrosis, recurrent urinary tract infections) may lead one to consider reconstructive surgery.

Type AD: This variation is due to the persistence of the left and right posterior cardinal veins. We have already alluded to this condition in quoting Gladstone's acardiac monster.

Type AB: Periureteric venous ring. This anatomic variation is due to the persistence of the right posterior cardinal vein and of the right supracardinal vein, together forming the postrenal segment of the inferior vena cava and thus a periureteric venous ring. This type was first described (Lepage and Baldwin 1972) much later than type A, the retrocaval ureter. Conversely to what is seen in type A, in this type the ureter passes through the venous ring, it is not always deviated medially, and the site of obstruction may be either very caudal or very cranial. Consequently, when there is ureteral obstruction, even if the ureter is not markedly displaced, a congenital vascular anomaly cannot be ruled out as cause of the obstruction. It is important to be aware of this variation, since its surgical treatment is much more simple than that of retrocaval ureter: it suffices to suppress one of the two branches of the venous ring.

Type B: Type B corresponds to persistence of the right supracardinal vein as prerenal segment of the inferior vena cava.

Type BC: The right and left subcardinal–supracardinal anastomoses and the intersubcardinal anastomosis persist. Communication at the level of the iliac vein is most often present, but may be absent. The frequency of type BC is about 2.2% to 3%. It consists in duplication of the postrenal segment of the inferior vena cava (Fig. 3.6). At the renal level the left caval trunk courses ventral to the aorta and joins its right mate. As could be expected from the embryology, the ureters remain lateral to the venae cavae.

Though it is rare, the possibility of persistence of both supracardinal veins (double inferior vena cava) should be kept in mind when ligature or plication of the inferior vena cava is considered. Similarly, recurrent thromboembolisms following caval flow interruption should lead one to suspect duplication.

Catheterization of one iliac vein may opacify an apparently normal vena cava, while a second one passes undetected: Therefore cavography should always be performed with bilateral femoral puncture.

A single case of type BC has been described with no anastomosis between the two trunks at the level of the renal veins (i.e., absence of the intersubcardinal anastomosis). In this case the left inferior vena cava was seen to drain downward to join the right inferior vena cava via iliac anastomoses. There existed also an anastomosis between the left renal vein and the hemiazygos vein.

Type C: Left postrenal inferior vena cava. This anatomic variation (Figs. 3.7 and 3.8) is due to the persistence of the left supracardinal vein. It is the mirror image of the normal vena cava. The two common iliac veins form a large ascending lumbar vein which drains the left kidney at the level of the second lumbar vertebra, then crosses sharply, ventral to the aorta, and continues cranially as a normal prerenal segment of the inferior vena cava. It then receives the drainage of the right kidney. The left renal and suprarenal veins drain directly into the inferior vena cava.

Type C is to be differentiated from a complete situs inversus. In spite of its rarity, (0.2% to 0.5%), this variation deserves to be known, on account of surgical incidences which are discussed later on.

3.3 Congenital Anomalies of the Retrohepatic Segment

There are two types, namely absence of the retrohepatic segment, known as azygos continuation of the inferior vena cava; and other anomalies, including atresias and abnormal diaphragms.

3.3.1 Absence of the Retrohepatic Segment (Azygos Continuation)

This malformation (Fig. 3.9) corresponds to complete absence of the right subcardinal vein, associated with absence of fusion with the right vitelline vein. When isolated, azygos continuation is usually asymptomatic, and for this reason very few cases are reported in the literature. The malformation is usually seen on a chest roentgenogram as a small, right laterotracheal opacity at the level of the fourth thoracic vertebra, corresponding to a dilatation of the arch of the azygos vein.

Catheterization and angiography with approach from below (since there is a risk of failing to recognize this malformation when catheterization is performed from above; Fig. 3.10) show the lack of opacification of the retrohepatic caval segment with the opaque blood being diverted most often via the azygos system.

Most often the collateral circulation follows the pathway of the great azygos vein, which empties into the superior vena cava at the level of the fourth thoracic vertebra. As seen on a frontal projection, the course of this vein is usually median in the lower part of the thoracic spine and then slightly to the right side of the spine. Very infrequently the blood flow follows the pathway of the hemiazygos vein (Figs. 3.11 and 3.12), which courses along the left side of the spine, and may join a persistent left superior vena cava (Fig. 3.13). A lateral view at angiography would confirm these findings and show a quite characteristic "candy cane" image with a vertical, posteriorly ascending, dilated azygos vein and an anteroinferior concavity of the arch.

Usually, this type of malformation is accompanied by hepatic veins that drain into the right atrium, either via a common trunk or separately. Injection into the right atrium shows readily the reflux into these upper hepatic veins.

The azygos continuation of the inferior vena cava is sometimes part of a complex syndrome, termed the asplenia syndrome, which results from a teratologic disturbance involving symmetry of the viscera. It comprises asplenia, visceral symmetry, and congenital cardiac anomalies. Azygos continuation of the inferior vena cava is often associated with this syndrome.

Absence of the retrohepatic segment is much more rarely associated with a double or left-sided postrenal segment of the inferior vena cava.

3.3.2 Other Anomalies of the Retrohepatic Segment

Cases may be observed either of hypoplasia or atresia, or of abnormal diaphragms and valves, in the terminal segment of the inferior vena cava.

Atresias

Several case reports describe a fibrous tract replacing the retrohepatic segment of the inferior vena cava. It is difficult, however, or even impossible, to differentiate these congenital atresias from after effects of an earlier venous thrombosis. Only the histology would provide some indication; angiography does not allow differentiation. From a practical point of view, however, the distinction is uninteresting, since the therapeutic problems are the same in both cases.

Hypoplasias

These are very rare and must be differentiated from stenoses due to extrinsic compression, such as are encountered in severe ascites and in some hepatomegalies affecting predominantly the caudate lobe.

Abnormal Diaphragms and Valves

This pathology is rather rare, but seems to be more frequently encountered in Japan. Cases with obstructive hypertrophy of the Eustachian valve (the valve at the entrance of the inferior vena cava into the right atrium) have been described by Rossal and Caldwell. Though it is a congenital condition, this anomaly is studied in Chapter 4.

3.4 Anomalies of the Left Renal Vein and Persistence of the Periaortic Venous Ring

We have seen that in the embryo there is a complete periaortic venous ring in the interrenal region (Fig. 3.15). We have reviewed the complex origin of this ring (Fig. 3.17). The renal veins are double on both sides. On the right side the two renal veins empty into the supracardinal–subcardinal anastomosis of the periaortic venous ring. On the left side, the ventral renal vein drains into the supracardinal–subcardinal anastomosis, whereas the dorsal renal vein joins the cranial portion of the supracardinal vein, a posterior structure that gives rise to the hemiazygos system. On the left side, this retroaortic part of the venous ring and the dorsal renal vein atrophy, so that, in the normal subject, only one preaortic renal vein remains. This ventral renal vein receives the suprarenal and the sex vein (Fig. 3.16).

Let us recall that the right portion of the venous ring contributes partly to the formation of the interrenal segment of the inferior vena caval trunk. There are thus three possible anatomic variations of the left renal vein: (1) preaortic, which is the most frequent, (2) retroaortic, found in 2% to 3% of cases, or (3) persistence of the periaortic venous ring, found in 3% to 9% of cases. Much more rarely a supernumerary dorsal or ventral left renal vein may be seen.

In the case of persistent periaortic venous ring, several features are noteworthy (Fig. 3.18): Most often the two branches do not have the same caliber. The superior branch receives the suprarenal and the sex vein. It courses ventral to the aorta. The inferior branch usually joins rather caudally. It is dorsal to the aorta and sometimes has a clearly descending course; it empties into the inferior vena cava two vertebrae below the superior preaortic branch. Very rarely the left sex vein empties into the dorsal and inferior portion of the venous ring. The hemiazygos venous system and the lumbar veins always join the posterior portion of the venous ring.

3.5 Anomalies in the Termination of the Inferior Vena Cava; Terminations of Abnormal or Aberrant Vessels

Anomalous terminations are extremely rare. Two cases have been described with abnormal opening of the inferior vena cava into the left atrium. Somewhat more frequent, though also rare, is the persistence in the adult of the Arantius canal (Fig. 3.14a, b), which connects the left portal branch with the inferior vena cava. As to termination of a right pulmonary vein in the inferior vena cava, this is usually seen in the so-called scimitar syndrome, and corresponds to abnormal partial pulmonary venous return.

3.6 Radiosurgical Applications

3.6.1 Surgery on the Postrenal Segment of the Aorta

Three main types of venous variations and anomalies can complicate surgery at the level of the aortic bifurcation (Fig. 3.19).

a) Variations in the *lumbar veins* (for instance, confluence of several left lumbar veins crossing the midline, dorsally to the aorta, at the level of the third lumbar vertebra) are quite frequent. It is possible to avoid injuring them by dissecting the aorta immediately below the renal arteries.

b) Anomalies of the *postrenal (infrarenal) segment of the inferior vena cava* are as follows: left inferior vena cava – 0.2% to 0.5%; double inferior vena cava – 2.2% to 3%. It is rare for these not to be recognized, and there is thus little risk of their being injured during surgical procedures. But they may considerably impede close infrarenal dissection of the aorta, since the left inferior vena cava passes usually ventral to it to receive the left renal vein, and continues, as a normal prerenal (suprarenal) inferior vena cava, on the right side of the spine. When upward or downward retraction does not suffice, it may be necessary to resect it. This has no consequences when there is a double inferior vena cava, but there is a risk of thrombosis in the case of single left inferior vena cava. In this latter case section of the right renal vein is considered, provided it receives the right sex and suprarenal veins, which will then ensure the drainage.

c) Anomalies of the *left renal vein* seem frequent: retroaortic left renal vein – 2% to 3%; double left renal vein – 3% to 9%. The retroaortic renal vein, which has a larger or smaller caliber depending on whether it is associated with a renal vein in a normal preaortic position (forming thus a collar around the aorta), crosses the midline obliquely downward to empty into the inferior vena cava. It often receives one or several left lumbar veins. The readiness with which these anomalies are recognized during an operation varies. When the left renal vein is entirely retroaortic, the total absence of a preaortic vein rapidly draws one's attention. Moreover, this disposition makes it easier to approach surgically the superior mesenteric artery, the left renal artery, and the proximal portion of the right renal artery. When there is a periaortic collar, the preaortic portion can be mistaken for a single vein in normal position. The risk of injuring the retroaortic portion while checking the aorta is then particularly high and serious. Among 22 recognized retroaortic left renal veins, Brenner et al. report that 10 were injured, 6 of which were repaired, 2 necessitated nephrectomy because of hemostasis, and 2 led to death of the patient due to exsanguination and bilateral renal vein thrombosis. Restoration is always difficult and requires good exposure of the vein, which is only provided by complete section of the aorta.

3.6.2 Anomalies of the Left Renal Vein: Further Radiosurgical Applications

Anomalies of the left renal vein should be kept in mind above all when one performs an angiography; indeed, if they are not duly recognized, the reliability of phlebography is diminished. They must be recognized in the following situations (we have already mentioned the problems due to aneurysms of the abdominal aorta):

1) In suprarenal venograms they are important, in that the left suprarenal vein always opens into the superior part of the periaortic venous ring, where this persists.
2) When sampling renin in the renal vein, it is desirable to obtain samples from both renal veins, even if there is a venous ring. On the other hand, the sampling must be distal, at the level of the hilus, so as to avoid falsely low results due to the dilution flow from collateral channels opening into the single or double left renal vein(s).
3) When renal transplantation is considered, the venous drainage of the donor's kidney must be known.
4) The retroaortic portion of the venous ring may sometimes be compressed by an aneurysm of the aorta or by a markedly calcified aorta. This pseudo-obstruction (by extrinsic compression) should not be confused with neoplastic thrombosis in angiographic investigation of hypernephroma (study of the renal vein in carcinomas of the kidney).
5) Anomalies of the left renal vein are to be taken into account when a Warren-type, splenorenal radicular portocaval shunt is envisaged.

References

Anderson RC, Adams P, Burke B (1961) Anomalous inferior vena cava with azygous continuation (intrahepatic interruption of inferior vena cava): Report of 15 cases. J Pediatr 59:370–383

Berdon WE, Baker DH (1968) Plain film findings in azigous continuation of the inferior vena cava. AJR 104:452–457

Boutelier P, Couinaud C (1962) Les anomalies dites primitives de la veine cave inférieure. J Clin 82:199–222

Brener BJ, Darling RC, Frederick PL, Linton RR (1974) Major venous anomalies complicating abdominal aortic surgery. Arch Surg 108:159–165

Chuang V, Mena E, Hoskins P (1974a) Congenital anomalies of the inferior vena cava. Review of embryogenesis and presentation of a simplified classification. Br J Radiol 47:206–213

Chuang V, Mena E, Hoskins P (1974b) Congenital anomalies of the left renal vein: Angiographic consideration. Br J Radiol 47:214–218

Downing DF (1953) Absence of the inferior vena cava. Pediatrics 12:675–676

Dupuis C, Nuyts JP, Christiaens L (1964) "Continuation azygos" de la veine cave inférieure. A propos de cinq observations. Arch Mal Coeur 57:28–49

Edwards EA (1951) Clinical anatomy of lesser variations of the inferior vena cava and a proposal for classifying the anomalies of the vessel. Angiology 2:85–87

Ferris EJ, Hipona FA, Kahn PC, Philipps E, Shapiro JH (1969) Venography of the inferior vena cava and its branches. Williams & Wilkins, Baltimore

Field S, Chir B, Saxton H (1974) Venous anomalies complicating left adrenal catheterization. Br J Radiol 47:219–225

Gladstone RJ (1905) An acardiac foetus (acephalus omphalositicus). J Anat Physiol 40:71–72

Gryska PF, Earthrowl FH (1967) Left sited inferior vena cava. Arch Surg 94:363–365

Heller RM, Dorst JP, James AE, Rowe RD (1971) A useful sign in the recognition of azygous continuation of the inferior vena cava. Radiology 101:519–522

Hirsh DM, Chan K (1963) Bilateral inferior venae cavae. Am J Med 185:729–730

Huntington GS, McClure CFW (1920) The develop-

ment of the veins in the domestic cat (*Felis domestica*). Anat Rec 20:
Kottra JJ, Castellino RA (1970) The circumaortic left renal vein. Angiographic appearance. Radiology 95:141–143
Lepage JR, Baldwin GN (1972) Obstructive periureteric venous ring. Radiology 104:313–315
Pernot C, Worms AM, Stehlin H, Bourgeois JM (1969) La "continuation azygos" de la veine cave inférieure. A propos de six observations. Ann Med (Nancy) 8:5–16
Petersen RW (1965) Infrahepatic interruption of the inferior vena cava with azygos continuation (persistent right cardinal vein). Radiology 84:304–307
Ries RH, Esenther G (1953) Variations in the pattern of renal vessels and their relation to the type of posterior cava in man. Am J Anat 104:293–294
Rossall R, Caldwell R (1957) Obstruction of inferior vena cava by a persistent Eustachian valve in a young adult. J Clin Pathol 10:40–41
Royster T, Lacey L, Marks R (1974) Abdominal aortic surgery and the left renal vein. Am J Surg 127:552–554
Stackelberg B, Lind J, Wegelius E (1952) Absence of the inferior vena cava diagnosed by angiocardiography. Cardiology 21:583–584
Thomas T (1970) Surgical implications of retroaortic left renal vein. Arch Surg 100:738–740

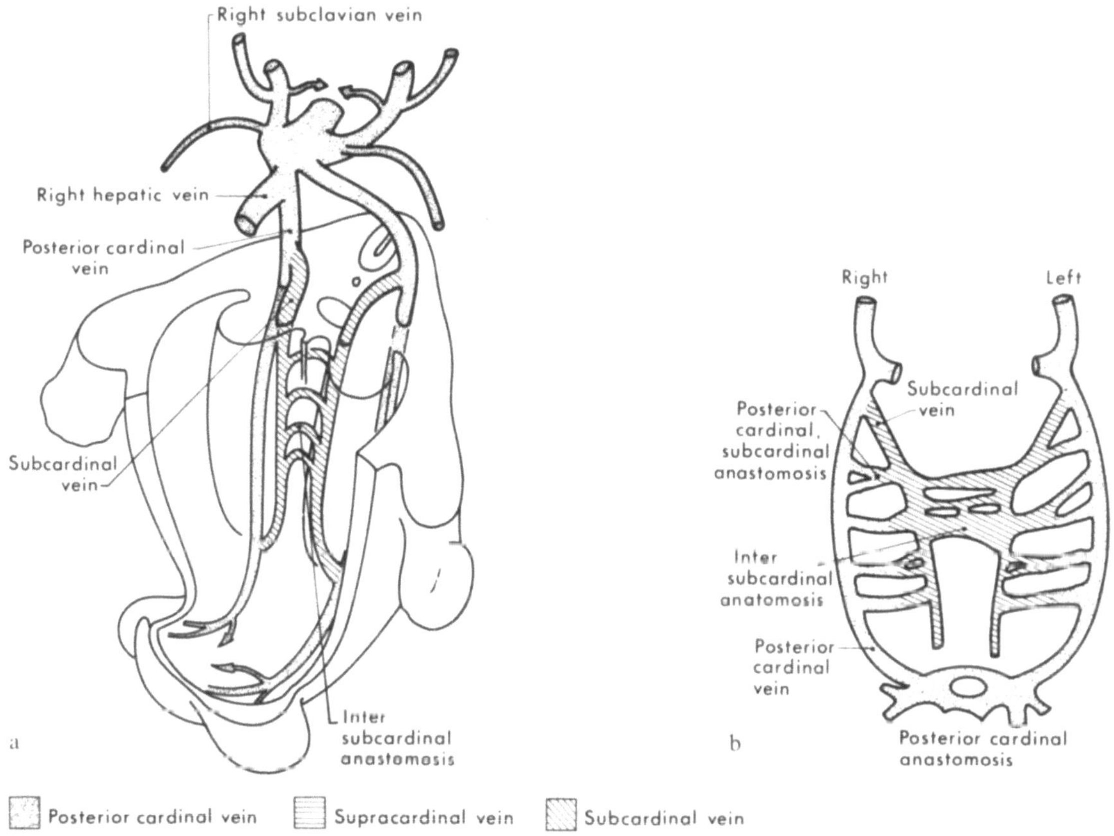

Fig. 3.1. a Transverse section of an embryo in the eighth week demonstrating the disposition of the venous network. b The paired posterior cardinal veins (*PC*) drain the blood from the dorsal part of the embryo to the duct of Cuvier. The paired subcardinal veins (*Sub.C*) develop medial to the posterior cardinal veins and gradually take over the drainage of the posterior cardinal veins

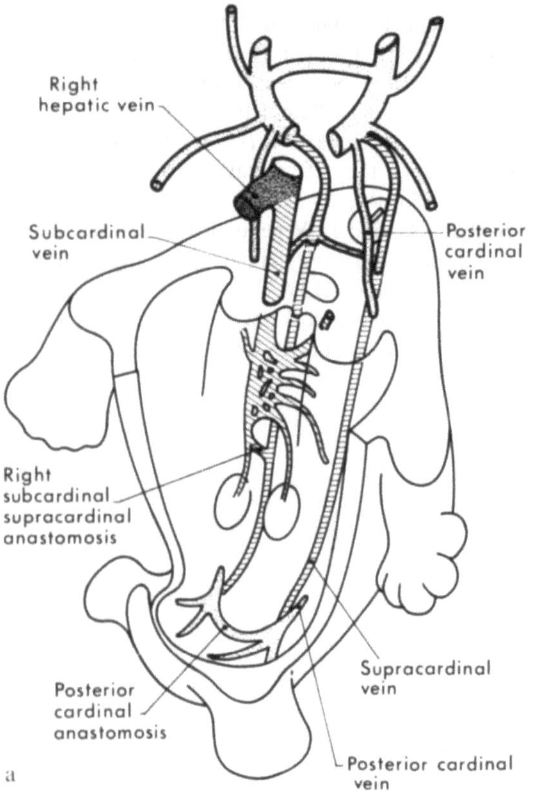

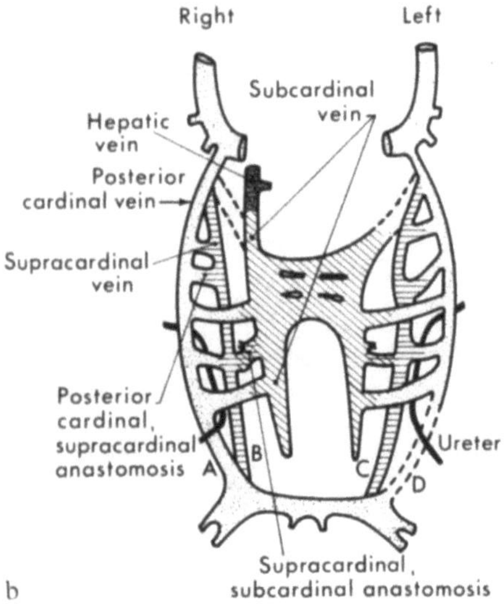

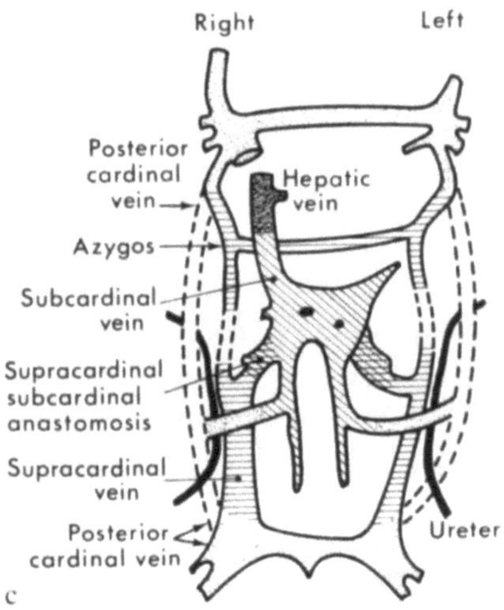

Fig. 3.2. a Transverse section of an embryo of nine weeks demonstrating the disposition of the venous network. b The right supracardinal vein anastomoses with the right hepatic vein which originates from the hepatic sinusoids to form the hepatosubcardinal channel. The paired supracardinal veins (*Supra C*) develop dorsal to the subcardinals and medial to the posterior cardinals. The ureter lies dorsal to the posterior cardinal vein in the region of the renal collar, but it descends medially and anteriorly. c The supracardinal and subcardinal veins anastomose to form the renal segment of the inferior vena cava. The caudal portion of the supracardinal veins persists as the postrenal segment of the inferior vena cava, while the cranial portion remains as the azygos and hemiazygos vein. After total regression of the posterior cardinal vein, the ureter parallels the inferior vena cava (the supracardinal vein) laterally

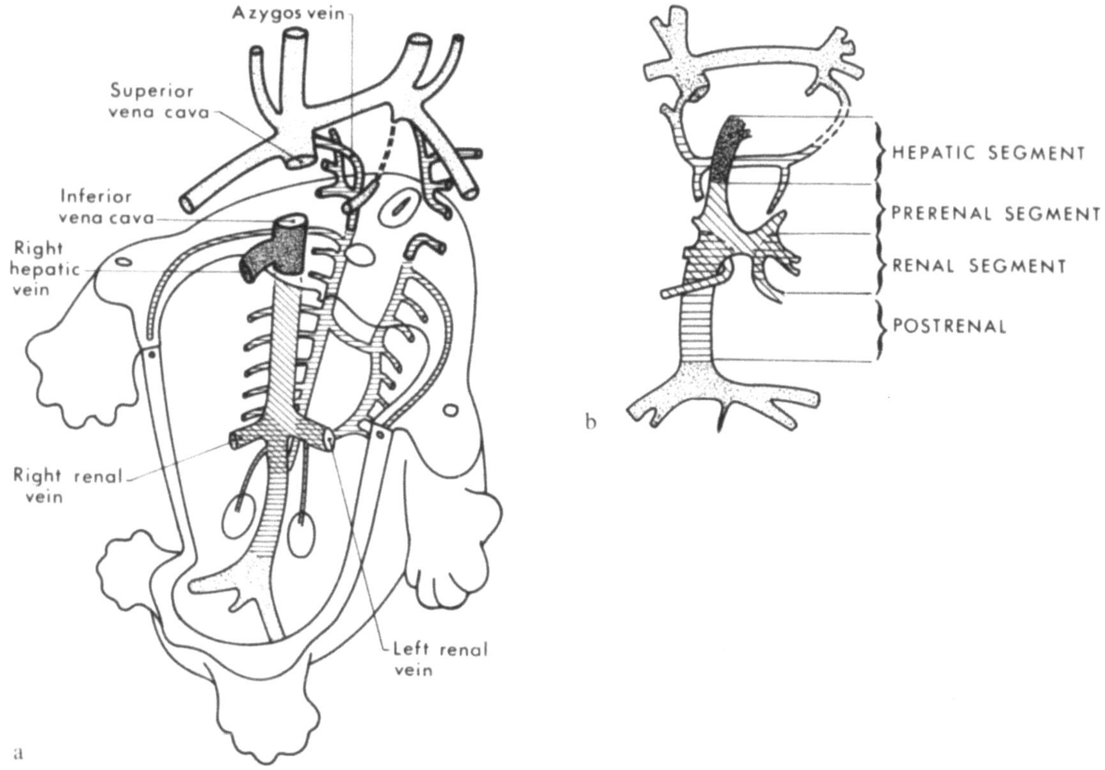

Fig. 3.3. a Transverse section of an embryo demonstrating the final disposition of the venous system of the inferior vena cava in an adult. The caudal portion of the left supracardinal vein decreases in size and eventually disappears. The paired channels are converted into a unilateral right-sided venous system of an adult which is composed of the right supracardinal vein, right sub-supracardinal anastomosis, right subcardinal vein, and right hepatic vein. b Divisions of the IVC

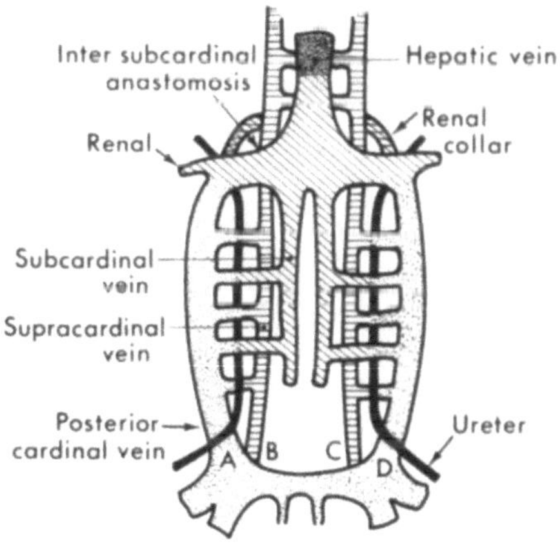

Fig. 3.4 Huntington and McClure's composite diagram of embryonic vessels allows interpretation of variations in the postrenal segment of the inferior vena cava: A: persistence of the right posterior cardinal vein. B: persistence of the right supracardinal vein. C: persistence of the left supracardinal vein D: persistence of the left posterior cardinal vein. Note relationship of the ureters to the right and left posterior cardinal veins and their parallelism with the supracardinal veins

Fig. 3.5a–c. Retrocaval ureter. a Pyelogram showing right ureteronephrosis with upwardly concave stop in the first portion of the ureter. Medial, hook-shaped deformation of the ureter. b Cavogram demonstrating the retrocaval position of the right ureter. c Retrograde ureteropyelogram demonstrates the medial course of the ureter in the lower lumbar area, its bayonet-shaped and, later, latero-caval course. Typical image of retrocaval ureter due to persistence of the right posterior cardinal vein

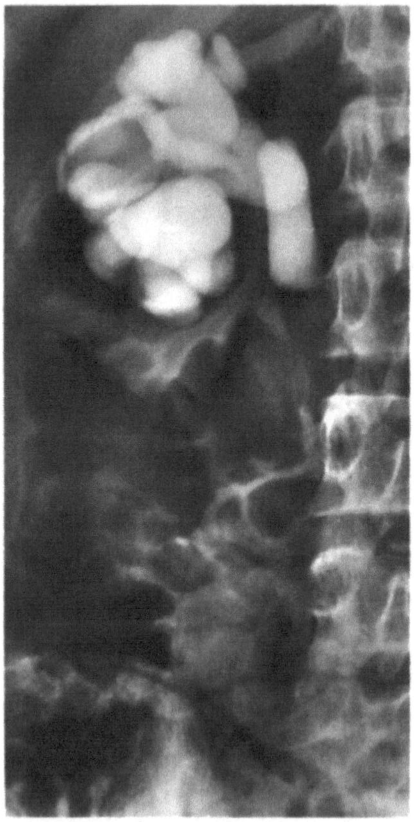

a

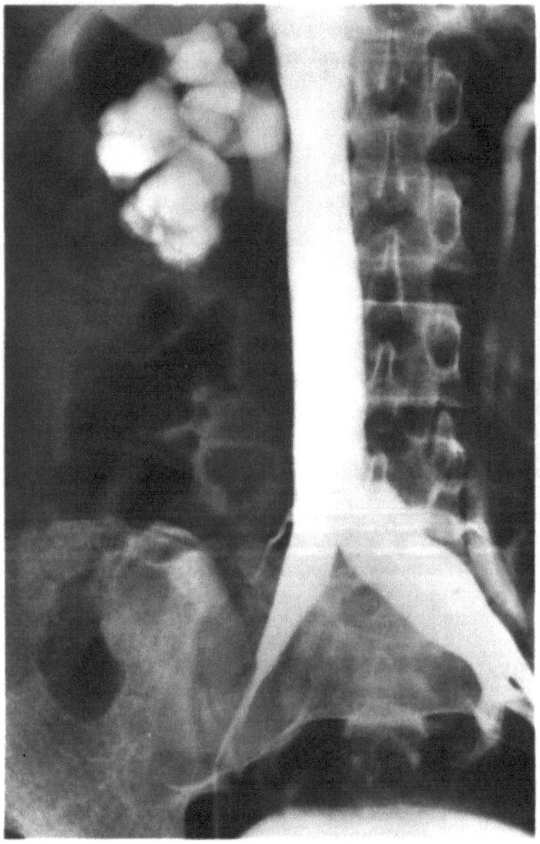

b

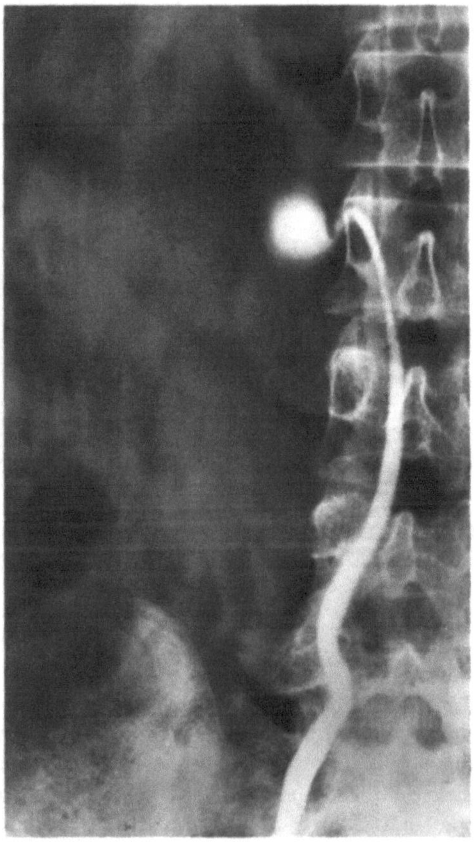

c

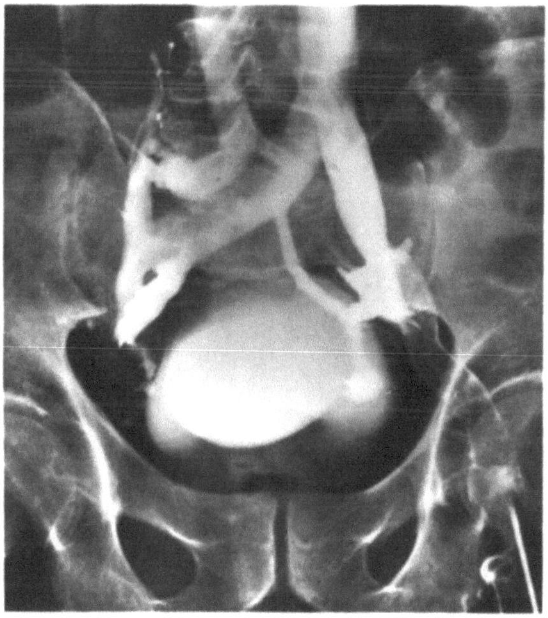

a

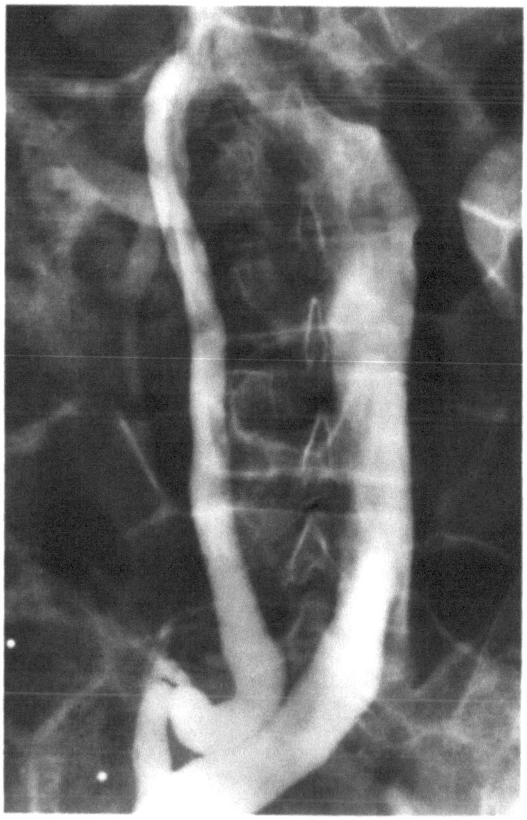

b

c

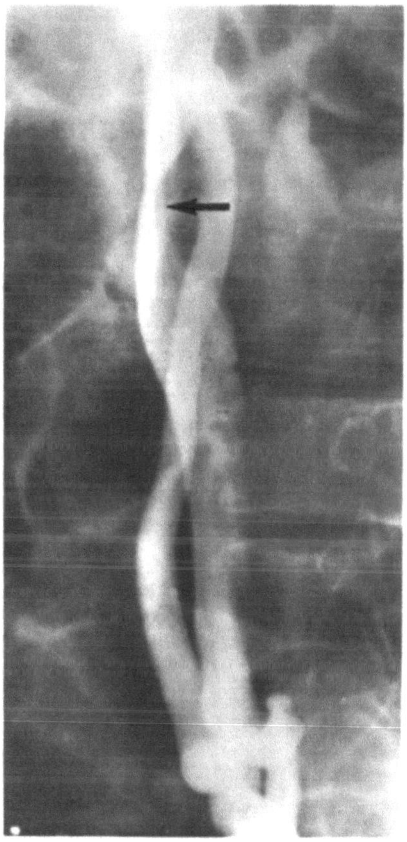

Fig. 3.6a–c. Double postrenal inferior vena cava. a Phlegmasia cerulea of the left lower limb. Left femoral puncture into a thrombus of the iliofemoral vein. Opacification of a double postrenal inferior vena cava. The left inferior vena cava is predominant and proceeds from the left iliac system and from the right common iliac and hypogastric system. The right inferior vena cava proceeds from the right ascending lumbar vein. b Frontal projection centered on the post- and prerenal segment of the inferior vena cava. Postrenal inferior vena cava duplication. The left is the larger of the pair. The right receives the right renal vein; the left receives the left renal vein, passes ventrally to the aorta and joins the right inferior vena cava. c Lateral cavogram in the same case showing the left inferior vena cava to be predominant, passing really ventral to the aorta (↗), and, finally, joining the right inferior vena cava at the level of the right margin of L1

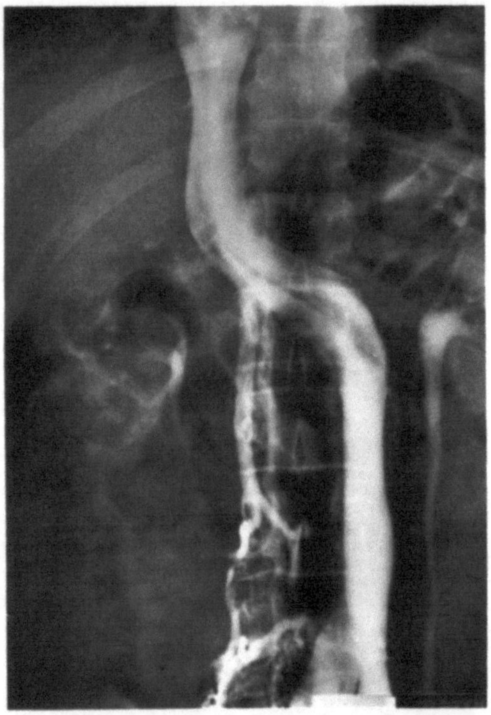

3.7a

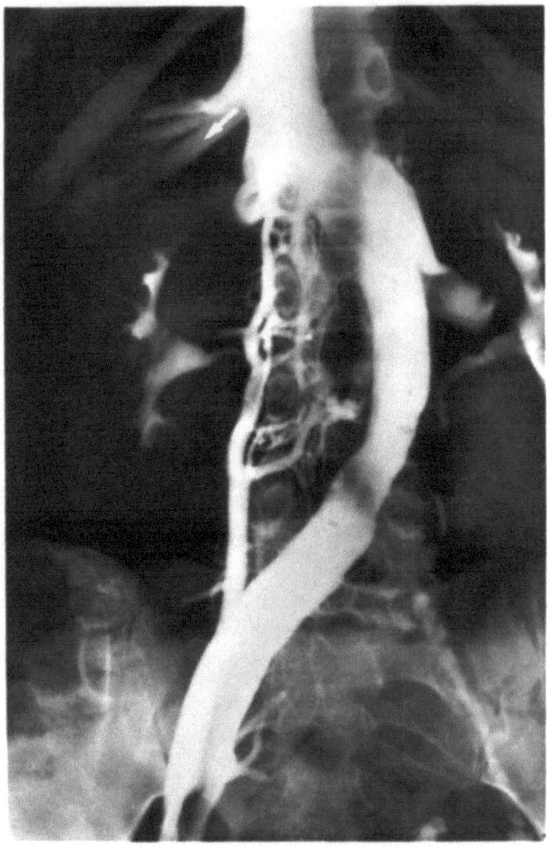

3.8

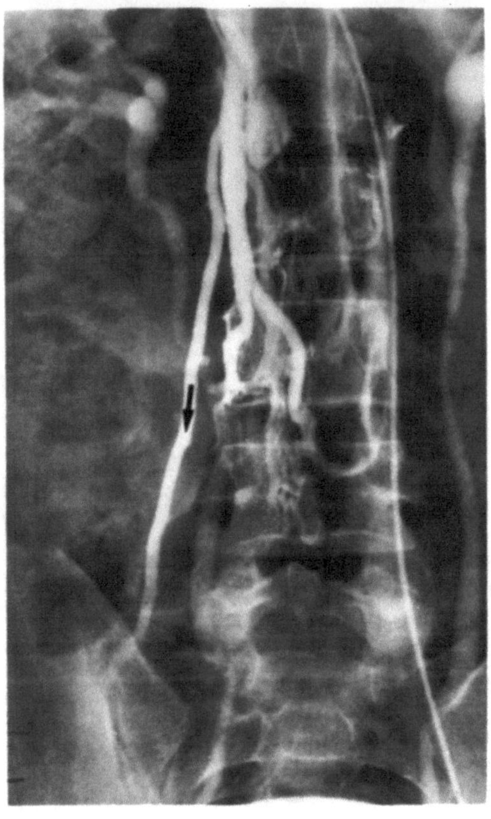

3.7c

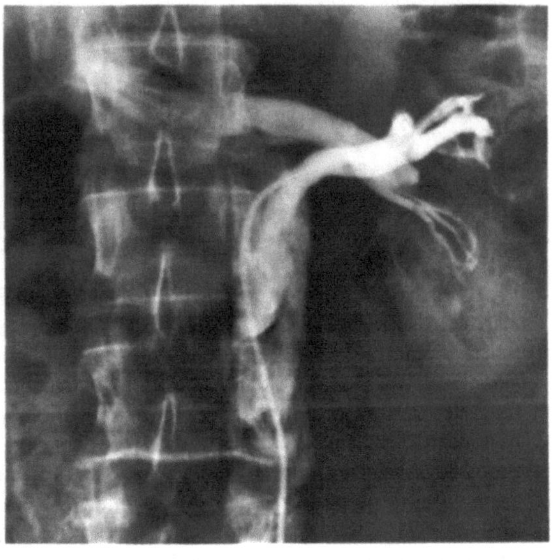

3.7b

Fig. 3.7a–c. Left inferior vena cava. a Bifemoral percutaneous cavography, frontal projection. Note the opacification of a right ascending lumbar vein and of an adjacent vein. b Left selective renal venogram showing a double left renal arch. c Retrograde catheterization of a common trunk from which arises the right ascending lumbar vein and the right spermatic vein (↗)

◁ Fig. 3.8. Left iliac phlebitis. Unsuccessful attempt at catheterization: left retrocrural extravasation of contrast material. Percutaneous right femoral iliocavography. Left inferior vena cava draining the left renal vein which theoretically crosses the aorta ventrally from left to right. Normal appearance of the prerenal segment with reflux into the accessory hepatic veins (↗)

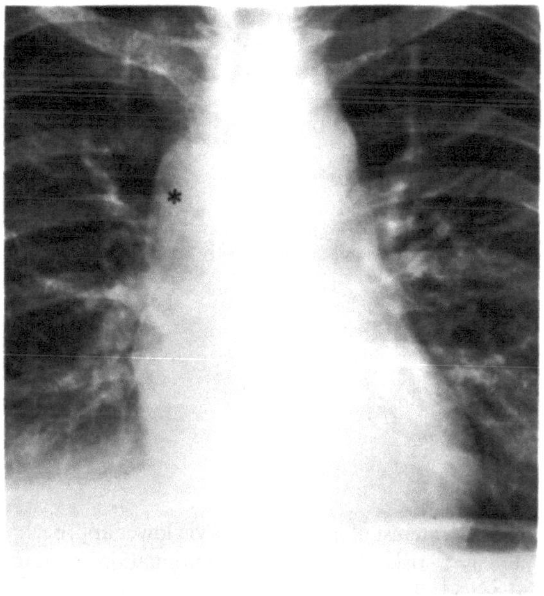

a

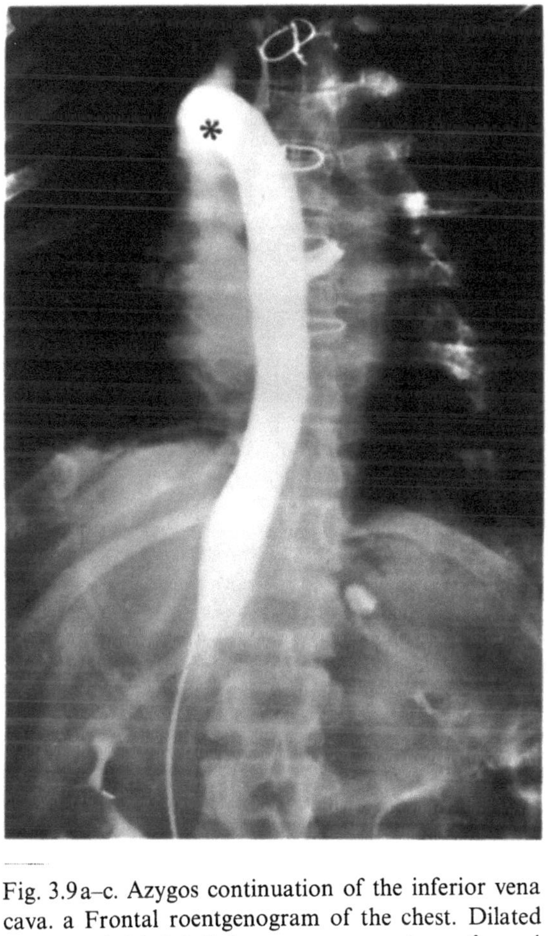

b

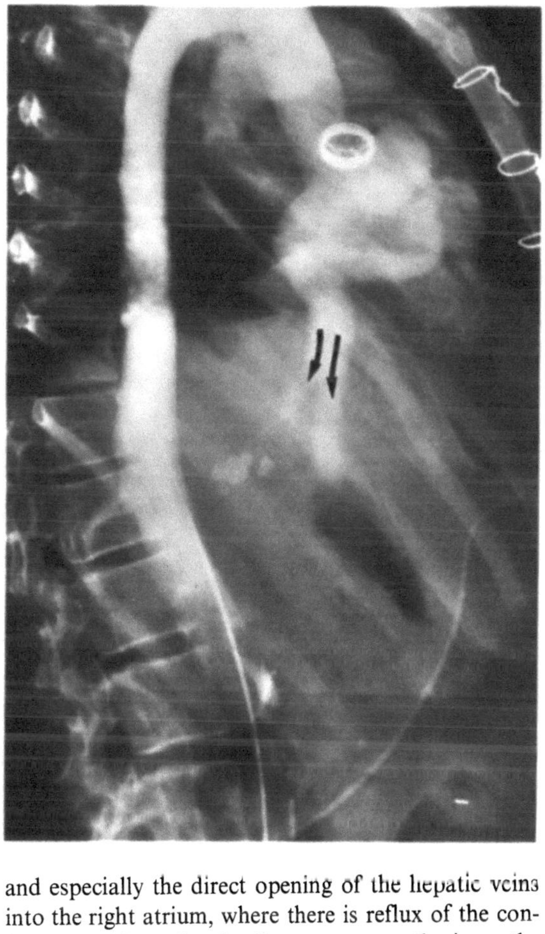

c

Fig. 3.9 a–c. Azygos continuation of the inferior vena cava. a Frontal roentgenogram of the chest. Dilated azygos arch (*). b Inferior vena cavography performed via a catheter inserted in the great azygos vein, which serves as continuation to the inferior vena cava above the level of the renal veins. c Lateral view of the same venography. Note the characteristic swan-neck image, and especially the direct opening of the hepatic veins into the right atrium, where there is reflux of the contrast (↙). Note also the Cutter-type prosthesis on the aorta. During extracorporeal circulation for the placement of this prosthesis the surgeon had not been able to cannulate the inferior vena cava from the right atrium on

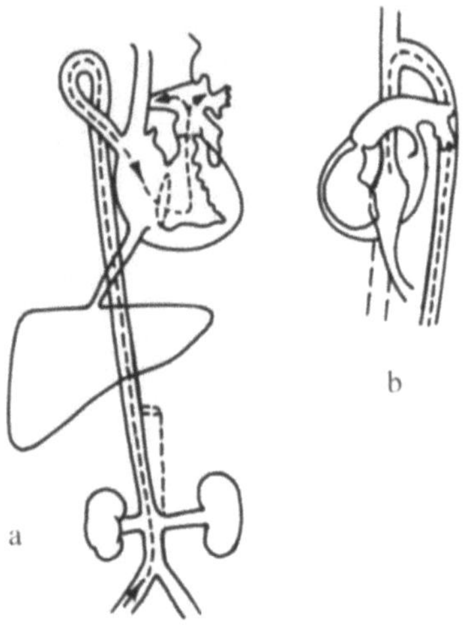

Fig. 3.10. Interest of investigations via lower approach. There is a risk of the azygos continuation passing undetected when the upper approach is used. a Frontal view. b Lateral view

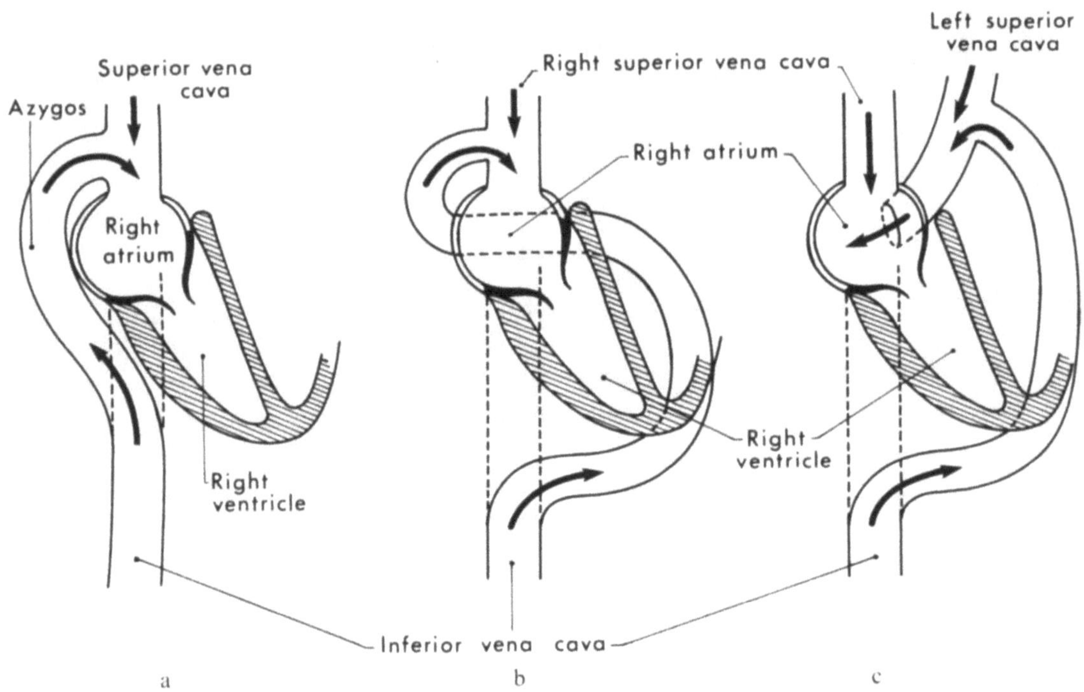

Fig. 3.11. a Azygos continuation of the inferior vena cava. b Hemiazygos continuation of the inferior vena cava into a right superior vena cava. c Hemiazygos continuation of the inferior vena cava into a left superior vena cava

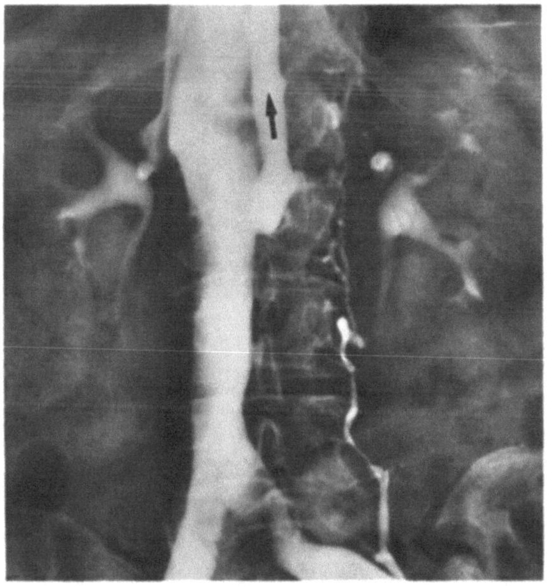

3.12a

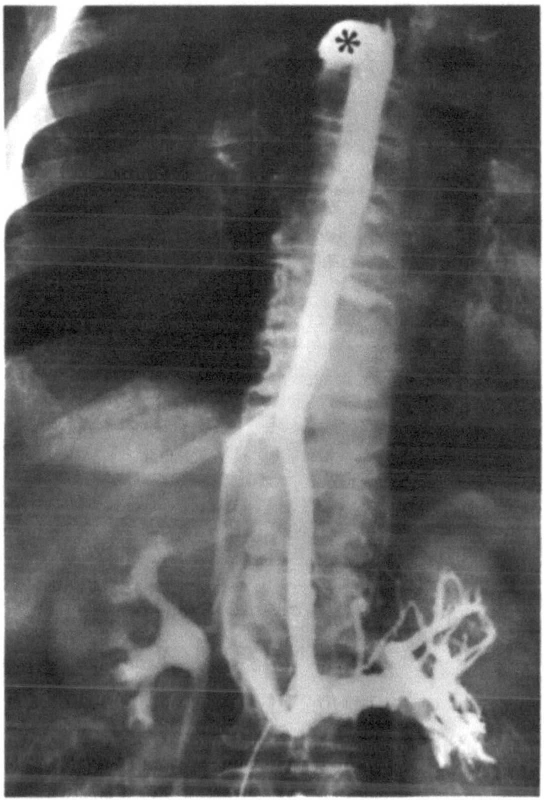

3.12b

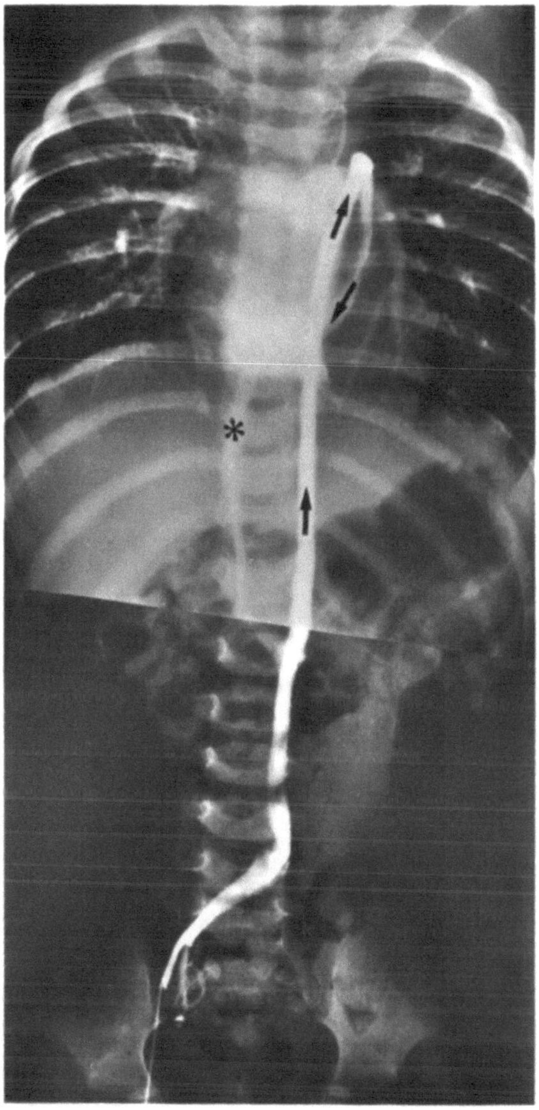

3.13

Fig. 3.12. a Percutaneous bifemoral inferior vena cavography. Extrinsic pressure defect on the left common iliac vein. Derivation via a left inferior hemiazygos vein (↗) at the level of the left renal vein. The retrohepatic segment of the inferior vena cava seems to be normal. b Left selective venography via the femoral vein. Filling of a large inferior hemiazygos vein which opens axially onto the great azygos vein at the level of T4 (*)

Fig. 3.13. Cavography in a child who had transposition of the large vessels. Right unilateral injection. Hemiazygos continuation of the inferior vena cava. This hemiazygos vein (↗) joins a persistent left superior vena cava which drains into the coronary sinus (↗). The retrohepatic segment of the inferior vena cava is partly patent (*). Note the medial location of the pulmonary artery trunk, which is characteristic for this type of cardiac malformation (transposition of the large vessels (by Courtory of P^{2}J Reing))

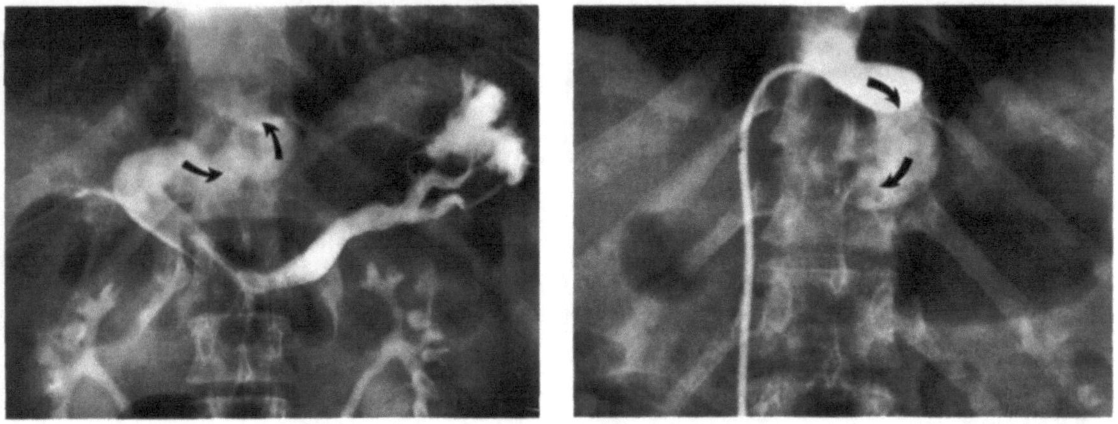

a b

Fig. 3.14a, b. Persistence of the Arantius canal. a Splenoportography showing the derivation of the portal flow via the Reix recess, which corresponds to the left portal branch (↗) and drains through a mediospinal venous canal (↗). b Cavography with catheterization of the Arantius canal. Moderate reflux due to the important blood flow in this canal. (By courtesy of Prof. J.L. Lamarque)

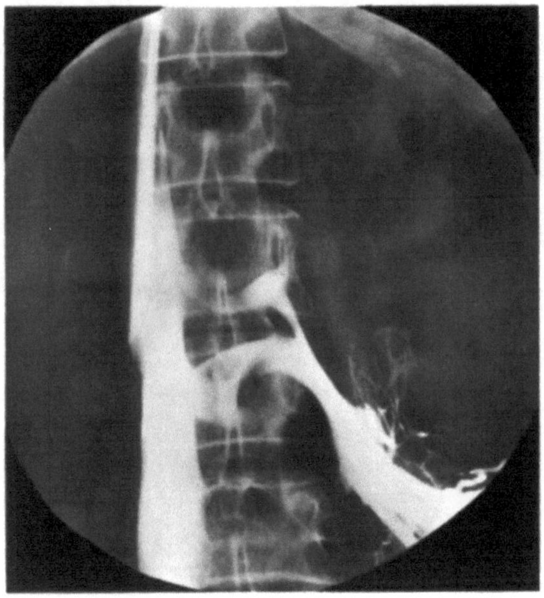

Fig. 3.15. Periaortic venous ring. Selective left inferior renal venography. The abdominal aorta passes through the center of the left renal venous ring. The retroaortic branch (which disappears normally) corresponds to the lowest located vein. It usually has a smaller caliber, not the case here. The two branches of the ring are anastomosed. The normal preaortic left renal vein lies just above. Note the presence of a left intrarenal expansive mass displacing downward the branches of the left renal vein

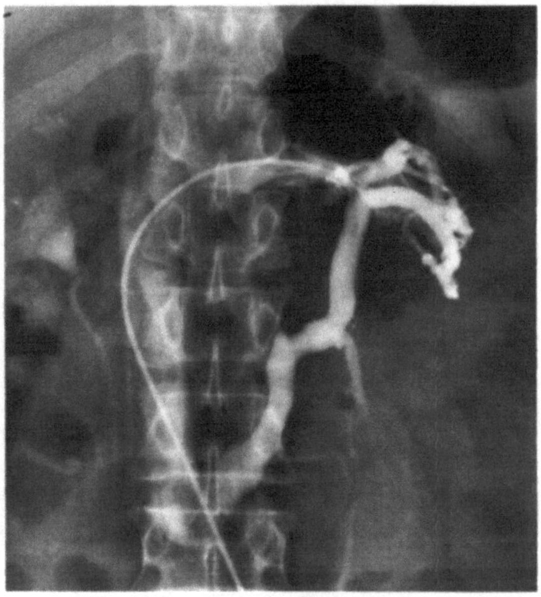

Fig. 3.16. Double left renal venous arch. Venography of the superior portion of the renal arch. Note that the left spermatic vein arises from the inferior portion of the renal venous arch

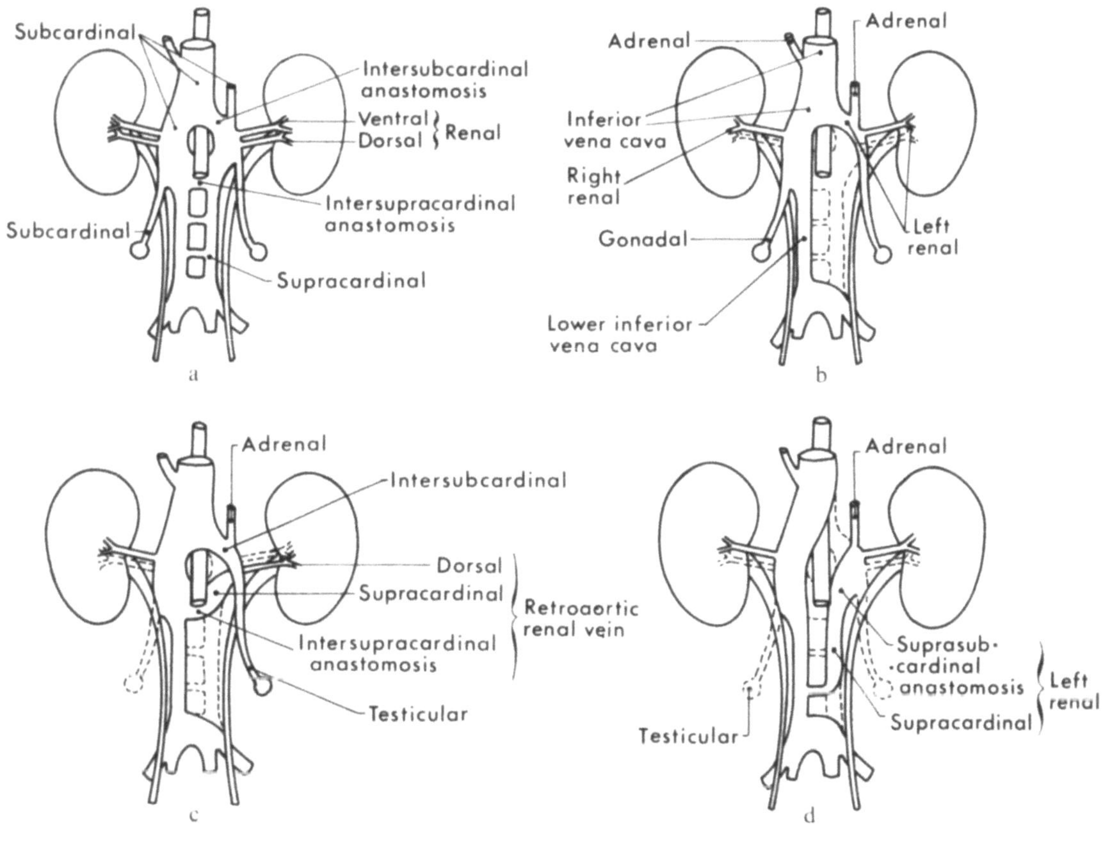

Fig. 3.17. a Simplified diagram to show the disposition of veins in the early embryo. The posterior cardinal veins have already disappeared, leaving the paired subcardinals which are ventral to the aorta and the paired supracardinals which lie dorsally. Anastomoses between these four trunks form a ring or collar at the renal level. The dorsal, retroaortic component atrophies together with the left supracardinal vein. b The changes mentioned above give rise to the normal adult pattern in which the subhepatic cava is formed from below upward from the right supracardinal vein, the right side of the renal collar, and the subcardinal vein. The left renal vein derives from the anastomosis between the subcardinal veins lying in front of the aorta. The stippled areas represent the parts of the primitive venous system which have atrophied. c Venous ring with left retroaortic renal vein. The preaortic renal vein receives the gonadal and suprarenal veins. d Retroaortic left renal vein with low junction level

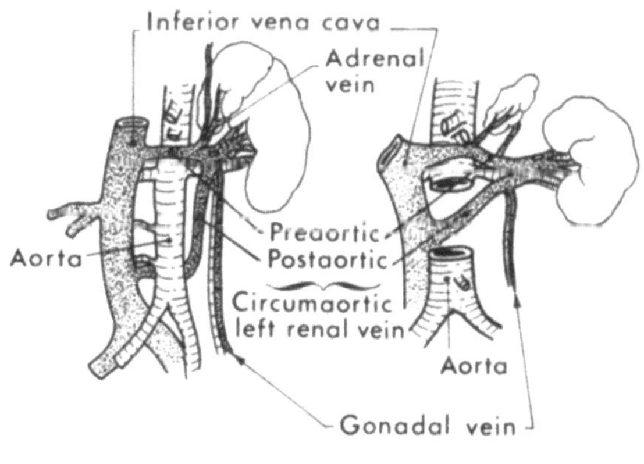

Fig. 3.18. Representation of the two types of periaortic left renal vein encountered in angiography

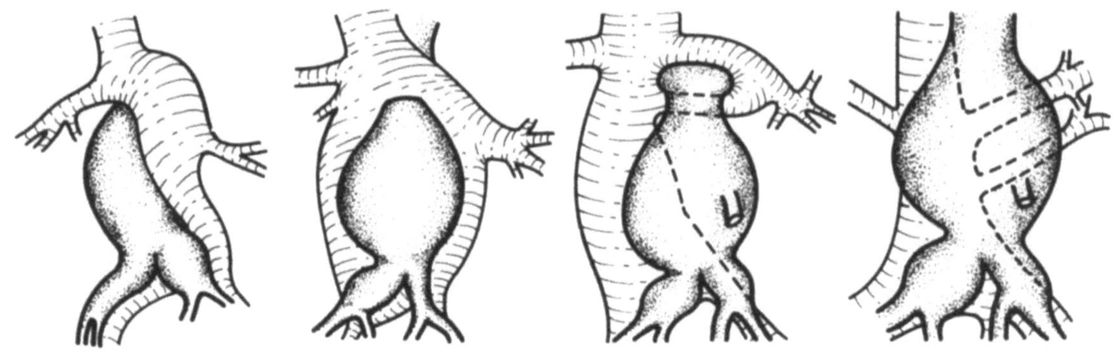

Fig. 3.19a–d. Aneurysm of the infrarenal abdominal aorta and congenital anomalies of the inferior vena cava. a Left inferior vena cava. b Double inferior vena cava. c Complete circumaortic venous ring. d Double left renal vein

Chapter 4. Intrinsic Iliocaval Pathology

Thromboembolic Disease of the Iliac Veins and of the Inferior Vena Cava

4.1 General Remarks

Thromboembolic disease is most often localized in the veins of the lower limbs but may also involve the iliac-inferior caval segment. Iliofemoral and iliocaval thrombosis is serious for two reasons: it is the origin of severe local or regional phenomena that produce important delayed sequels, and it causes a large number of massive pulmonary embolisms.

Phlebography plays an important role in this type of venous thrombosis. It allows accurate positive and topographic diagnosis, it guides the tactics of a surgical procedure, and may be used to evaluate early or delayed morphologic and functional results. Phlebography also has the merit of having demonstrated the frequency of thromboses without inflammatory signs of phlebitis, and of having shown how difficult it may sometimes be to establish a diagnosis of phlebitis on the strength of isolated clinical arguments. Classical thrombophlebitis is only a clinical form of venous thrombosis: all forms of it demand the same diagnostic procedures and the same inquiry into their etiology.

Iliofemoral thrombosis, including popliteal vein thrombosis, accounts for 75% of the cases of thrombosis of the veins of the lower limbs, according to Fontaine's statistics. On the basis of data from 100 cases we were able recently to demonstrate the importance of precise preoperative phlebographic diagnosis. This single technique, in iliofemoral thromboembolic disease, serves three ends: anatomopathologic, diagnostic, and above all, therapeutic. Iliofemoral thromboembolic disease can most often be treated surgically.

4.2. Thrombophlebitis of the Iliac Veins

4.2.1 Definition

The only definition to be retained is an anatomic definition: iliac thrombophlebitis involves a part or the whole of the venous segment between the junction of the deep femoral vein with the common femoral vein, and the termination of the common iliac vein on the inferior vena cava. This conception in terms of the iliofemoral segment treated as a single entity can best be understood using the notion of "critical points."

When the femoral bifurcation is occluded it constitutes a very dangerous area, since it is the level of convergence of the three collateral systems of the lower limb. Moreover, from this level originate the superficial subcutaneous and the deep hypogastric collateral pathways. Obstruction at this point of confluence causes total venous blockage in the lower limb and thus acute venous stasis.

The iliac venous bifurcation constitutes a second critical point: indeed, obliteration of the hypogastric vein partly cuts off the collateral circulation. Obstruction of the terminal segment of the common iliac vein is probably less dangerous, insofar as contralateral compensation is frequent and the homolateral ascending lumbar vein may suffice to circumvent the obstacle when only the common iliac termination is occluded. Finally, the clinical definition of iliofemoral thrombophlebitis cannot be retained for following reasons:

The symptomatology cannot always be ascribed to the occlusive or nonocclusive character of the thrombus, since there may be associated localized or diffuse inflammatory processes.

On the other hand, it is not possible to state, from the clinical data, whether a thrombosis in the iliac system is diffuse or segmental.

It would be the merit of noninvasive methods (velocimetry by Doppler effect, testing with labeled fibrinogen) to localize the occlusion to the iliofemoral segment and thus provide the indication for phlebography. But these methods are not entirely reliable, even at this level.

4.2.2 Clinical Symptoms

The lack of constancy and specificity of the symptoms accounts partly for retarded diagnosis. Iliac thrombophlebitis does not always realize the complete classical syndrome of pain in the thigh or groin with edema of the thigh and lower leg and dilatation of the superficial veins. Asymptomatic, mild, ambulatory, or latent forms are the main indications for phlebography, which should be systematically performed whenever venous thrombosis of the inferior limb is suspected. Strikingly, the most severe forms (phlebothrombosis, the cause of pulmonary embolism) have the least by way of clinical symptoms.

In a series of 100 iliac thromboses we found four clinical conditions:

1) Isolated venous thrombosis with edema of the thigh was observed in less than half of our cases; such clinical signs strongly point to iliac thrombophlebitis, but correspond often either to an acute phase of chronic phlebitis, or to very adhesive, hence quite evolved, inflammatory phlebitis.
2) Other cases showed clinical features of ischemic phlebitis, either the classical features of phlegmasia cerulea dolens, or, in four cases, the features of venous gangrene (moist gangrene with phlyctenae). Out of 100 cases of iliofemoral phlebitis we found 12 ischemic forms, i.e. 8 cases of phlegmasia cerulea and 4 of venous gangrene. These two forms belong in fact to the same clinicopathologic entity; they differ only in the degree of venous obstruction. All cases of iliac ischemic phlebitis examined in this series were late diagnosed (3 to 8 days after the occurrence of the first clinical signs).
3) Pulmonary embolism sometimes revealed the existence of iliac phlebitis.
4) In more than one-third of our cases, there were nonspecific clinical signs, which only systematic phlebography showed to be correlated with iliac phlebitis.

It is the lack of specificity of the symptoms and their late occurrence that lead us, after other authors (Haller, Fontaine), to reject the clinical definition of iliofemoral phlebitis.

4.2.3 Preoperative Angiographic Investigations (Phlebography of the Lower Limb and Iliocavography)

Technology has greatly simplified this investigation, which is now performed under quite satisfactory technical conditions. Improved contrast media provide better opacification and better tolerance, hence permit the injection of larger amounts. The harmlessness of this method has been affirmed in the literature, particularly by Fontaine, and is confirmed by our statistics: there is no pulmonary embolism secondary to phlebography in our series. Two patients developed scabs on the back of the foot secondary to extravasation of contrast material into the subcutaneous tissues. One of them had skin grafting performed.

As concerns phlebographic investigations in acute iliofemoral venous thrombosis, we observe the following imperatives:

1) A phlebography, with all its modalities, can be performed in extreme emergency at any time of day or night.
2) Bifemoral percutaneous iliocavography has always been attempted.
3) Ascending phlebography of the leg (by puncture of a vein in the back of the foot) is also carried out, as far as possible.

The ideal would be to achieve opacification of the entire venous system of the diseased lower limb, with complete study of the iliofemoral axis and above all of the inferior vena cava, in order to localize the upper extent of the thrombus, which is fundamental for surgery.

Phlebography of the Lower Limb

Since iliofemoral phlebitis is frequently accompanied by edema, it is in numerous cases necessary to apply an Esmarch bandage, so as to reduce the edema and hence render visible the superficial veins. All injections have been performed with an automatic injector with constant delivery rate. The contrast medium is always a product containing 380 mg iodine/ml injected at a rate ranging from 3 to 6 ml/s.

We have always injected 80 to 100 ml contrast, so as to opacify at once not only the collateral circulation of the lower limb but also the homo- or contralateral collateral circulation. Physiologic, ascending opacification of the iliofemoral system, or, when this is obliterated, of its collaterals, may readily be obtained with ascending, nonpressurized phlebographies, provided a sufficient amount of contrast material is injected at a constant rate. Manual injection never permits one to obtain the same amount of morphologic and hemodynamic information, especially in iliofemoral phlebitis; furthermore, it has the drawbacks of irradiation. At the end of injection the superficial and the deep veins are rinsed with physiologic saline solution with heparin.

Bilateral Percutaneous Iliocavography

We have always made a point of attempting percutaneous puncture of both femoral veins in all patients, even when the ascending phlebography had shown one of them to be thrombosed (Fig. 4.1 a, b). We have never observed migration of embolus during phlebography. Puncture of the thrombosed femoral vein is possible and there is a very slight reflux of blood, very different from the normal physiologic reflux. The injection moulds the thrombus perfectly (Fig. 4.1 c) and usually allows its head to be opacified. Occasionally the puncture was not possible but it was nevertheless possible to catheterize a small superficial vein draining the collateral system (usually a branch of the arch of the internal saphenous vein) and to demonstrate the homolateral and contralateral derivation routes. In other cases, we have performed a left anterior oblique cavographic projection so as to localize some intracaval thrombi located on the posterior wall of the inferior vena cava when the patient is supine. The oblique projection provides a good visualization of such thrombi.

Descending Retrograde Cavography

Descending retrograde cavography is performed to demonstrate the head of an intracaval thrombus (Figs. 4.2a, b and 4.3). The technique is simple: A catheter with side holes is introduced, with the help of a Desilets introducer, at the level of the bend of elbow and pushed through the superior vena cava, via the right atrium, into the inferior vena cava. Continual test injections make it possible to stop 2 to 3 cm above the head of the thrombus. A high-rate injection (20 ml/s at least) permits perfect outlining of the inferior vena cava, and in certain cases of the common iliac veins up to the external iliac valve. It also demonstrates the renal veins, if this is necessary. This technique provides less contrasted pictures than occlusive inferior vena cavography, but allows nevertheless very precise radioanatomic diagnoses, which have always been confirmed by surgery.

Retrograde Iliac Phlebography

This additional technique (Fig. 4.4) localizes precisely the upper level of an iliofemoral thrombus. It opacifies the homolateral iliac system in a retrograde fashion, thanks to contralateral venous Seldinger procedure. A high-rate injection moulds the head of the iliofemoral thrombus. The upper level of the thrombus should not be confused with the image of the external iliac valve, which is usually located at the termination of the external iliac vein: the valve is convex downward, whereas the head of the thrombus is generally convex upward. This technique has the advantage of permitting partial opacification of the homolateral hypogastric system when it is patent.

4.2.4 Radioanatomic Forms

Radioanatomic and Topographic Type of Iliac Thrombophlebitis

Topography. There is a clear prevalence of left iliac thrombophlebites. The left iliac venous compression syndrome may give evidence, at least partly, of this prevalence. Among a series of 60 patients with iliac thrombosis, Lea Thomas et al. found three radioanatomic and topographic types:
Group 1: external iliac thrombosis (9 cases)
Group 2: common iliac thrombosis (11 cases)
Group 3: diffuse iliac thrombosis (external iliac and common iliac vein; 37 cases)

Three patients of their series had bilateral iliac obstruction.

In our series of 100 patients with iliac phlebitis, we found the topographic features indicated in Table 4.1. Table 4.1 calls for the following comments:

Table 4.1.

Iliac phlebitis	Right	Left
Unilateral (92)	29	63
Segmental		
Common iliac vein	1	4
External iliac vein	10	8
Diffuse	18	51
Thrombosis of the deep veins of the lower limbs	8	30
Free thrombus in the postrenal segment of inferior vena cava	5	3

Table 4.2. Radioanatomic type (phlebographic diagnosis)

	Iliac phlebitis	Caval phlebitis
Phlebothrombosis	31	9
Thrombophlebitis	69	3

As many authors, we find a clear predominance of unilateral left iliac phlebitis (63 of 92).

We have noted the two common topographic types of iliac phlebitis:

1) Segmental iliac phlebitis, especially external iliac, corresponds usually to the head of a femoral thrombus and represents the greater part of our cases with segmental phlebitis; however, we had 5 cases with segmental common iliac thrombi (Fig. 4.12), most often free thrombi, in the terminal segment of the common iliac vein. These can be located above a patent iliofemoral system, or above an ancient iliofemoral phlebitis. This is a fundamental notion, since three of our five cases correspond to acute phases in chronic iliac phlebitis in patients treated with heparin. Thus, it seems that a thrombus may develop above chronic iliac phlebitis in patients receiving anticoagulant treatment. This particularly emboligenic thrombus passes undetected when cavography is not systematically per-

formed in addition to phlebography of the lower limb.

2) Diffuse iliac phlebitis represents the greater part of our series (69 of 92 unilateral phlebites). In this group the predominance of left-sided involvement is very clear (51 left, 18 right).

There exists a frequent misunderstanding according to which thrombosis of the iliac veins results from an ascending progression from a thrombus located in the veins of the leg. In our series, isolated iliac vein phlebitis, i.e., without involvement of the subjacent segment, is very frequent: 58% of the cases. While it is true that such a progression may be encountered, most of the cases with iliac phlebitis nevertheless show patency of the veins of the leg and of the popliteal vein.

Among our series of 100 patients, high-situated extensive thrombosis of the deep veins of the lower limb was found in 42 cases; 38 times it was associated with unilateral iliac vein phlebitis, and 4 times with bilateral iliac vein phlebitis.

Bilateral iliac phlebitis is rare, but far from being exceptional, since we found it in 8 cases, of which 4 were associated with inferior vena caval thrombosis.

Radioanatomic Type. Classically, the semiologic data provided by phlebography allow one to determine the radioanatomic type of the phlebitis. A floating thrombus, with a "snake head" image, is classically attributed to a very emboligenic and poorly adhesive phlebothrombosis. In inflammatory and adhesive thrombophlebitis, phlebography shows a very faint opacification of the iliac system and, especially, derivation via the collateral circulation. Table 4.2 shows the radioanatomic types of phlebitis in our series of 100 patients as diagnosed from the phlebogram.

Adhesive thrombophlebitis predominates in our series, since we found 69 cases with iliac vein phlebitis of this type. Iliac vein phlebothrombosis is less frequent, but our group includes 9 cases with associated floating thrombus in the inferior vena cava, which is a strongly emboligenic form.

In the literature, numerous publications point out the discrepancy between the phlebographic findings and the surgical verification. A rather poor angiographic technique very likely accounts for this fact. Obviously, precision in the radioanatomic diagnosis is only possible with exhaustive and complete phlebographic investigations. Simple phlebography of the lower limb is insufficient to identify the radioanatomic type of iliac phlebitis. Another factor has also to be taken into account with regard to the radiosurgical discrepancies, namely the delay between phlebography and the surgical procedure. The rapidity of the inflammatory phenomena may very quickly change phlebothrombosis into adhesive phlebitis, thus rendering unreliable a diagnosis of recent or long-standing phlebitis.

Iliac Phlebitis and Congenital Anomaly of the Ilio-Inferior Caval System

Systematic phlebograms of iliac vein phlebitis allowed us to find among our 100 cases several congenital anomalies of the iliac veins and three anomalies of the inferior vena cava (two cases with left inferior vena cava, and one case of double inferior vena cava) (Fig. 4.5). Anomalies of the inferior vena cava are dealt with in Chapter 3.

4.2.5 Evolutive Forms

Acute Iliac Thrombophlebitis

This is the most often encountered radioclinical feature. Of our series, 84 patients have been examined in the 24 h following the occurrence of the first clinical symptoms. We have already pointed out the lack of specificity of certain clinical symptoms. Since the respective indications for treatment with heparin or thrombolytic drugs or for surgery depend largely on the phlebographic data, it seems necessary to perform phlebography as soon as phlebitis is suspected. This attitude implies that angiographic investigations, with all technical modalities, were carried out as said previously. We must admit that in daily practice, and apart from some main hospitals, phlebographic investigations can only rarely be performed at any time of day or night.

Chronic Iliac Phlebitis

During treatment, the phlebogram shows a more or less complete recanalization with a stenosed "laminated" appearance of the iliac axis as evidence of the recanalization of the thrombosis (Figs. 4.13 and 4.14). Collateral circulation depends on the degree of recanalization of the main iliac axis. A postphlebitic syndrome is frequently encountered in chronic iliac phlebitis: more than half of them after the fifth year. The disturbances are more severe, the more extensive the anatomic lesions are.

One peculiar feature must be pointed out: the existence of acute phases on chronic phlebitis. The clinical signs are particularly misleading and real phlebothrombosis may develop above a femoral or iliac pathway involved by chronic phlebitis. One may thus understand the occurrence of pulmonary embolism in chronic phlebitis (Fig. 4.8).

Forms Revealed by Pulmonary Embolism

Iliac phlebitis is the most emboligenic of the phlebites (Fig. 4.6). In our series of 100 cases, pulmonary embolism has been the predominant revealing sign of iliac phlebitis in eight cases. There were almost no underlying clinical signs in four of these eight cases. The phlebitis was of the phlebothrombotic type in four cases, two of which with a floating intracaval thrombus, and of the adhesive phlebitis type in four cases. Iliocavography made it possible in the same investigation, to carry out pulmonary angiography via the retrograde femoral approach and through the contralateral iliac system, which was patent, since the eight cases had unilateral iliac phlebitis.

The incidence of iliofemoral thrombosis in angiographically confirmed pulmonary embolisms varies between 12% and 15%. Fontaine recorded 12% of pulmonary embolisms, with 7.2% having caused death, among 249 cases of iliofemoral thrombosis. Our figure of 8% of revealing pulmonary embolisms is certainly below the actual proportion insofar as we have only taken into account patients who had a phlebography performed.

Ischemic Phlebitis

This type of phlebitis does not perhaps deserve to be treated separately, since in our series it always corresponds to very advanced, untreated cases of iliac phlebitis. Extensive upstream thrombosis of the veins of the lower limb was a constant finding. This has been reported by several authors in this type of ischemic phlebitis.

4.2.6 Etiologic Forms

Primary Iliac Phlebitis

In our series of 100 patients this condition represents the greater part of the cases (64%) for which no general or local cause has been found. Our statistics thus comprise a very large proportion of "primary" iliac phlebitis whereas previous publications report percentages ranging from 10% to 33% (Lenegre, Barker)

Secondary Iliac Thrombophlebitis

Locoregional causes are diverse and more detailedly dealt with in later chapters. Usually there is an abdominopelvic tumoral etiology causing extrinsic compression or even invasion of the vein, producing stasis and then thrombosis. It must be pointed out how difficult it is to differentiate on a phlebogram some signs of venous invasion from a real iliac thrombosis, the more so since association of the two is possible. Among our series of 100 patients there were six cases with signs of true left iliac venous compression associated with iliac phlebitis (Figs. 4.7 and 4.15). Among the locoregional favoring factors there is also the iliofemoral venous catheterization performed for right cardiac catheterization, for placement of a pacing catheter, or for selective venography of one of the branches of the inferior vena cava.

General causes: among our series of 100 patients, 14 presented a general cause which could have accounted for the occurrence of phlebitis. These causes are classic: cardiac insufficiency with decompensation, cachexia, evolutive neoplasia, hemopathy, and, finally, postoperative phlebitis.

4.3 Left Common Iliac Compression Syndrome

4.3.1 History – Definition

As early as 1854, l'Aulnoye reported the presence of a "membrane" in the lumen of the left common iliac vein (LCIV).

This was confirmed in 1954 by Fellus in his thesis. In 1965 Cockett and Lea Thomas published a study bearing on 35 patients with a major obstruction of the left common iliac vein; they described this syndrome which has since been known as the "Cockett syndrome."

More recently, in 1969, Sztankay noted 20.6% of anomalies in a series of 500 dissections.

The Cockett syndrome comprises two clinical stages, an acute and a chronic, associated with three main phlebographic findings.

1) Thrombosis obstructing the more or less recanalized LCIV.
2) Marked collateral circulation (Fig. 4.16).
3) Cockett insists on a third and purely anatomic criterion which would correspond to fibrous stenosis involving the LCIV at the point where it crosses below the right common iliac artery (RCIA). This stenosis would be secondary to chronic compression by the artery.

The actual definition has also been applied to cases satisfying the above-described cardioanatomic criteria, but examined prior to the thrombosis stage.

4.3.2 Radioanatomy of the Junction of the LCIV with the Inferior Vena Cava

The LCIV results from the union of the hypogastric vein with the external iliac vein.

The LCIV is situated anteriorly and medially to its artery (LCIA) and courses obliquely upward and to the right. It bends medially, emerges between the common iliac arteries, crosses the right common iliac artery (RCIA) dorsally to unite with the right common iliac vein (RCIV) on the right side of the midline and form the inferior vena cava.

The length of the LCIV ranges between 69 and 78 mm. It is 16 to 18 mm wider than the RCIV.

Noteworthy is the fact that it is usually valveless at the level of its crossing with the RCIA.

The main relations of the LCIV are as follows.

At its origin, i.e., at the junction of the hypogastric with the external iliac vein, the LCIV is behind and somewhat below the iliac arterial bifurcation. Several types of relations are encountered, depending on the relative levels of the arterial bifurcation and of the venous confluence. The LCIV is thereafter related with the LCIA, which is in front of and above it, covering it partly and coursing more or less close to it; then it crosses dorsal to the RCIA, usually just before the caval confluence. Thus, the origin of the inferior vena cava is normally situated below, behind, and to the right of the aortic bifurcation.

But these relations may vary. On the basis of 97 dissections, Negus describes three types: (1) the classical type, as seen above, 75%; (2) a higher type, in which the RCIA crosses the inferior vena cava anteriorly, and courses along the left aspect of the RCIV, 22%; and (3) a lower type, in which the RCIA crosses the LCIV prior to its termination, and courses along the left aspect of the RCIV before also crossing it anteriorly to join its right aspect.

The second main relation of the caval confluence is the lumbar spine. The inferior vena cava is related to its right aspect, most of the time at the L4–5 disk level, but sometimes higher, at the L4 vertebral body, or lower, at the L5 body.

Louis and Maresca, from 105 dissections, described five types of variation, depending on the level of the aortic bifurcation with regard to the spine and with regard to the caval confluence.

What mainly matters is the level at which the RCIA crosses in front of the iliocaval junction. Thus there may be either crossing in front of the vena cava alone, or crossing in front of both the inferior vena cava and the RCIV, both the LCIV and the RCIV, or, finally, of the LCIV alone, which is the most common occurrence. This depends moreover on the relative levels of the arterial and venous bifurcations, and would account for the existence of bilateral or even isolated right compressions.

A third relation is to be noted in this area: the relation with the lymphatic system which courses closely alongside the LCIV, forming a plexus at its side and ascending with it toward the caval confluence.

Finally, the LCIV is also related to the branches and especially to the collateral routes followed by the blood flow in case of interruption of the normal routes. Angiography has made it possible to make numerous anatomic descriptions by providing a true "functional anatomy" of the iliofemoral and common iliac collateral circulation (see Chap. 5).

4.3.3 Pathologic Anatomy

Compression of the LCIV by the RCIA has been known for a long time and reported by numerous anatomists: MacMurrich in 1906, Ehrich and Kumbhaar in 1943, May and Thurner in 1957, and Negus in 1968 have all described this compression. Numerous surgeons had also noted the compression, in particular Cockett, who reports a number of cases to show true fibrous stenosis of the LCIV at the point where it crosses dorsal to the RCIA. In his thesis, David reports about nine patients presenting such a compression, and in whom the vein was seen to be flattened against the spine by the artery.

The frequency of such compressions is very high compared to that of clinical signs of venous insufficiency, which raises the problem of the physiologic limits of such a syndrome.

Negus deduced from measurements of LCIV diameters that a markedly reduced AP diameter is often compensated by an increased transverse diameter, so that, apart from the cases with endovenous synechiae, the cross-sectional area is minimally reduced, and, hence, the venous flow only slightly diminished.

According to David's peroperative findings, the LCIV is, on the contrary, very often completely flattened. Moreover, even if the total cross-sectional area at this point is not diminished, changes in its shape would in any case provoke turbulence and stasis and hence favor thrombosis.

Nevertheless, the large proportion of patients with an LCIV stenosis without other symptoms does not allow one to conclude that the stenosis is pathologic by itself.

Perhaps more significant is association of iliac compression and endovenous lesions.

A number of anatomists have dissected the LCIV and have discovered anomalies. David summarizes the percentage of anomalies found on 2,229 LCIV dissections. The different authors report an average of 22.3% of endovenous anomalies of the LCIV. The different types described concern parietal hypertrophic lesions, sometimes joining within the lumen to form true endovenous synechiae. The anatomists give various descriptions, but all point out marginal or central obstacles. Histologically it is fibrous sclerosis of the intima with parietal hypertrophy. Junction of two hypertrophic sites facing each other forms an endovenous synechia (Fig. 4.18), developing the more easily, the more the AP diameter is reduced by extrinsic compression.

The presence of hypertrophic stenoses and/or synechiae raises the problem of their etiology.

4.3.4 Etiology: Congenital or Acquired?

The embryology, as well as the existence of other malformations of the LCIV related to the embryologic development, would suggest a congenital origin. As a matter of fact the LCIV derives for a large part from the anastomosis of the two posterior cardinal veins, dorsal to the aorta: the interiliac anastomosis. During embryogenesis the left posterior cardinal vein disappears and the blood flows through this anastomosis. Right at its origin the LCIV is thus formed by the left posterior cardinal vein, but for its main part it is formed by the posterior intercardinal iliac anastomoses, whereas the RCIV results entirely from the right posterior cardinal vein, the iliocaval confluence resulting from the entry of the anastomosis into the right posterior cardinal vein.

Thus a certain number of congenital malformations concerning mainly the LCIV have been described: pure and simple aplasia, obstruction of the inferior vena cava associated with bone malformations, and duplication of the LCIV (Fig. 4.17). Is it not conceivable that anastomoses that should theoretically disappear during the embryologic development might persist and small duplications (Fig. 4.20) along the course of the anastomoses account for the presence of these endovenous malformations?

However, other arguments exist, in favor of an acquired origin. The major argument is the fact that the percentage of endovenous lesions increases with the age of the patients: in 88 autopsied fetuses, May and Thurner found no endovenous anomaly. On 127 autopsies of children and newborns, Ehrich and Kumbhaar found only 4.7% of endovenous anomalies, whereas they found 33% in adults.

Finally, according to Cockett, it is the intima that is affected by hypertrophic perivenous fibrosis with thickening when there is a compression, whatever the site. Indeed, though compression of the LCIV by the RCIA is the most frequent, other areas of crossing may be the site of compressions; we shall see these later on. The existence of other perivenous lesions similar to that of the LCIV would be in favor of an acquired, reactional origin of the endovenous lesions, though, to our knowledge, no endovenous synechiae have been seen in these cases.

4.3.5 The Angiographic Features of the Syndrome

Technique

Several venographic techniques are available. We always carry out one or both of (a) and (b) below:

Upstream phlebography of the lower limb. 80 to 100 ml contrast medium is injected in order to opacify at once the collateral circulation of the lower limb as well as the iliopelvic homo- and contralateral superior collateral circulation. This technique demonstrates well the iliofemoral system (Fig. 4.24a).

When a doubt remains, we use an additional technique (Fig. 4.24b).

Bilateral percutaneous iliocavography by percutaneous puncture of both femoral veins. Unilateral injection would provide a more reliable study of the possible collateral circulation, but anomalies on the right iliac system would be mistaken.

Finally, when a defect is seen in the course of a vein, and when there is doubt as to whether it could be an arterial impression, it is possible, as Lea Thomas does, to couple phlebography and aortography, and superimpose the two (Fig. 4.26).

Recording the pressures. The phlebographic investigation terminates with measurement of the pressures: it is useful to evaluate the pressure gradient of the inferior vena cava and the LCIV. According to Negus and to Cockett a gradient superior to 2 mm Hg corresponds to obstruction. During exercise the increase of the gradient is considerable with regard to values measured in normal subjects. This explains for a large part the venous claudication described by Cockett.

But, what is most important, the gradient is low or nonexistent when there is an important collateral circulation, i.e., in cases of severe obstruction.

It seems thus that measurement of pressures has only a minor value for the study of the iliac compression syndrome.

Results

We study successively compression with or without synechiae, the possible collateral circulation, and finally the recording of pressures, which can be performed at the end of the angiographic examination.

Compression with or without synechiae. From the morphological point of view, three compression patterns may be described from the phlebogram. There may be a linear strip traversing the vein over its entire length, the artery seeming to be moulded by the contrast material.

Sometimes, one sees only a simple lateral spur, with its base on the wall of the vein and the tip becoming blurred within the lumen.

Finally, there is sometimes a central defect, separating two channels. This feature seen on the LCIV corresponds to a synechia (Fig. 4. 19). The arterial impression is most often located on the LCIV: in 11 of 12 cases with a defect seen on the phlebogram, Lea Thomas and Fletcher found the impression of the RCIA on the very terminal part of the LCIV. They note, however, six other images which could be consistent with arterial impressions, and one could imagine that in some cases compressions exist elsewhere, for instance on the inferior vena cava when the aortic bifurcation is in a higher position, or on the RCIV when this is crossed anteriorly by the RCIA, which explains the presence of a bilateral or solely right compression syndrome.

For all that, a defect due to the passage of the RCIA should be a pathological sign, but this is not the opinion of most authors: impression of the RCIA on the LCIV is a frequent, even a constant occurrence. Negus reports 17% of dilated LCIV without defect, 62% of dilatation with arterial impression, and 4% of dilatation with an image indicating synechiae.

According to Cockett, compression is commonly seen but adherences are rare.

Collateral circulation. Association of collateral circulation and phlebographic defects is more significant. This is invariably seen in thromboses. Visualization of the collateral channels (the anatomic appearances of which have been described above) is sometimes associated with images of defects though the patient has no, or had never had, signs of thrombosis (Fig. 4.21).

These results should be critically considered: indeed, according to some authors, filling of the ascending lumbar vein would be virtually constant, as well as minimal reflux into the hypogastric trunk, during iliocavography. However, according to most of the authors, collateral circulation allowing a left-to-right pelvis shunt seems highly pathological (Fig. 4.23). There is however one exception: passage via the presacral plexuses, which seems to be very frequent. This may be explained quite adequately by the fact that the presacral plexuses are valveless, so that it is easy for the flow to take this route.

It should also be pointed out that the results may vary with the position of the patient during the investigation. In particular, a certain number of images seem to disappear when the patient is prone and reappear when the patient is supine (Fig. 4.25). Thus a phlebogram performed with the patient prone seems preferable, since the persistence of compression and derivation images would be an additional sign of the severity of the compression. According to David, the variations in the degree of compression are due to the fact that the RCIA is not the only cause, and that the degree of lumbar lordosis also plays a role, the lumbar vertebra together with the RCIA acting like pincers on the LCIV. This accounts for the accentuation of the signs with the patient supine or upright. In the latter case, moreover, the pressure increases due to the orthostatism, whereas the prone position diminishes the importance of the signs.

4.3.6 Common Iliac Compression Syndrome

It is not our purpose to develop all pathologic problems raised by this syndrome. We shall only quote the main ones among them:

The First Problem

The first problem, which seems fundamental, is that of the boundaries between the physiologic and the pathologic aspects of the iliac compression syndrome. As a proof we would like to point out the chance diagnosis of this syndrome by phlebographic investigations carried out for other indications than thromboembolic disease. The existence of an isolated venous compression seems insufficient for diagnosing a Cockett's syndrome and must be considered physiological. On the other hand, the presence of venous synechiae and of collateral circulation (left to right) seems an unquestionable sign. The presence of one of these latter signs is not sufficient.

The Second Problem

The second problem concerns the association of a left iliac compression syndrome with phlebitis of the subjacent lower limb. Among 100 cases of iliac phlebitis we have found 58% of isolated iliac phlebitis without subjacent involvement (63% of these cases were on the left side). Of the total 100, only 30% had extensive thrombosis of the subjacent deep veins. In this series, six patients had a Cockett's syndrome with synechiae of the LCIV confirmed by surgery (Fig. 4.27). It seems thus that the Cockett syndrome explains partly the left preponderance of phlebites and, on the other hand, that phlebites of the lower limbs do not always affect the whole length, but may correspond to isolated segmental iliac phlebites (Fig. 4.22), integrated or not in the Cockett syndrome.

Correlations Between the Cockett Syndrome and Pulmonary Embolism

It is actually proved that iliofemoral phlebites are the most emboligenic. According to Cockett, however, the iliac compression syndrome diminishes the risk of pulmonary embolism insofar as the embolus could only with difficulty pass the narrow pathway at the compression site.

There is still another unsolved problem: it concerns the patients who had a bilateral phlebographic and a cavographic complete investigation after pulmonary embolism. When these investigations are entirely negative, when they display no signs of recent or long-standing thrombophlebitis, and when they do not give evidence of a Cockett syndrome, is it possible to incriminate the latter in the genesis of the embolism?

Association of an Iliac Compression Syndrome and Varicocele

Ponthieu and Huguet in 1976 reported six cases of left varicocele with an iliac compression syndrome in man. Among these six cases, left selective spermatic phlebography showed no renospermatic reflux in three cases. The authors make the following hypothesis: the left iliac venous compression syndrome would at least partly explain some left varicoceles by an anastomosis between the spermatic vein and the left common iliac vein via the epigastric vein. In the female, Cockett has shown the existence of phlebitis of the left lower limb secondary to hysterectomy. Suppression of some pelvic varices in females may suppress efficient collateral circulation and thus provoke either phlebitis, or chronic venous insufficiency of the lower limb.

4.4 Thrombosis of the Inferior Vena Cava

Obliteration of the inferior vena cava by a fibrinocruoric thrombus may be considered the most severe manifestation of thromboembolic disease. Paradoxically for this large vessel, it often remains unknown and is particularly formidable since it causes massive pulmonary embolism in one case in two. Inferior vena cavography becomes here a screening method and is the only investigation to affirm its presence (Fig. 4.28). Malignant intracaval thrombi extend sometimes from a renal vein (malignant tumor of the kidney) (Figs. 4.32 and 4.33).

4.4.1 Frequency, Etiology, Radioanatomic Localization

Factors Favoring Thrombosis

Thrombosis of the inferior vena cava represents, according to the statistics, 5% to 15% of the venous thromboses of the lower limbs. It was the merit of iliocavography to show the frequency of this localization of thromboembolic disease. Among our series of 100 iliac phlebites we have 12 cases with associated thrombosis of the postrenal segment of the inferior vena cava (Fig. 4.30). In four cases there was evidence of adhesive-type caval thrombosis, with nonopacification of the inferior vena cava and derivation via the collateral circulation. Inferior vena cava thrombosis sometimes reflects a thromboembolic disease the primary character of which can only be attested by the elimination of any local or regional cause. Sometimes it results from nonphlebitic obliteration by benign or malignant, invasive or expansive retroperitoneal processes, which compress, invade, or infiltrate completely the inferior vena cava, thus being responsible for true fibrinocruoric thrombosis secondary to compression or invasion of the inferior vena cava.

The diagnostic process is clearly not simple and it may sometimes be difficult, even with the help of multiple projections, absolutely to rule out extrinsic compression or invasion of the cava by a retroperitoneal process.

Moreover, association of the two is possible, since the fibrous or neoplastic inflammatory changes in the pericaval tissues favor the occurrence of adjacent thrombophlebitis, which could provide a clue for the diagnosis as we have seen with some cases of seminoma of the testicle, in which inferior vena caval thrombosis was the first clinical sign of a cancer of the testicle. The clinician should indeed always fear the presence of a latent neoplasia when discovering a thrombosis of the inferior vena cava, since some statistics show one-third of the cases to have a neoplastic etiology.

Initial Localization of the Thrombosis

Isolated thrombosis of the inferior vena cava is relatively rare. In the great majority of cases the thrombus originates from the iliac system and extends into the inferior vena cava.

Extension of the Thrombus

This depends on anatomic and hemodynamic factors. The inferior vena cava may be divided into two segments:

1) The initial or postrenal segment is very large and communicates almost only with the spinal plexuses, which have a low capacity. It is commonly involved in iliac phlebitis.
2) The other, visceral segment, with the renal pedicle at its origin, and the confluence of the hepatic veins at its termination, which all act as hemodynamic barriers impeding the extension of the thrombus.

Another factor intervenes in the extension of the thrombus: namely the collateral circulation, when it is markedly developed, which accounts very well for the latency of these caval thromboses. The chapter dealing with the collateral circulation provides a detailed study of these derivation routes.

4.4.2 Radioclinical Diagnosis

The long clinical latency of this localization of thromboembolic disease explains the difficulty of making an early diagnosis. Most often the inferior vena cava involvement follows more or less typical peripheral signs, which form part of the symptoms of a sometimes bilateral iliac phlebitis. The inferior vena cava involvement itself is usually silent, and only systematically performed iliocavography will demonstrate a caval lesion. Finally, in some cases it is the pulmonary embolism that draws one's attention, and the complete phlebographic investigation demonstrates thrombosis of the inferior vena cava (Fig. 4.29).

There is a technical point that seems fundamental: the entire iliocaval system must be studied when iliofemoral phlebitis has been diagnosed, even on one side only (Figs. 4.31 and 4.34). A low-centered film that does not include the origin of the renal veins and the retrohepatic portion of the inferior vena cava could fail to detect a fibrinocruoric or neoplastic inferior vena caval thrombosis. Good visualization of some intracaval floating thrombi is only achieved with a left anterior oblique projection performed with the patient supine. A last point deserves to be stressed: there are inferior vena caval thromboses, most often of a phlebothrombotic type with floating thrombus, that are totally asymptomatic and are discovered during the preoperative investigations for retro- or intraperitoneal masses.

We have observed unquestionable examples of this situation, in which only cavography has allowed us to consider the diagnosis of inferior vena caval thrombosis.

4.5 Membranous Occlusions and Stenoses of the Inferior Vena Cava Termination (Fig. 4.36)

Our knowledge of congenital membranes responsible for a form of obstruction of the segment of the inferior vena cava lying between the hepatic veins and the heart is relatively recent: Bennet's original observation dates back only to 1951, and it was only in 1963 that Kimura published his first three surgical reports.

4.5.1 Etiology

For most authors the congenital origin of these membranes is unquestionable. This theory is based on numerous arguments:

1) Even though the average age at treatment is relatively high (37 years, with extremes of 15 and 56), it should be noted that the first symptoms most often occur rather early: the average age is 26 years, with extremes of 9 and 43.

2) The absence of another demonstrated etiology, particularly thrombosis, has in

our opinion no great value, since thrombosis may complicate congenital membrane, as we shall see.

3) Also, the anatomopathologic study of the rare anatomic or surgical specimens is not absolute. Though the macroscopic aspect is not different from that of a normal endovein, the histology shows a trivial fibrous structure which does not allow one to eliminate with certainty an organized thrombosis: the case published by Eguchi is particularly disconcerting in that respect.

4) The embryologic studies are much more convincing: Boutelier and Couinaud, who published an accurate study in 1962, and Kimura in 1963 point out that the site of the membranes of the inferior vena cava is exactly at the junction of the two last segments of different embryologic origin that form the inferior vena cava. They insist on the complexity of the embryology of the inferior vena caval system, which would account for the frequent occurrence of anomalies at this level, as opposed to the clearly rarer involvement of the superior caval system, the embryology of which is much more simple.

5) Finally, the frequency of associated venous anomalies is an argument in favor of a congenital etiology. It is most often the hepatic venous system that is affected: Kimura and Yamamoto insisted on this peculiarity and considered these anomalies to be constant. Their involving mainly the left hepatic vein is not uninteresting: as a matter of fact, in the fetus this vein is very closely related to the Arantius canal. Kimura believes that obliteration of the left hepatic vein may be considered an extension of the process obliterating normally the Arantius canal; he even compares caval obliteration to coarctation of the aortic isthmus, and the remnant of the Arantius canal to the arterial ligament.

4.5.2 Pathologic Anatomy

Anatomic study of the lesions is particularly important since it orientates the therapy.

Site

The site of the lesions is relatively constant: Obliterations of the inferior vena cava are usually located in its hepatocardiac segment, most often where it perforates the diaphragm, sometimes between the diaphragm and the opening of the vein into the right atrium. However, in three cases the membrane was seen to be subdiaphragmatic and inserted at the level of the hepatic veins, the right one opening below the membrane, and the left above it.

Lesions of the superior vena cava would be located on the initial segment of the vein above the termination of the azygos veins, as it seems.

Type of Lesions

The type of lesion, in contrast to the site, varies greatly. Most often it is a thin, almost pellucid membrane, sometimes incomplete, inserted at right angles on the internal aspect of the vein, without any stenosis of this vein.

More rarely, the membrane is as thin as in the previous case, and is accompanied by mild stenosis of the inferior vena cava.

Finally, the membrane is sometimes thick and associated with tight stenosis of the inferior vena cava. Watkins employs the term "coarctation" to designate these forms.

Associated Venous Lesions

Such lesions are frequent, as we have already said, and apart from Johansson's case, they involve mainly the hepatic veins. These lesions are of the same type as the vena caval lesions. They produce either tight stenosis or complete obliteration of the embouchment of the vein into the inferior vena cava.

Obliterations

The consequences of the obliterations of the terminal segment of the inferior vena cava are interesting to study since they explain the clinical picture and the evolution.

As in any vascular obliteration, the normal compensatory phenomenon is development of a collateral circulation, which tends to diminish the direct consequences of the obliteration, both above and below it.

The collateral venous routes are well known as concerns isolated obliterations of the inferior or superior vena cava: they comprise the three main longitudinal axes, apart from the vena cava: the parietal veins, particularly the epigastric and the internal mammary veins, the azygos system with the lumbar veins, and the intra- and extraspinal plexuses.

But in case of double caval obliteration, collateral circulation is hardly conceivable. Two facts are to be pointed out: in neither of our two cases has the obliteration been simultaneously complete, which allowed the above-mentioned longitudinal collateral routes to function at a reduced rate through the incomplete obliteration. On the other hand, below the obliteration, the caval veins receive important branches: inferior phrenic veins, the azygos vein, even the left hepatic vein when the membrane is inserted astride the termination of the hepatic veins.

Obviously, the more or less marked and rapid development of the collateral circulation plays an important role in the date of appearance of the syndromes: a certain number of obliterations of a single vena cava, in the event of a well-developed circulation, remain very likely asymptomatic throughout the patient's life. Conversely, it is logical that double obliterations, especially when they are complete, should cause earlier symptoms. Thus, in our second case, in which one obliteration was complete and the other incomplete but very tight, severe manifestations occurred as early as age 28 years, whereas in the first case, with incomplete and not very tight obliteration, the patient has lived to the age of 52 without great discomfort.

When the collateral circulation proves insufficient, which, as we have seen, is not always the case, there occurs a repercussion involving mainly the lower limbs, the kidneys, and especially the liver, with appearance of a postsinusoidal block of suprahepatic type.

Besides this mechanical phenomenon there may be additional and often extensive thrombosis of the subjacent segment due to stasis, menacing particularly the hepatic veins. It is easily conceivable that in this case the syndrome should become indistinguishable, apart from the chronology, from a Budd-Chiari syndrome complicated by inferior vena caval thrombosis.

From all these considerations, two aspects deserve in our opinion to be pointed out as particularly important: (1) For prognosis, the main problem in all these cases is the hepatic repercussion, of which we have seen the possible triple origin, i.e., congenital anomaly of the hepatic veins, hypertension and stasis below the obstacle on the inferior vena cava, and finally, extensive thrombosis. (2) For therapy, the technical possibilities depend directly upon the type of lesion, so that it seems appropriate to describe the four quite different types.

Type 1: thin membrane, complete or incomplete, without associated caval stenosis

Type 2: thin membrane, complete, not very tight caval stenosis

Type 3: thick membrane, complete, with tight stenosis of the cava

Type 4: stenosis in addition

4.5.3 Clinical Symptomatology

Although certain forms may remain asymptomatic in the event of there being good collateral channels, most obstructions of the caval veins by a membrane quite rapidly produce a striking clinical symptomatology and may lead to death, unless a suitable therapy is applied.

The clinical picture characteristic of obliterations of both vena caval terminations consists of the elements of both syndromes, i.e., superior vena caval syndrome and the suprahepatic obstruction syndrome of the inferior vena cava, of which Corcos and Caroli provided an accurate description in 1960. The first syndrome is well known and we do not dwell upon it, the more so since in our two cases its signs were far less important than the inferior vena caval symptoms. In our first case there were no signs at all, since the superior vena caval stenosis was not tight enough to be hemodynamically significant. Also, in the second case, almost complete obliteration of the superior vena cava produced only venous turgor and upper thoracic collateral circulation.

It thus appears justified to dwell mainly upon the signs of the inferior vena caval syndrome and to draw attention to the peculiar features suggesting an associated superior vena caval obstruction.

These signs may be divided into two groups:

1) The signs of inferior caval hypertension are usually the first to occur. They dominate for a long time the evolution of the clinical syndrome. Their frequency is quite remarkable: a) Varices of the lower limbs. b) Edema of the lower limbs, which may be quite extended and reach the flanks, or consist only of simple malleolar edema c) Chronic ulcers of the lower extremities which do not respond to the usual symptomatic treatment. d) Peripheral collateral circulation, which has a quite significant semiologic value: in case of isolated occlusion of the inferior vena cava, characteristic filling of the parietal veins of the trunk from below upward occurs, a feature that is of course not present in case of associated superior vena caval obstruction e) Proteinuria, which is hardly ever mentioned in the literature but must be added to the list.

2) The signs of portal hypertension are usually more discreet and occur later. a) Hepatomegalia is very frequent: the liver is first moderately hypertrophic, slightly painful, has an increased consistency. A long-standing evolution may be responsible for severe hepatic repercussions and ensuing cirrhosis. Besides retention of sulfobromophthalein (SBP), which is present in the early stages, hepatic function tests are clearly disturbed only in later stages. b) Ascites may be present but usually not in large amounts. Caroli insists on its high protein concentration, allowing one to distinguish it from ascites in Budd-Chiari syndrome or in trivial cirrhosis. c) Splenomegaly, digestive tract hemorrhage, and jaundice are less common. These are in fact later symptoms or rather complications indicating severe involvement of the liver, with fatal issue. The films often give evidence of esophageal varices.

Associations between these two groups of signs produce various clinical pictures, so that clinical diagnosis is often difficult.

Most often, inferior caval hypertension signs are predominant, at least during the initial period, so that many of these patients undergo stripping or sclerosing of their varices or symptomatic treatments for edema and ulcers of the lower limbs.

Sometimes the symptoms of portal hypertension are the more important, suggesting a diagnosis of liver cirrhosis, as was the case for our first observation. We are sure that a better knowledge of the above-reported features would make it possible to avoid some erroneous diagnoses of cirrhosis.

When the two groups of symptoms are found to be associated at the first examination, they most often evoke the diagnosis of cardiac insufficiency or constrictive chronic pericarditis: it is easy to understand how difficult it will be to rule out these two diagnoses when there is also a superior vena caval obstruction.

Whatever the case, the preoperative diagnosis can only be based on the complementary investigations. Two of them are decisive: catheterization with determination of the pressures and, above all, angiography.

Catheterization has a double interest since it permits one, first, to demonstrate the pressure gradient of the inferior vena cava and of the right atrium. This gradient is dependent on whether the obstruction is complete or incomplete, but it has always been significant enough to leave no doubt as to the presence of an obstacle. And second, it permits one to survey the course of the catheter: in the event of complete obstruction the phlebographer does not succeed in traversing the obstacle and entering the right atrium.

Angiography makes these data precise and moreover provides anatomic clues that are essential for the choice of therapeuthic procedure: It demonstrates the lesion, identifies its site and the shape of its distal contours. Kimura insists on the interest of a double angiography – superior and inferior vena cava – allowing demonstration of both limits of the obstacle and thus appreciation of its extent. The collateral circulation is opacified, in particular the azygos vein. It is important to know whether the azygos vein terminates above or below any superior vena caval obstruction; it is sometimes dilated to the point of becoming visible on a plain X-ray of the chest as a rounded opacity occupying the right tracheobronchial angle. Finally, it is not uninteresting to study the state of the hepatic veins. The high frequency of left hepatic vein obstruction was first demonstrated by angiography.

These are the diagnostic data in obstruction of the terminal segment of the venae cavae. Apart from the two large series reported by Kimura and by Yamamoto, the exact diagnosis of the nature of the obliteration has only rarely been made prior to operation. A better knowledge of these abnormal membranes should mean that this eventuality can be considered more frequently.

4.5.4 Evolution

The spontaneous evolution is catastrophic and consists of acute hepatic insufficiency and hemorrhage of the digestive tract.

The importance of an early diagnosis, and hence early surgical procedure, should be understood, the more so since a longstanding condition carries the risk of making surgery dangerous and chancy.

4.6 Surgery in Iliofemoral and Iliocaval Phlebitis

Half a century elapsed between the first venous thrombectomy carried out by Schepelman in 1910 in a case of humero-axillo-subclavian thrombosis, and the present-day development of this procedure. It was mainly Fontaine who promoted thrombectomy as the only procedure capable of preventing pulmonary embolisms and the sequelae of iliofemoral phlebitis. Several techniques are available: either thrombectomy by phlebotomy and removal of the thrombi with tweezers, or thrombectomy with Fogarty's technique with a balloon. The major problem is to maintain the patency of the iliofemoral system under operation. One may perform either a local injection of fibrinolytic agents, or (more often nowadays) create a temporary arteriovenous fistula in Scarpa's triangle.

Early postoperative angiographic survey is carried out by antegrade iliac arteriography after placement of a catheter at the aortic bifurcation with the help of a contralateral Seldinger. Opacification of the homolateral iliac artery continues with opacification of the arteriovenous fistula (most often a reversed internal saphenous vein) and then occurs opacification of the external iliac and common iliac venous axis on the same side as the fistula. After that occurs filling of the inferior vena cava (Fig. 4.37).

It seems advisable to perform prior to this a phlebography of the lower limb on the side of the operated iliac phlebitis, in order to appreciate the status of the deep veins of the subjacent lower limb, which has not always been done preoperatively. This upstream phlebography is particularly important for demonstrating that the veins which were patent prior to the operation (isolated iliac phlebitis) remain patent after thrombectomy with arterialization.

In our series of 100 cases of iliac phlebitis, 78 patients have been operated and immediate postoperative controls have shown 58 perfectly patent thrombectomies (with arterialization). Two patients had recurrent thrombosis of the arterialized iliac vein, and two others had diffuse bi-iliac and inferior vena caval thrombosis below a caval clip (Fig. 4.38).

Surgical procedures in case of chronic iliac phlebitis consist most often of a Palma operation, possibly followed by arterialization at Scarpa's triangle. This latter type of procedure may also be controlled, like the previous one, by a homolateral iliac arteriography via a contralateral Seldinger (Fig. 4.40). Palma operations without arterialization can be controlled by ascending nonpressurized phlebography with a large amount of contrast material.

4.7 Surgical Prevention of Embolic Migration

Several surgical techniques are available: ligature of the inferior vena cava, partial interruption of the inferior cava by plication (Fig. 4.41), filter operation with nonresorbable thread (Fig.4.42), and finally, placement of Teflon clips. Besides being effective, the last-mentioned procedure has the advantage of not requiring a rupture of the endovein and hence of not favoring thrombosis in situ. More recently, endocaval septation by placement of umbrella filters has been performed, and other items of apparatus have been inserted into the vein via distant venous catheterizations.

The choice between these different methods depends upon the indications. But three factors have to be taken into account:

1) The immediately postoperative severity of this surgical procedure
2) The effectiveness in preventing immediate and recurrent pulmonary embolisms
3) The effect on the postphlebitic disease: incomplete interposed obstruction may be preferable to ligature.

In our series of 100 cases with iliac phlebitis, we were able to control the result of the prophylactic therapy of pulmonary embolism by placement of a Teflon clip on the inferior vena cava in 12 patients (Fig. 4.39). Of these incomplete interruptions, 95% were seen to be patent and functional on a postoperative angiogram. This figure is slightly higher than Demester's; he reports 60%. Nevertheless two patients had diffuse bi-iliac and inferior caval thrombosis below the clip, demonstrated in one case by arteriography and in the other by retrograde catheterization with passage of the catheter below the clip into the thrombosed lower segment of the inferior vena cava.

None of the patients who had had placement of a clip on the inferior vena cava developed early or delayed postoperative pulmonary embolism.

It seems thus that incomplete interruptions of the inferior vena cava have proved their effectiveness in preventing migration of emboli and have at the same time eliminated the dangers of serious hemodynamic perturbations such as were observed after ligations.

References

Bennet JL Jr A unique case of obstruction of the inferior vena cava. Bull Johns Hopk Hosp 87:290–298

Boutelier B, Couinaud Cl (1962) Les anomalies dites "primitives" de la veine cava inférieure. J Chir (Paris) 82:199–222

Brodelius A, Loring P, Nylander G (1973) Phlebographic techniques in the diagnosis of acute deep venous thrombosis of the lower limb. Am J Roentgenol 794–801

Buecheler E, Weber KW (1974) Membranous occlusion of the inferior vena cava. Br J Radiol 47:444–447

Calnan J (1962) Unilateral idiopathic lymphoedema with obstruction of the common iliac vein by the common iliac artery. Lancet 2:537–539

Chermet J (1979) Left Common Iliac Compression Syndrome. Anatomia Clinica 1, 347–355

Chermet J, Tubiana JM, Monnier JP, Rouanet JP, Wesley C, Chalut J (1977) Les phlébites iliaques. A propos de 100 observations. Valeur de l'angiographie pré- et post-opératoire. Ann Radiol 20 7:649–666

Cockett FB (1966) The iliac compression syndrome alias "iliofemoral thrombosis" or white leg. Proc R Soc Med 59:360–361

Cockett FB (1967) Venous causes of swollen leg. Br J Surg 54:891–894

Cockett FB, Lea Thomas M (1965) The iliac compression syndrome. Br J Surg 52 10:816–821

Cockett FB, Lea Thomas M, Negus D (1967) Iliac vein compression: its relation to iliofemoral thrombosis and the post-thrombotic syndrome. Br Med J 2:14–19

Corcos V, Caroli J, Paraf A, Couinaud Cl, Bonneville B (1960) Les obstructions mixtes des veines cave inférieure et sushépatique. Rev Med Chir Mal Foie 35:315–317

Corcos V, Valla A, Caroli J, Paraf A, Bonneville B (1960) Le syndrome d'obstruction supra-hépatique de la veine cave inférieure. Rev Med Chir Mal Foie 35:295–296

David G (1976) La réalité du syndrome de Cockett. Thèse, Marseille

Dodd H, Cockett FB (1976) The pathology and surgery of the veins of the lower limb. Livingstone, Edinburgh London New-York

Dubost Ch, Piwnica A, Carpentier A, Kieffer E (1969) Traitement chirurgical des oblitérations membraneuses du segment terminal des veines caves. Ann Chir Thorac Cardiovasc 8 4:433–443

Edwards WH, Sawyers JL, Foster JH (1970) Iliofemoral venous thrombosis reappraisal of thrombectomy. Ann Surg 171:961–970

Ehrich WE, Krumbhaar EB (1974) Frequent obstructive anomaly of the mouth of left common iliac vein. Am Heart J 59/10:533–537

Fellus (1954) Malformation de la configuration interne de la veine iliaque primitive gauche. Thèse, Paris

Fontaine F, Tuchmann L (1963) Les indications et résultats de la thrombectomie dans les thromboses veineuses récentes d'après 74 observations personelles. Lyon Chir 161–191

Fontaine R, Kieny R, Tuchmann L, Suhler A, Babin S (1965) Quelques réflexions sur les embolies pulmonaires d'après une statistique personnelle de 409 thromboses veineuses récentes. Ann Chir Thorac Cardiovasc 4:628–632

Fontaine R, Kieny R, Tuchmann L, Suhler A (1965) Contribution à l'étude clinique et thérapeutique de la Phlegmasia Cerulea dolens. A propos de 32 observations personnelles. Lyon Chir 61: 321–334

Haimovici H (1965) Ischemic form of thrombo-phlebitis. Thomas, Springfield

Johnsson KA, Cothman B, Norstrom J (1974) Iliac compression syndrome. Acta Radiol [Diagn] (Stockh) 15/5:539–545

Kimura C, Shirotani H, Kuma T, Miroka M, Hayashi K, Tsunekawa K, Matsuda S (1962) Transcardiac membranotomy for obliteration of the inferior vena cava in the hepatic portion. J Cardiovasc Surg (Torino) 3:393–404

Kimura C, Shirotani H, Hirroka M, Terrada M, Iwahashi K, Maetani S (1963) Membranous obliteration of the inferior vena cava in the hepatic portion. J Cardiovasc Surg (Torino) 4:87–98

Lea Thomas M, Fletcher E, Cockett FB, Negus D (1967) Collaterals in external common iliac vein obstruction. Clin Radiol 18:403–411

MacMurrich JP (1906) The valves of the iliac vein. Br Med J 2:1699–1700

Mavor GE, Galloway JM (1967) The iliofemoral venous segment as a source of pulmonari emboli. Lancet 1:871–874

Meester TR de, Rutherford RB, Blazek JV, Zuidema GD (1967) Plication of the inferior vena cava for thromboembolism. Surgery 63:56–65

Miles RM (1973) Some surgical implication of the anatomy of the cava-iliofemoral system. Ann Surg 177:740–747

Negus D (1969) The iliac veins in relation to lymphoedema. Br J Surg 56:481–486

Negus D, Cockett FB (1967) Femoral vein pressures in post-phlebitic iliac vein obstruction. Br J Surg 54:522–524

Negus D, Fletcher EWC, Cockett FB, Lea Thomas M (1968) Compression and band formation at the mouth of the left common iliac vein. Br J Surg 55/5:369–374

Ponthieu A, Huguet JF (1976) Varicocèle gauche et stase veineuse iliaque. J Urol Nephrol (Paris) 3: 187–200

Powell EDU, Mullaney JM (1960) The chiari network and the valve of the inferior vena cava. Br Heart J 22:579–584

Rigas A, Womocoyennes A, Tasardakos E (1970) Iliac compression syndrome. Report of ten cases. J Cardiovasc Surg (Torino) 11:389–392

Rossall RE, Caldwell RA (1957) Obstruction of the inferior vena cava by a persistent Eustachian valve in a young adult. J Clin Pathol 10:40–45

Serradimigni A, Mercier C (1973) Les thromboses veineuses profondes des membres. Masson, Paris

Sztankay C (1969) Iliocaval dysplasia: studies on the pathogenesis of venous diseases in the lower extremity. J Cardiovasc Surg (Torino) 10:16–21

Weese JA de (1969) Management of acute iliofemoral venous thrombosis including the role of thrombectomy. Heart Bull 18:55–57

Weese JA de, Jones TI, Lyon J, Dalew A (1960) Evaluation of thrombectomy in the management of iliofemoral venous thrombosis. Surgery 47: 140–144

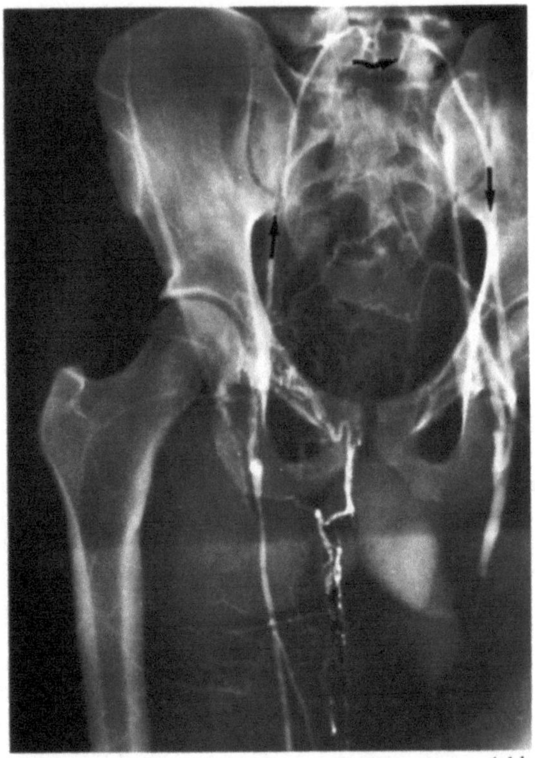

4.1b

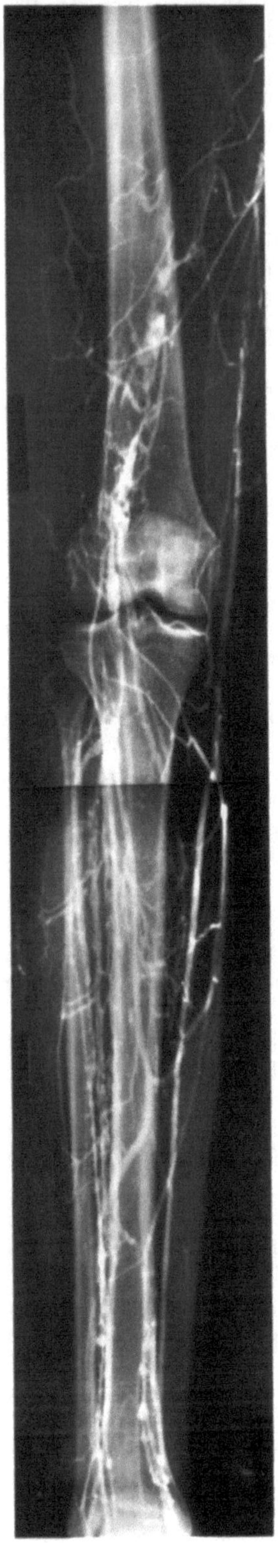

4.1a

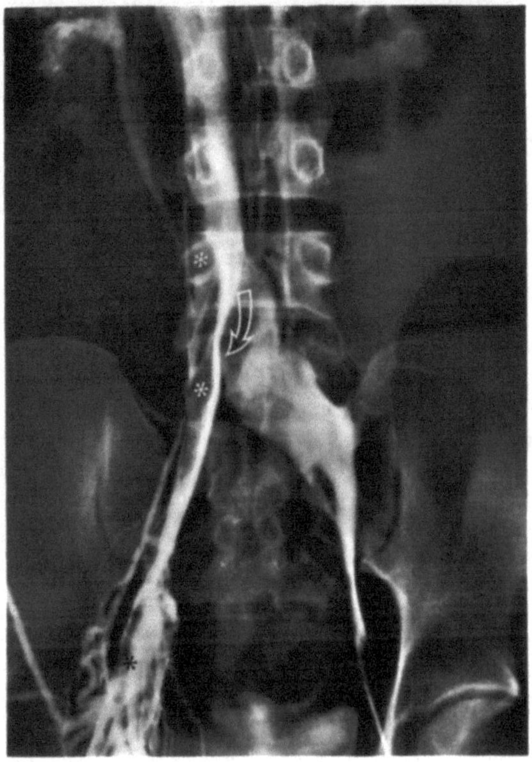

4.1c

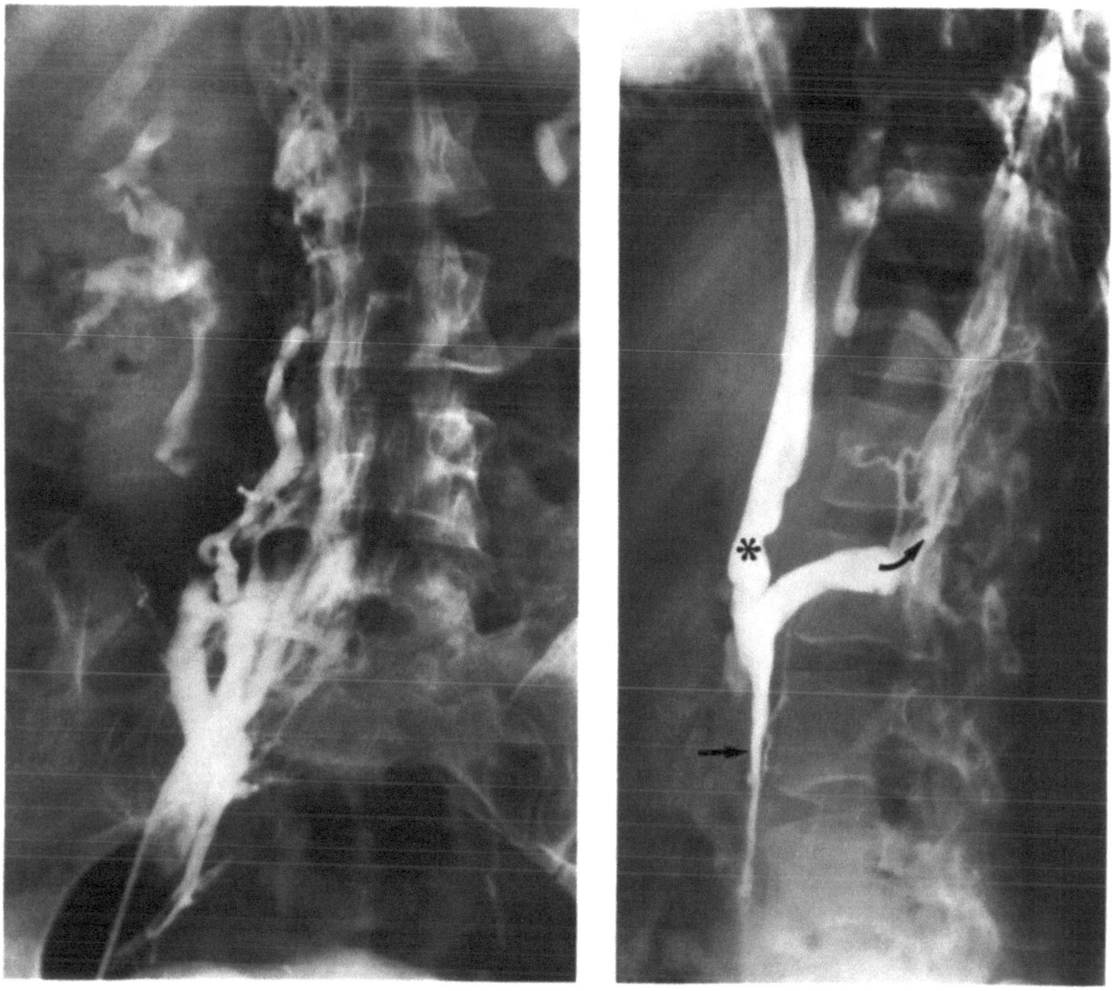

a b

Fig. 4.2. a Right unilateral cavography. Ill-defined obstruction at the level of the common iliac vein and probably of the inferior vena cava. By means of this injection alone it is impossible to identify precisely the upper level of the thrombus or to affirm the existence of interrenal or even suprarenal thrombosis. b Descending cavography by percutaneous brachial approach. The catheter is in the interrenal segment of the inferior vena cava (*). Postrenal caval thrombosis, like flakes of fire (→); opacification of the left renal vein and of the inferior hemiazygos system (↗). This additional technique (b) permits one to determine the upper level of the iliocaval thrombosis

◁ Fig. 4.1. a Venogram of the right lower limb. Floating thrombi in some deep veins of the leg. Femoropopliteal obstruction. b Venogram centered on the pelvis. Contralateral drainage over subcutaneous abdominal veins. Left reflux in the deep femoral vein. c Bifemoral percutaneous cavography with deliberate puncture of the thrombus on the right (same patient). Cockett's syndrome with flattening of the left common iliac vein in the frontal plane (↙). Adhesive type thrombosis of the external iliac vein. Iliocaval thrombosis with intracaval floating thrombus (*). Only cavography systematically associated with venography demonstrates the intracaval floating thrombus above adhesive phlebitis of the external iliac vein

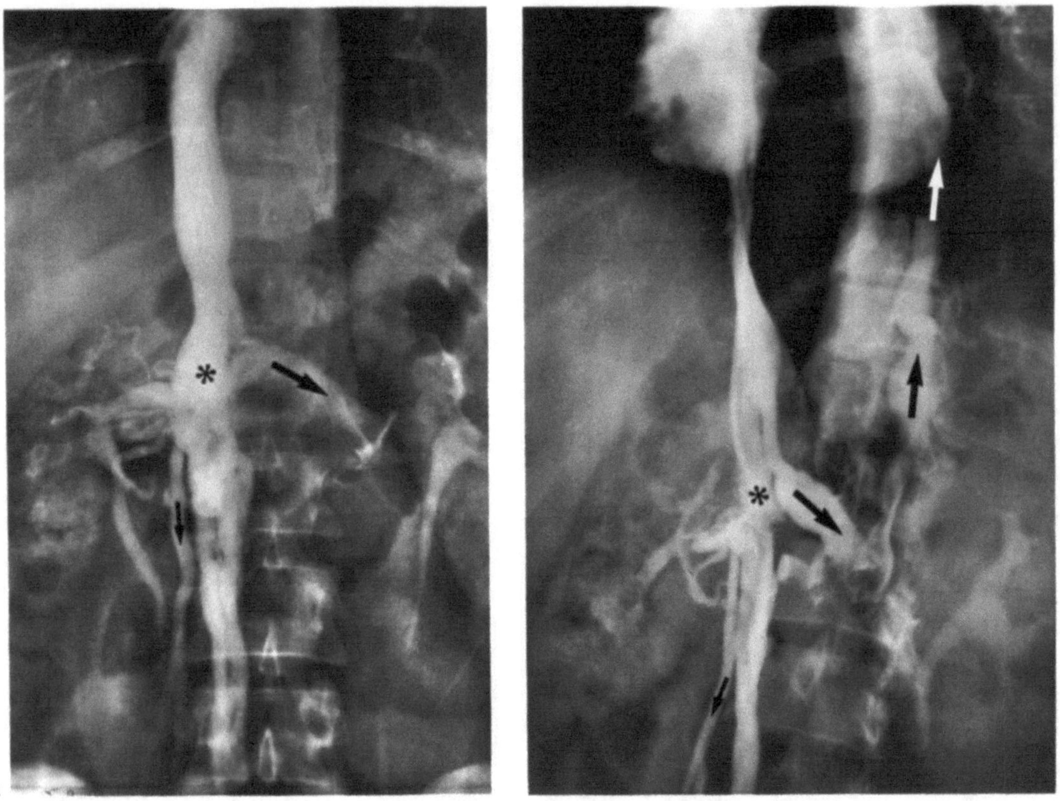

a b

Fig. 4.3. a Frontal retrograde cavogram. b Lateral retrograde cavogram. Note the long-standing obstruction of the postrenal segment of the inferior cava, which has a laminated aspect. Reflux in the right gonadic vein (↙). Opacification of collateral channels over the left renal vein (↘) and the inferior hemiazygos system (↗) readily visible on the left anterior oblique projection. (*) catheter tip in the vena cava

---

Fig. 4.5. Congenital anomaly of the inferior vena cava: double vena cava. Left iliofemoral thrombosis (left unifemoral cavography with puncture into the thrombus). Postrenal left inferior vena cava. The inferior vena cava on the left is predominant. The left unifemoral cavography opacifies both inferior venae cavae. In conclusion: iliac phlebitis associated with a congenital anomaly of the inferior vena cava ▷

Fig. 4.6. Phlebitis of the entire length of the right iliac, external iliac, and common iliac veins, with a huge intracaval free thrombus (*). The phlebitis was discovered on the occasion of pulmonary embolism. Right femoral puncture into the thrombus. Left femoral puncture shows the left iliac system to be normal

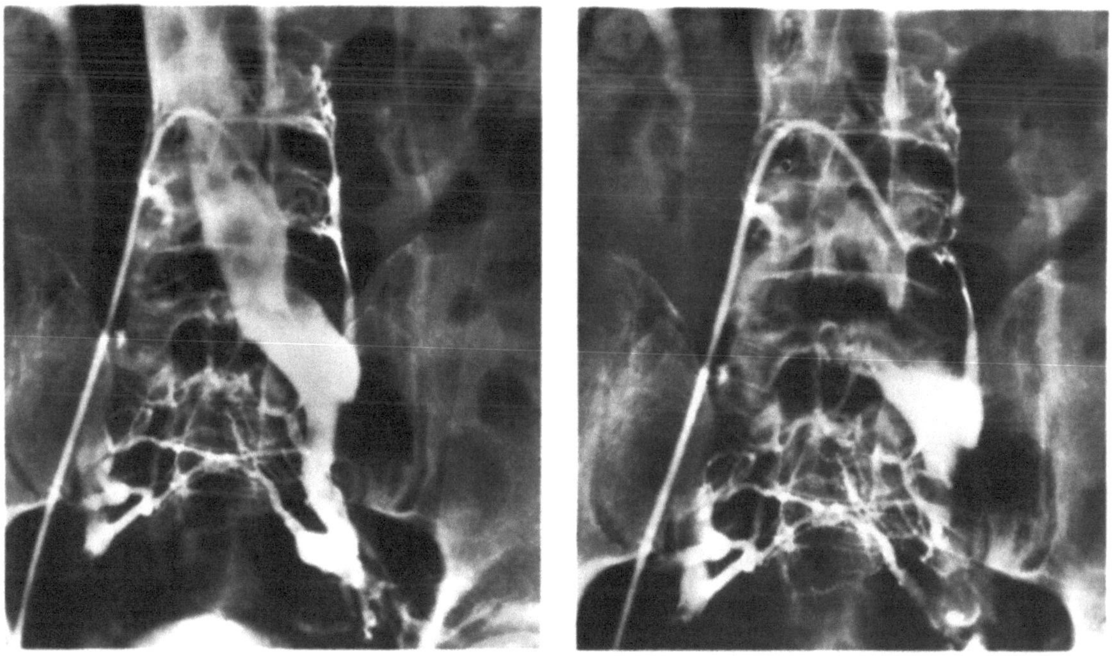

a b

Fig. 4.4a, b. Left iliofemoral phlebitis. Search for the upper level of the thrombus. Retrograde iliac phlebography with right femoral approach. Anterograde phlebography of the left lower limb had shown a large iliofemoral obstruction but did not allow precise determination of the superior level of the thrombus. a Retrograde opacification of the left common iliac vein and of the left hypogastric vein. The cul-de-sac is cranially concave. b Late phase of retrograde iliac phlebography. No washout and persistence of the upwardly concave opaque cul-de-sac. In (a) this feature could have been taken for a valvule of the external iliac vein; it corresponds in fact to the head of a left iliofemoral thrombus, because the contrast medium has not been washed out

4.5

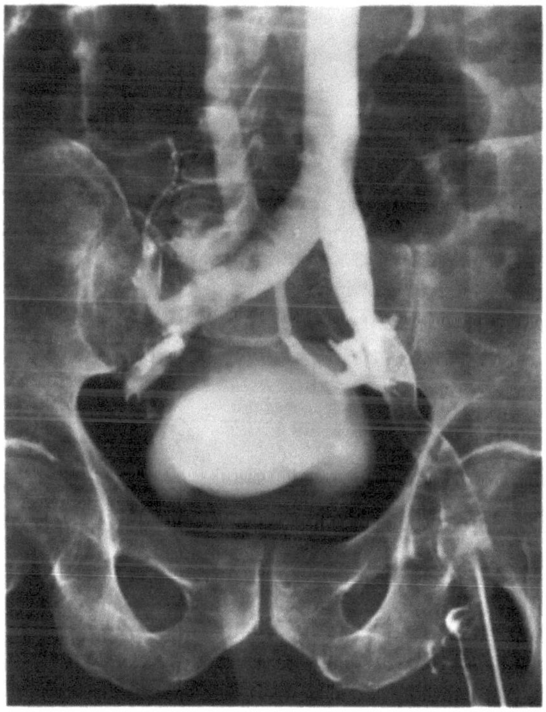

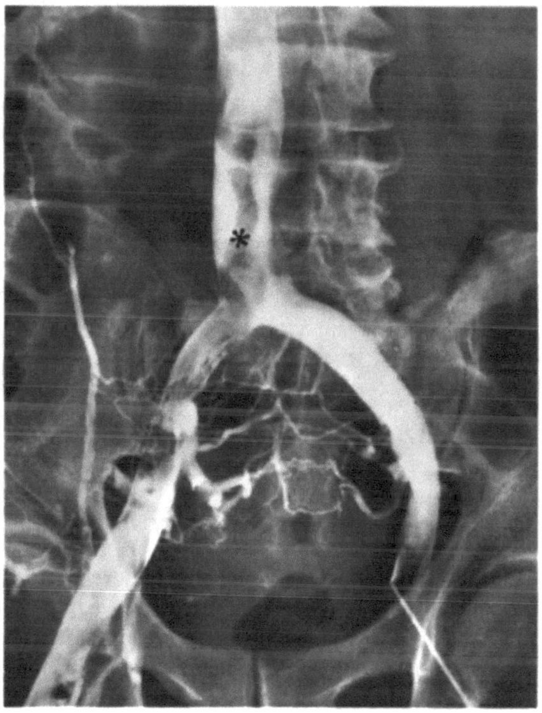

4.6

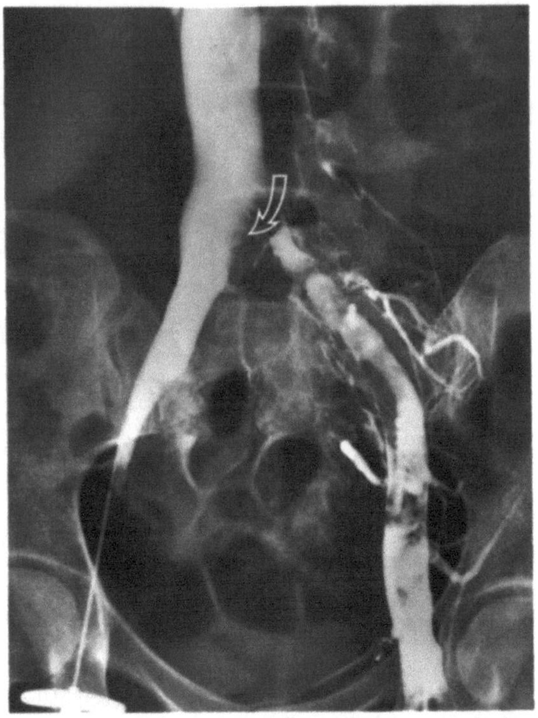

Fig. 4.7. Bifemoral percutaneous cavography. Left femoral puncture into a thrombus. Complete left iliac phlebitis caudally to a Cockett syndrome (↙)

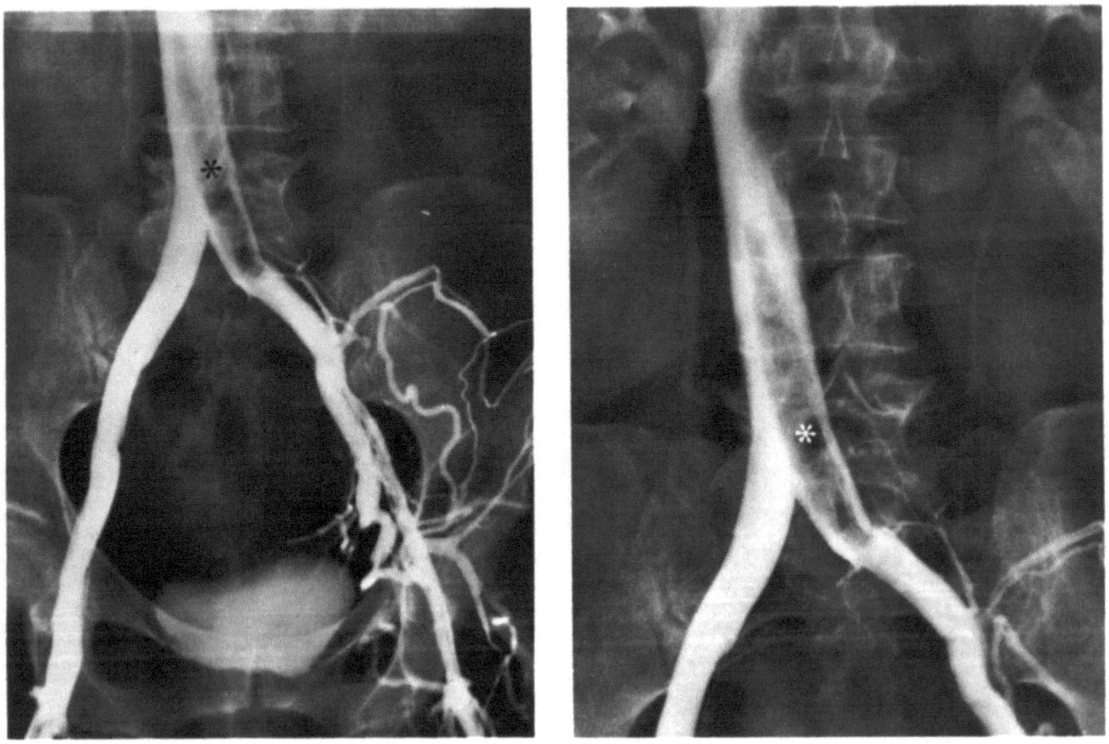

a b

Fig. 4.8a, b. Phlebothrombosis above the level of chronic phlebitis. Importance of systematic cavography in the study of lower limb phlebitis. a Bifemoral percutaneous catheterization. Long-standing left iliofemoral chronic phlebitis with laminated aspect of the iliac system, which is being rendered permeable with heparin. The left common iliac vein is permeable but shows at its termination a huge intracaval free thrombus (*). b Higher focused film: note the intracaval free thrombus (*). Value of systematic cavography for the study of even chronic phlebitis of the lower limbs

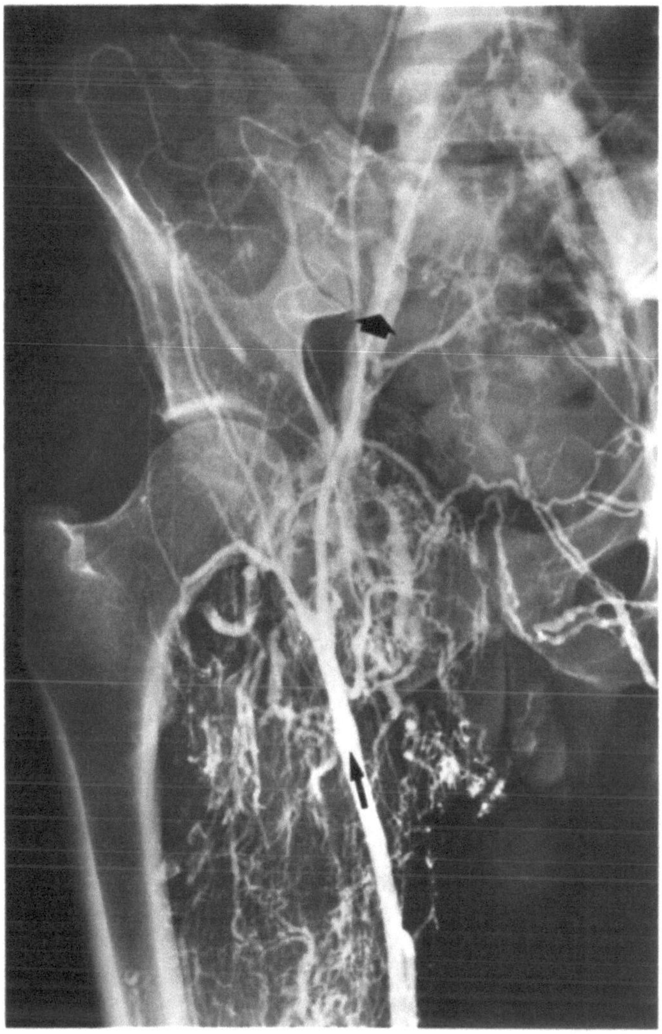

4.9a

Fig. 4.9a, b. Emergency phlebography and emergency iliocavography. a Phlebography of the right lower limb. Complete thrombosis of the femoropopliteal deep system and even of the deep femoral vein, which fails to opacify. The only collateral route is the internal saphenous vein (↗). Opacification of the right hypogastric vein (↗), contralateral derivations toward the left iliac system through the Retzius space

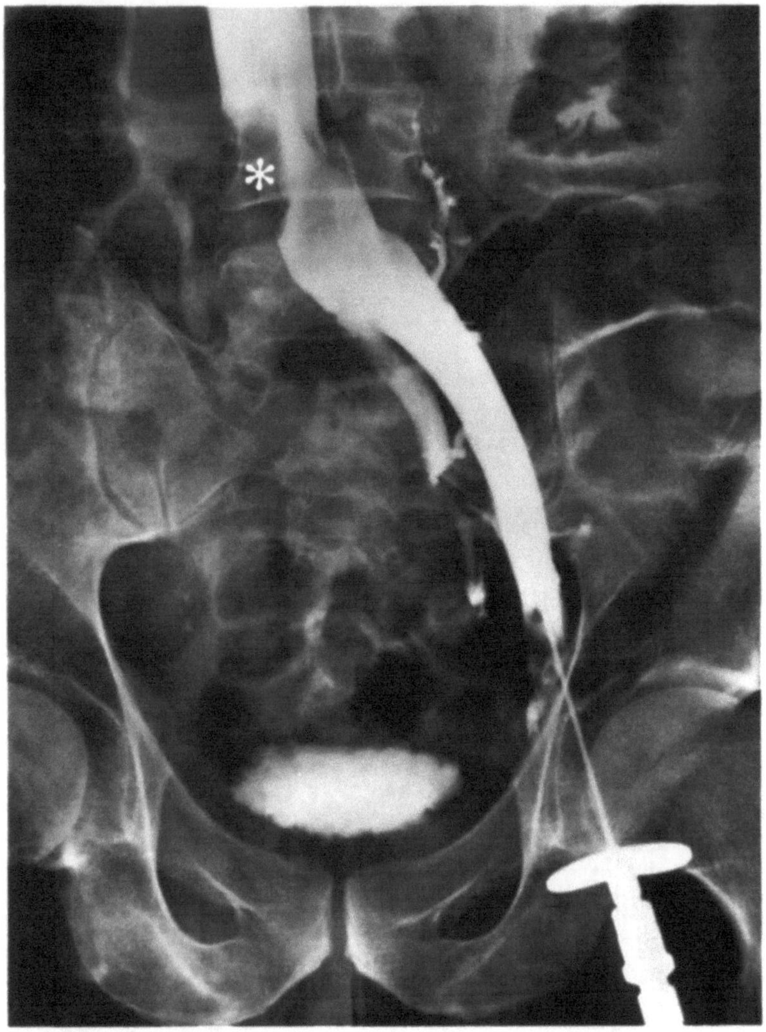

4.9b

Fig. 4.9b. Left unifemoral cavography. The left iliac system is patent. A Valsalva maneuver allows one to visualize the head of the thrombus which extends into the inferior vena cava (*). This emergency examination allows one to determine the extent of the phlebitis and visualize the superior level of the thrombus (in the present case, it is situated at the origin of the inferior vena cava)

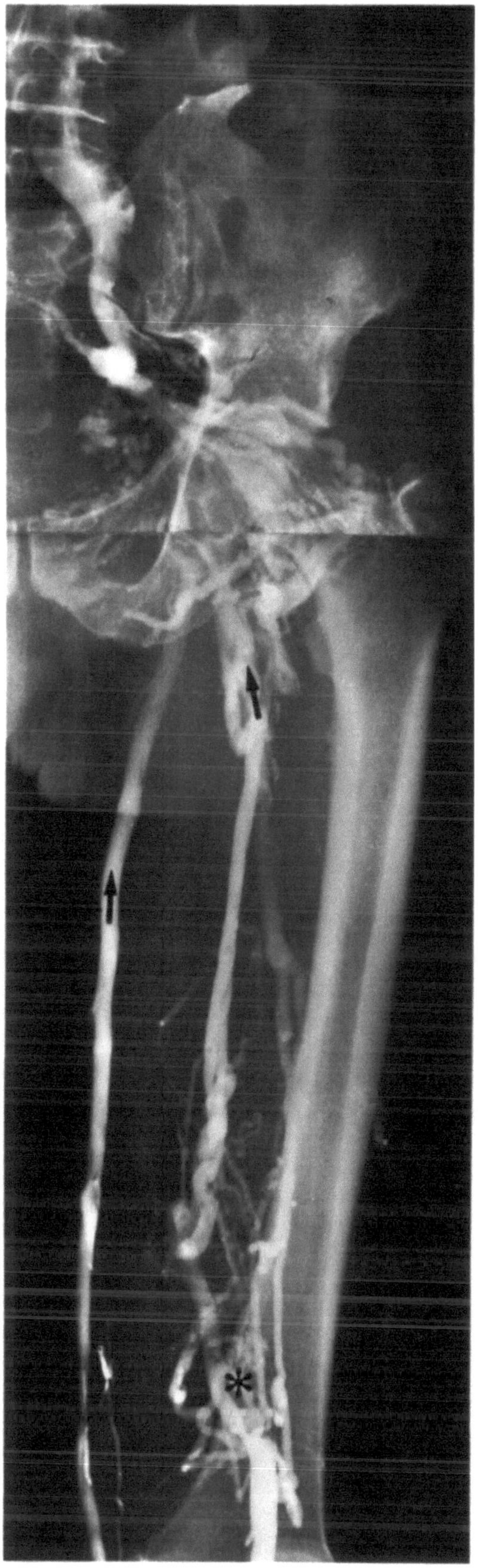

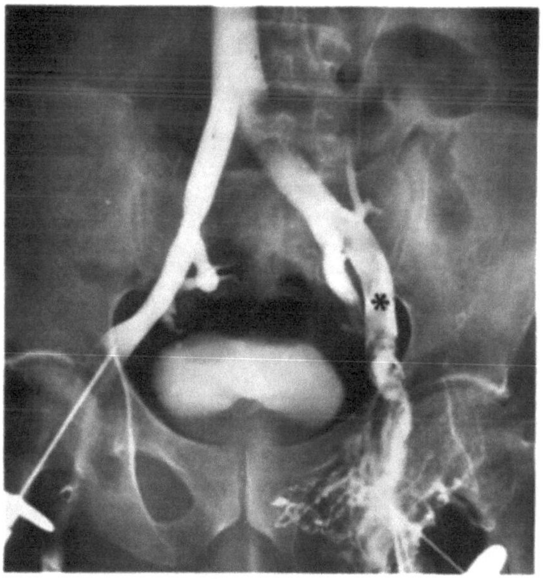

Fig. 4.11. Bifemoral percutaneous cavography. On the left, puncture of the femoral thrombus. Note the free thrombus extending all along the left external iliac vein (*)

◁ Fig. 4.10. Phlebography of the left lower limb. Large iliofemoral obstruction. The superficial femoral vein is thrombosed at its origin (*). Collateral circulation over a retro-adducting vein which drains into the deep femoral vein (↖). Note the large internal saphenous vein (↑), which serves also for the collateral circulation. Left iliofemoral occlusion with collateral circulation in the manner of a medusa head, over the sciatic veins, opacifying the left hypogastric system and the left common iliac vein. In this patient we performed retrograde iliac venography in order to identify the head of the thrombus (see Fig. 4.4)

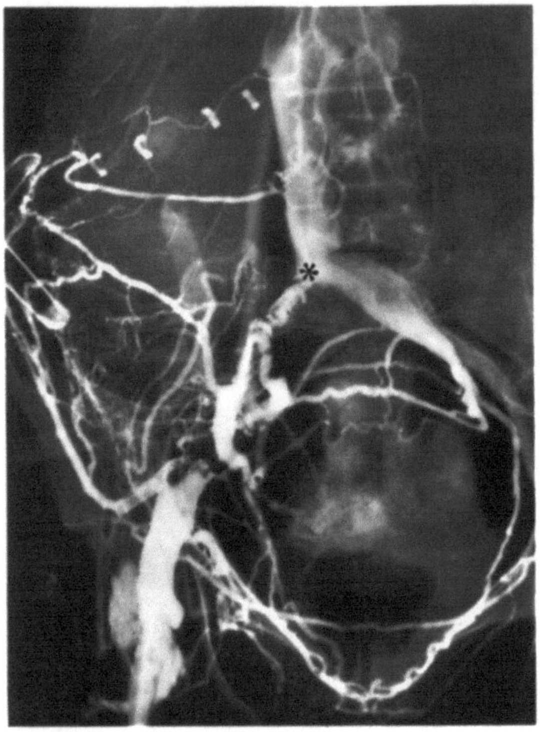

Fig. 4.12. Right segmental phlebitis of the common iliac vein. Right unifemoral injection. Perivenous extravasation. Opacification of the collateral channels with contralateral drainage and reopacification of the upper part of the thrombus, which does not reach the inferior vena cava (*). Postsurgical iliac phlebitis: digestive tract surgery

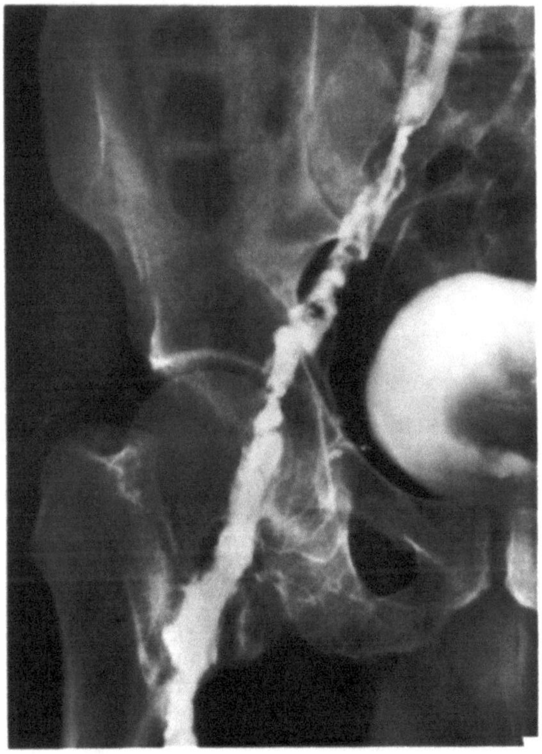

Fig. 4.13. Right iliac chronic phlebitis. The patient was treated with fibrinolytics. Note the very irregular, laminated and gridlike aspect of the iliac vein

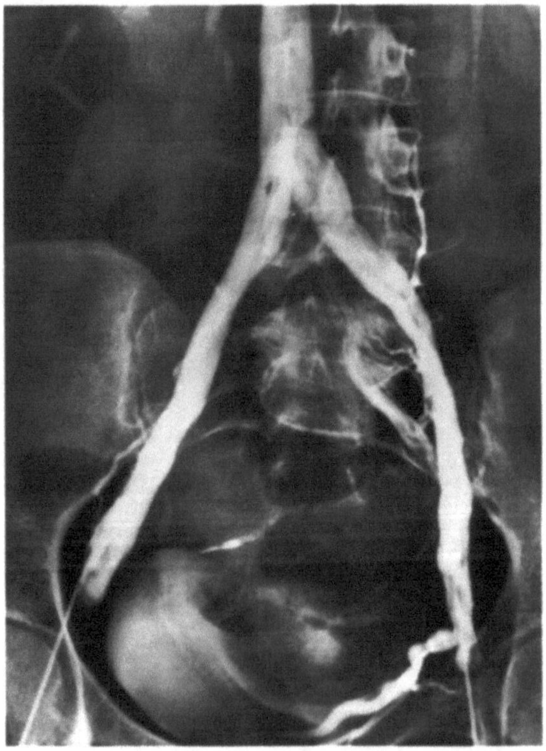

Fig. 4.14. Bilateral chronic iliac phlebitis. Laminated aspect of both iliac systems which become patent again

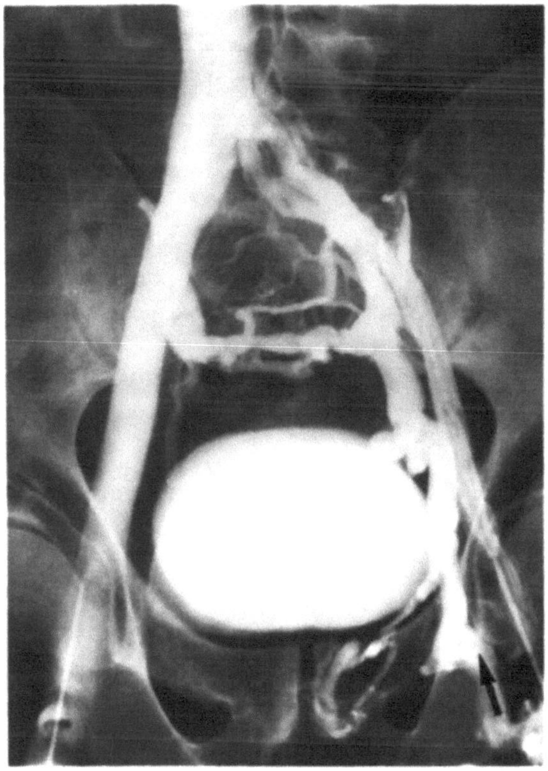

Fig. 4.15. Chronic left iliac phlebitis becoming patent with heparin treatment. Note the collateral circulation over the obturator and sciatic veins (↗) draining into the left hypogastric system. The left external iliac vein is laminated. Cockett syndrome with fenestration of the left common iliac vein. Iliac phlebitis below a preexistent Cockett syndrome

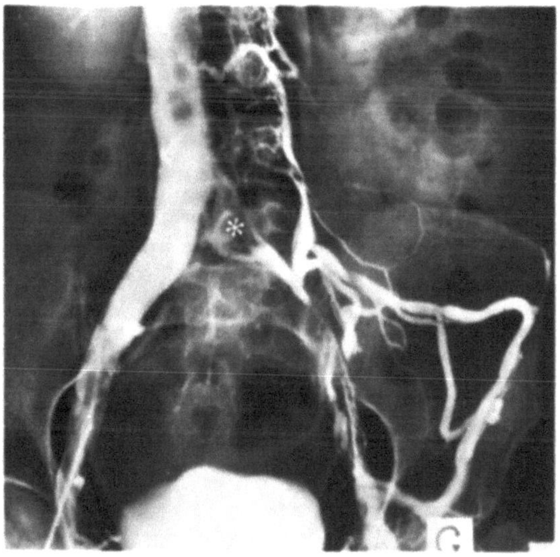

Fig. 4.16. Bifemoral percutaneous cavography. Left femoral puncture into a thrombus. Chronic phlebitis with narrowed left external iliac vein. Collateral circulation through the deep iliac circumflex vein, opacifying, on the one hand, the left ascending lumbar vein and, on the other hand, a short segment of the left common iliac vein, which shows synechia of its extremity and extrinsic compression (*): chronic phlebitis below a Cockett syndrome. No inferior vena cava thrombosis. A phlebography of the left lower limb (not shown here) demonstrated upstream extensive thrombosis of all deep veins of the lower limb. (G = left side)

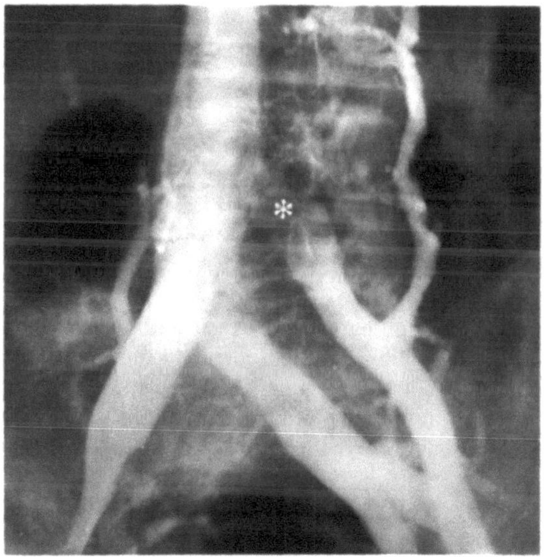

Fig. 4.17. Duplication of the left iliac vein. Bifemoral cavography. The inferior branch drains the hypogastric system. The superior branch drains the left ascending lumbar vein, which opacifies the spinal plexuses. Extrinsic pressure (*) on the superior branch due to the right common iliac artery

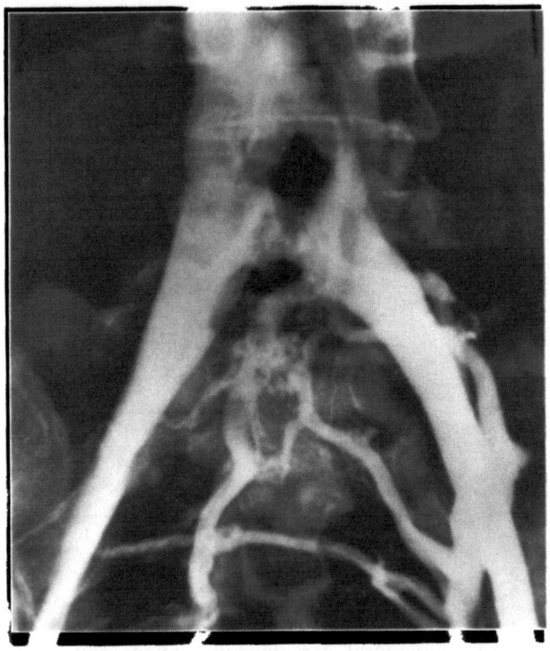

Fig. 4.18. Cockett's syndrome. Synechia responsible for a quite large lacuna at the level of the left common iliac vein. Left to right collateral circulation through the presacral plexuses

Fig. 4.20. Duplication of the right and left common iliac veins. Additional iliocavography was performed after ascending phlebography had shown left femoropopliteal thrombosis. Duplication of the right iliac vein: the inferior vein forms a venous arch which anastomoses with a right hypogastric system caudally, and with the left common iliac vein cranially. A synechial-type septum divides up the terminal part of the left common iliac vein; associated extrinsic compression: Cockett's syndrome ▷

Fig. 4.21. Short cutoff of the extremity of the left common iliac system: Cockett's syndrome. Large derivation through a left ascending lumbar vein which reanastomoses early at the level of L3 with the trunk of the inferior vena cava. Extrinsic pressure deformity upon the termination of this vein caused by the aorta (*)

Fig. 4.19. Cockett's syndrome with radiolucent synechia of the extremity of the left common iliac vein. Homolateral collateral circulation through the ascending lumbar vein, and contralateral collateral circulation through the presacral plexuses

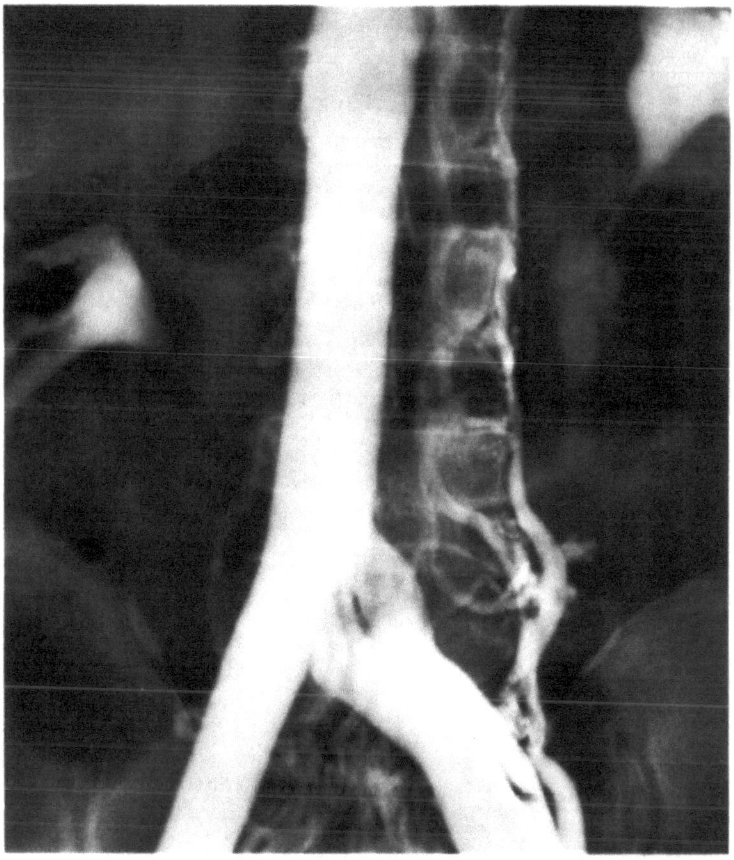

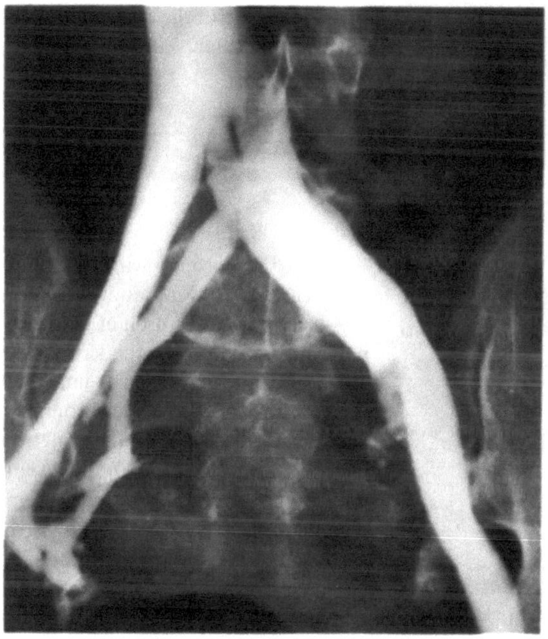

4.20

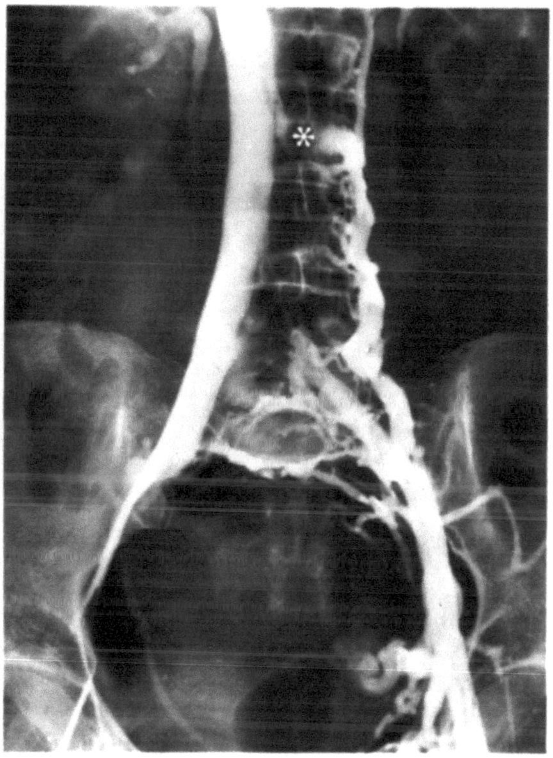

4.21

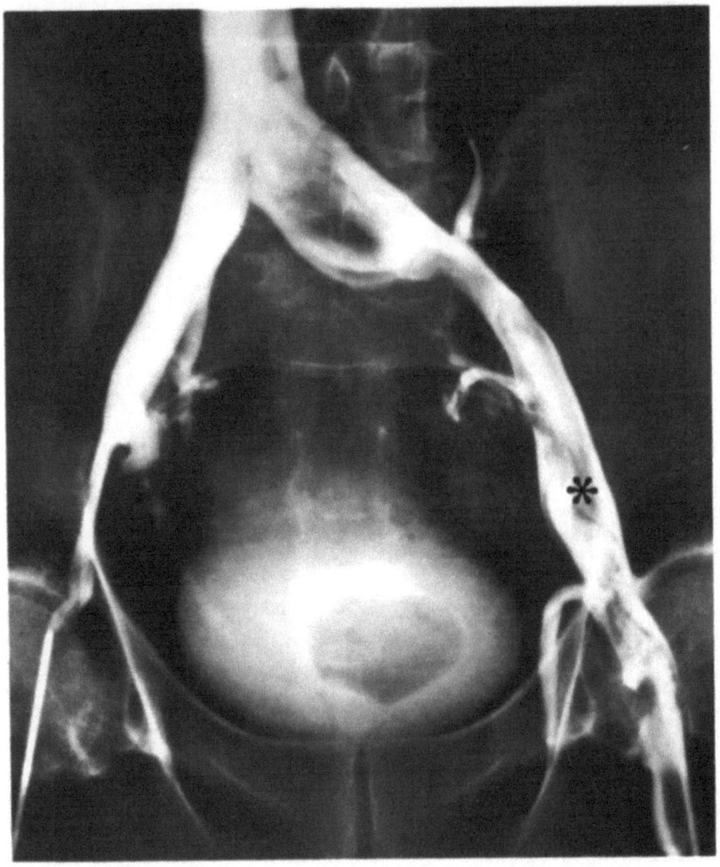

Fig. 4.22. Cockett's syndrome with flattening of the left common iliac vein in the frontal plane. Underlying iliac phlebothrombosis (*). Bifemoral percutaneous cavography. Puncture into the thrombus on the left

Fig. 4.24a–c. Cockett's syndrome. a ▷ Ascending phlebography of the left inferior limb. Perfect patency of all deep veins. b Higher centered projection shows opacification of the inferior vena cava through the presacral plexuses, deriving the opaque flow from left to right. c Complementary bifemoral percutaneous cavography in the same patient confirms the presence of Cockett's syndrome. Complete flattening of the extremity of the left common iliac vein (*)

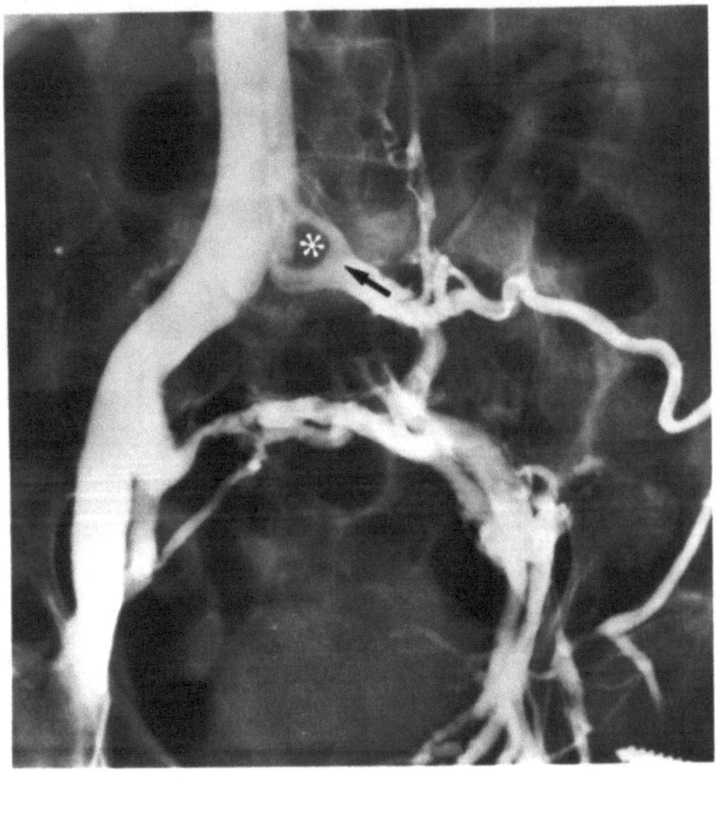

Fig. 4.23. Cavography with right femoral catheterization and injection into a branch of the arch of the internal saphenous vein on the left. Cockett's syndrome with lacunar image on the termination of the left common iliac vein (*). Collateral circulation over the deep iliac circumflex vein, and mainly over the obturator vein, which reopacifies the left hypogastric system and then the left common iliac vein at its origin (↖). Left and right contralateral derivation. Cockett's syndrome with extensive iliofemoropopliteal obstruction

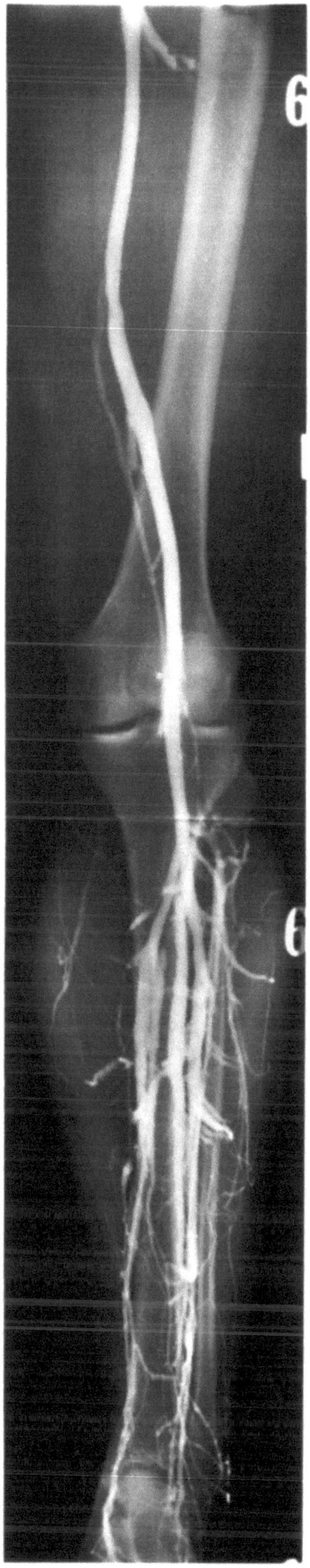

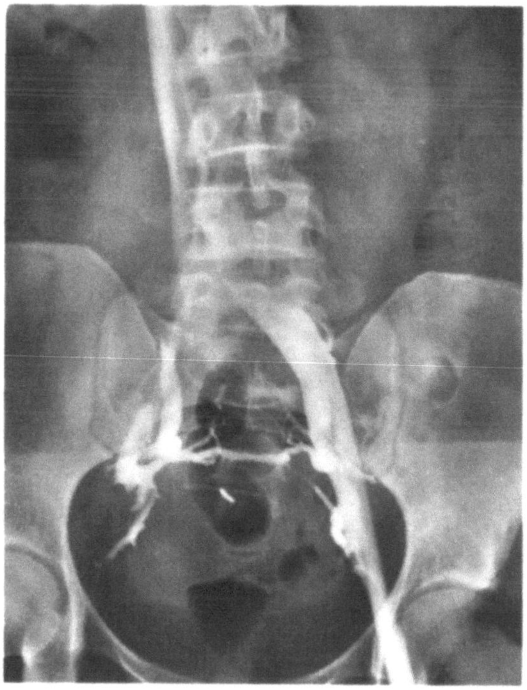

△ 4.24b

◁ 4.24a

▽ 4.24c

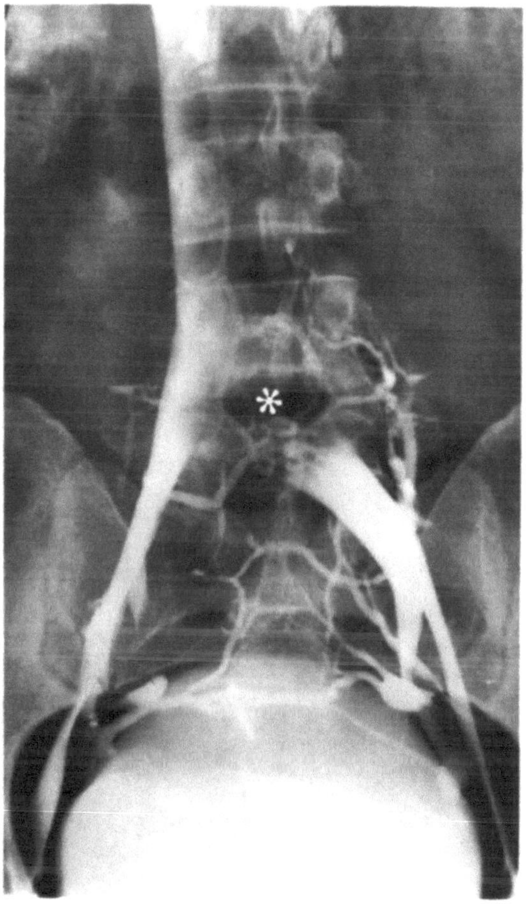

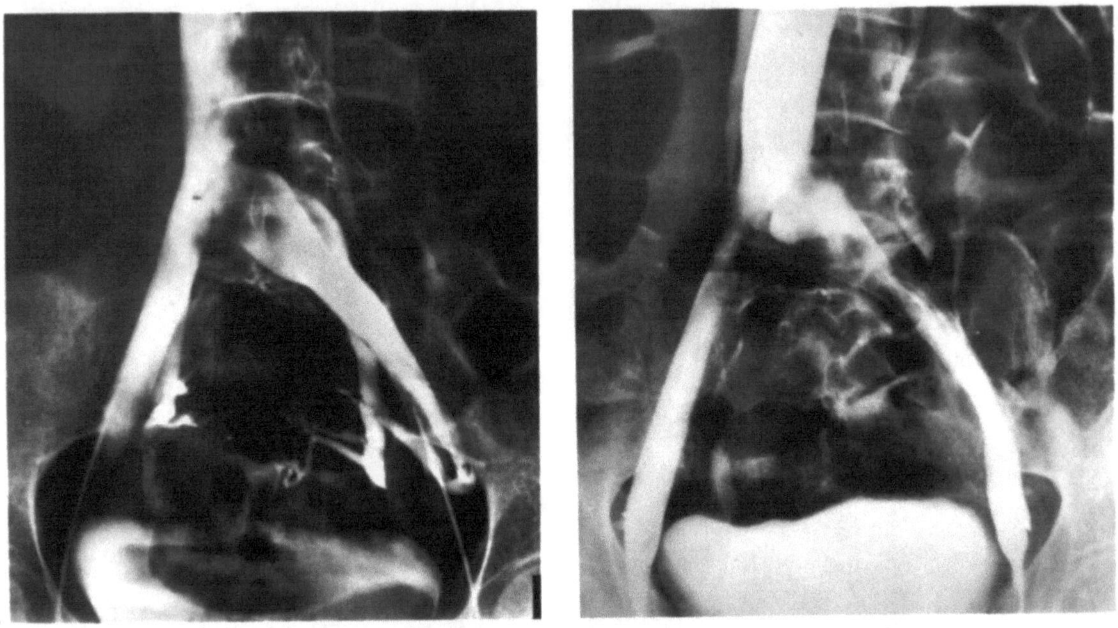

a b

Fig. 4.25a, b. Cockett's syndrome in a patient who had a confirmed pulmonary embolism. The venogram (a) gives no evidence of thrombosis in the lower limbs. The only visible anomaly is a Cockett syndrome with a well-displayed compression on an X-ray taken with the patient supine. b Cavography has been performed with the patient prone, which considerably diminished the images due to the Cockett syndrome and abolished the left-right collateral circulation over the presacral plexuses

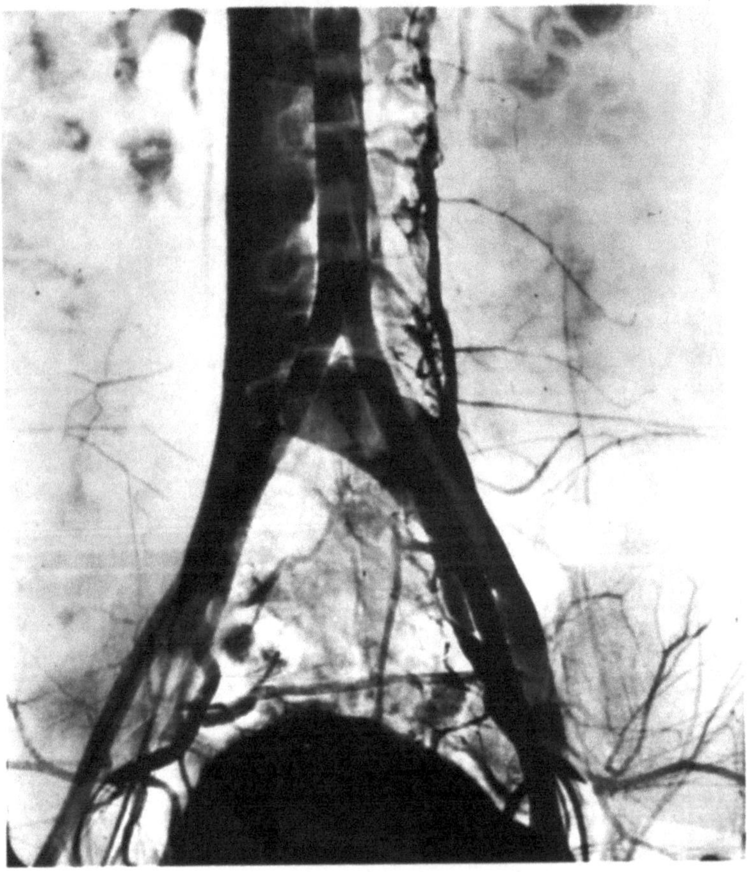

Fig. 4.26. Subtraction: Bifemoral percutaneous iliocavography combined with aortography. This simultaneous injection readily displays the correlations of the right common iliac artery which crosses the terminal segment of the left common iliac vein. Note the left to right collateral venous circulation through the presacral plexuses as well as through the left ascending lumbar vein

a

b

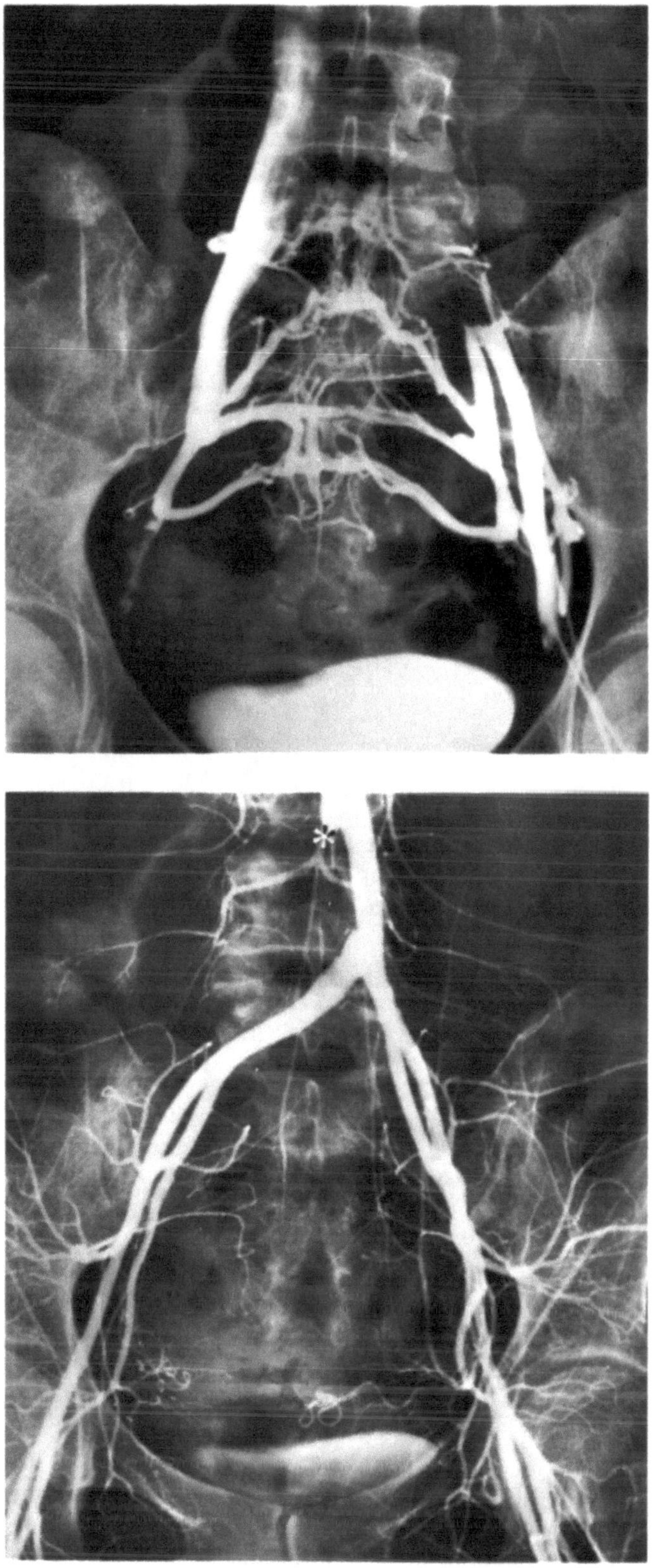

Fig. 4.27. a Left unifemoral iliocavography following prophylactic surgery on Cockett's syndrome (surgery report: thrombectomy plus venous enlargement patch) Complete failure with occlusion of the entire left common iliac vein. Left to right contralateral derivations. b Aortographic control in the same patient, in whom, besides operation upon the left common iliac vein, arterial uncrossing had been performed. Note the low reinsertion of the right common iliac artery into the left common iliac artery and the sutured stump of the right common iliac artery origin (*) on the aorta

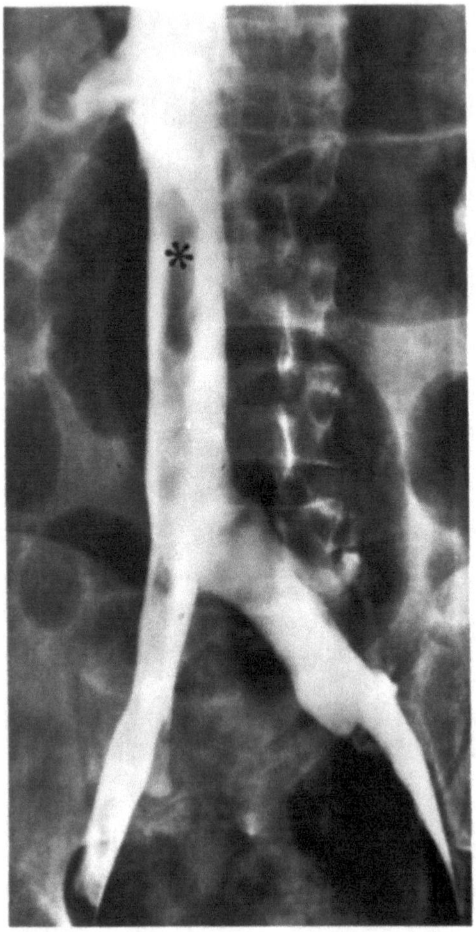

4.28

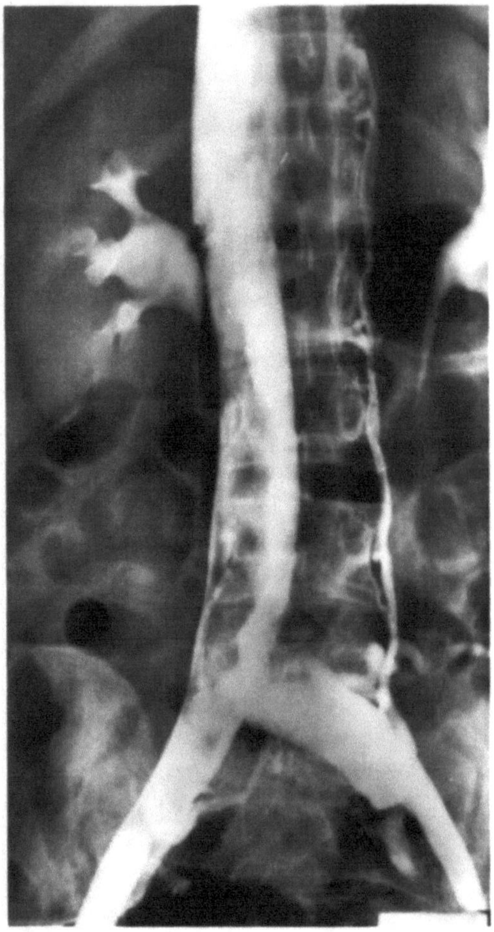

4.29

Fig. 4.28. Bifemoral percutaneous cavography. Cancer of the right kidney. Systematic preoperative cavography. Huge iliocaval thrombus originating in the right iliac vein and extending up to the postrenal segment of the inferior vena cava (*). The thrombus is not a malignant but a fibrinocruoric thrombus. Totally asymptomatic caval thrombosis with floating thrombi in a patient with renal cancer

Fig. 4.29. Floating iliocaval thrombus in a female with pulmonary embolism secondary to gynecologic surgery. Caval thrombosis revealed by pulmonary embolism

Fig. 4.30. Free thrombus (*) in the postrenal segment of the inferior vena cava following iliac phlebitis of the phlebothrombotic type, on the left. Phlebography of the lower limb confirms the obstruction of the right iliac route (not shown here)

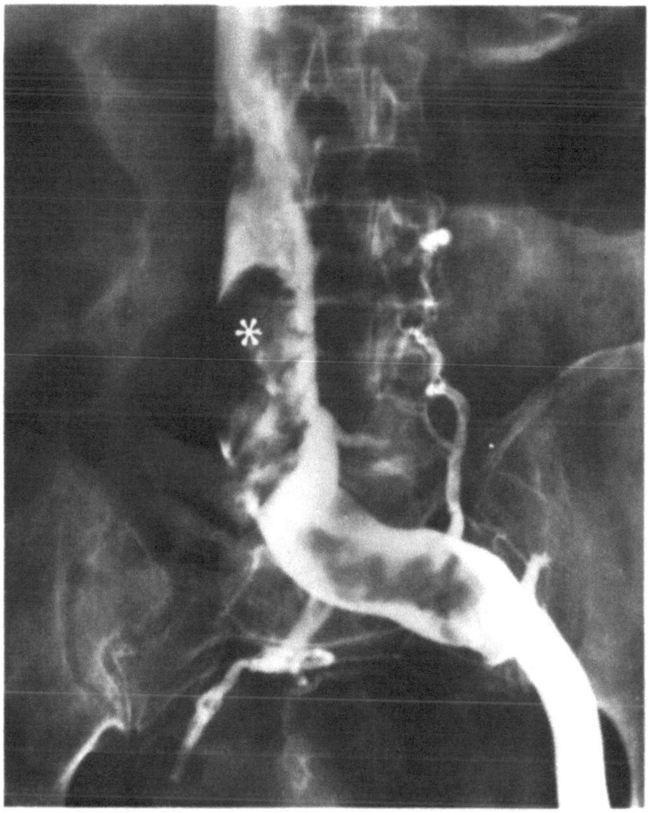

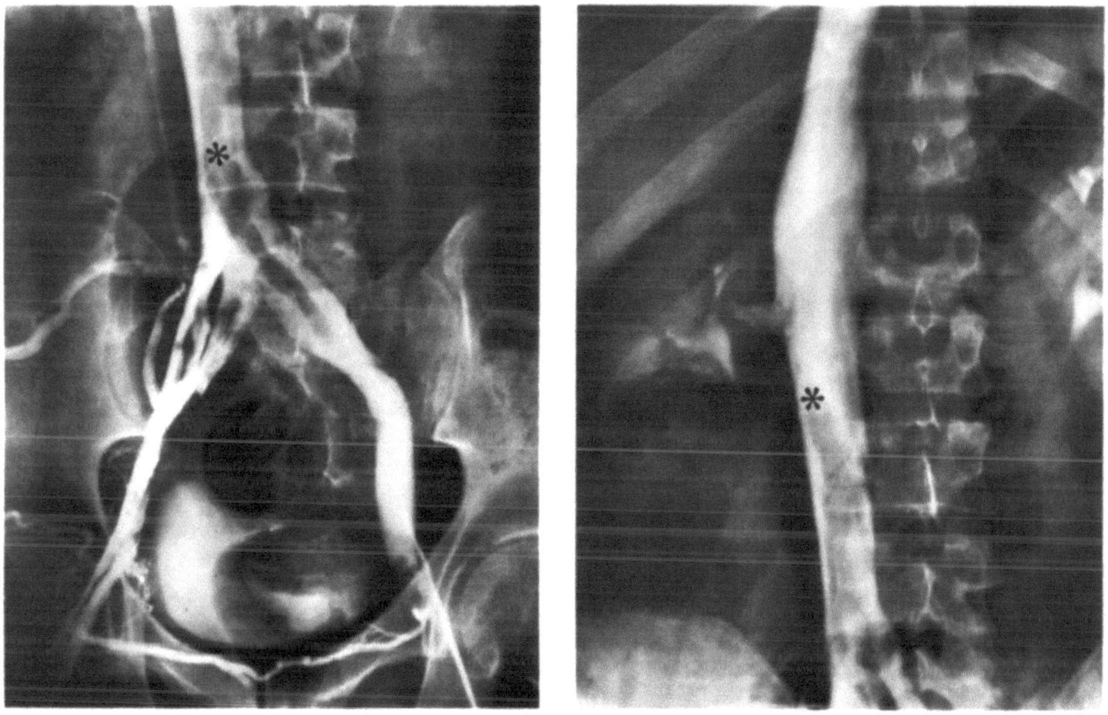

a b

Fig. 4.31 a, b. Long-standing phlebitis of the right iliac vein: a lower focusing; b higher focusing. Bifemoral percutaneous cavography. Duplication of the right common iliac vein. Asymptomatic left free iliocaval thrombus (*) extending up to the renal veins, well visible on the higher focused film (b). Note the interest of performing bilateral cavography for unilateral phlebitis

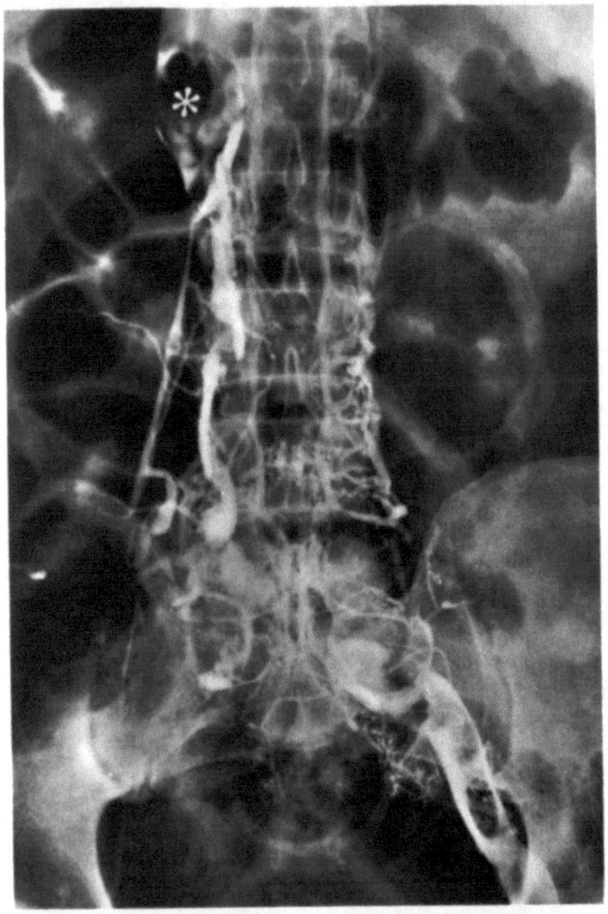

Fig. 4.32. Fifty-year-old male with clinical signs of bilateral blue phlebitis and superficial thoracoabdominal circulation. Inferior cavography by left femoral percutaneous puncture. Filling defects in the left common and external iliac veins consistent with phlebothrombosis. Occlusion of the terminal segment of the left common iliac vein. Opacification of the intra- and extraspinal plexuses. Faint reopacification of the interrenal segment of the inferior vena cava with a huge defect (*). Subjacent perfusion of the retrohepatic inferior vena cava which is patent. Surgical report: cancer of the right kidney with malignant intracaval thrombus in the area of the right renal vein. Thromboembolic disease related to the interrenal inferior caval obstacle

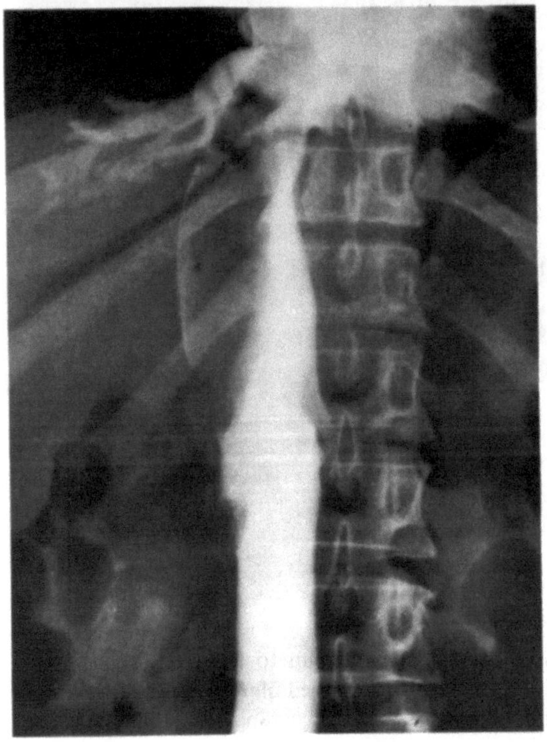

◁ Fig. 4.33. Cancer of the right kidney. Cavography. Malignant thrombus propagated to the retrohepatic segment of the inferior vena cava and to the right atrium

---

Fig. 4.35 a, b. Behcet's disease. Inferior caval thrombosis in a 30-year-old male. a Bifemoral percutaneous inferior vena cavography. Important inferior caval thrombosis with marked abdominopelvic collateral circulation. b Retrograde cavography by brachial approach. Patency of both renal veins. "Radish root" appearance of the postrenal segment of the inferior vena cava, which is obliterated at L3 level ▷

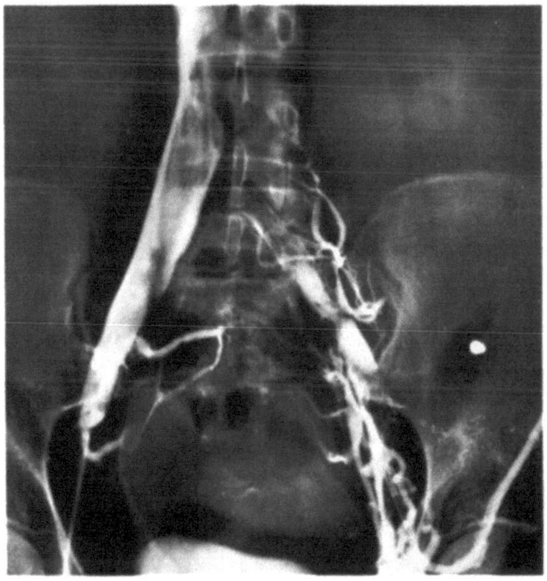

a

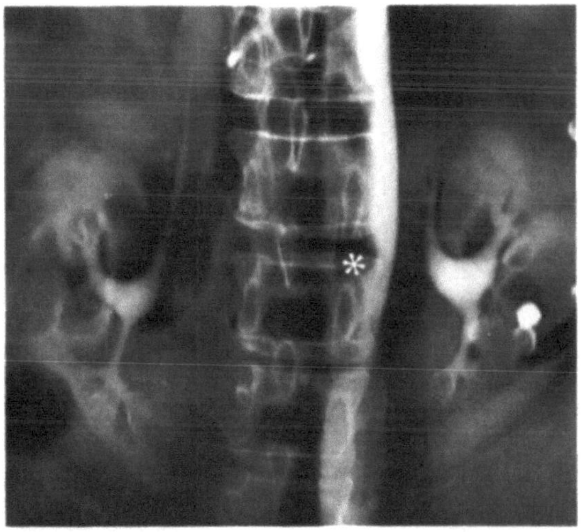

b

Fig. 4.34a, b. Left iliac phlebitis. Bifemoral percutaneous cavography. Left iliac adhesive phlebitis with very faint opacification. Bifemoral percutaneous cavography shows on a higher focused film (b) a huge ilio-inferior caval thrombus of the phlebothrombotic type extending up to the renal veins (*). This intracaval floating thrombus would have passed undetected if only unilateral left injection had been performed. Note some residual barium in colon diverticulosis

4.35a

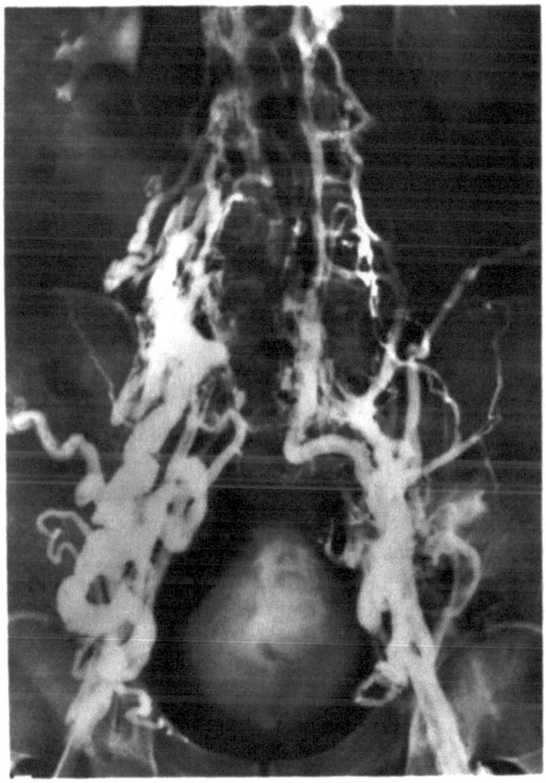

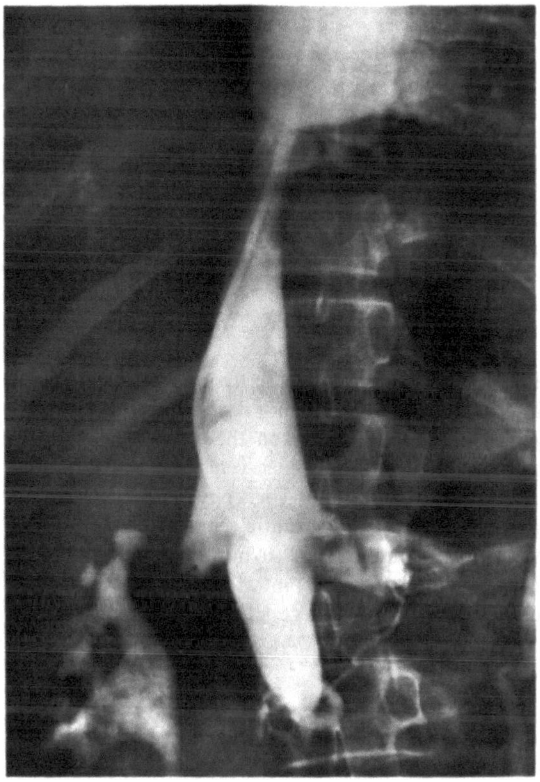

4.35b

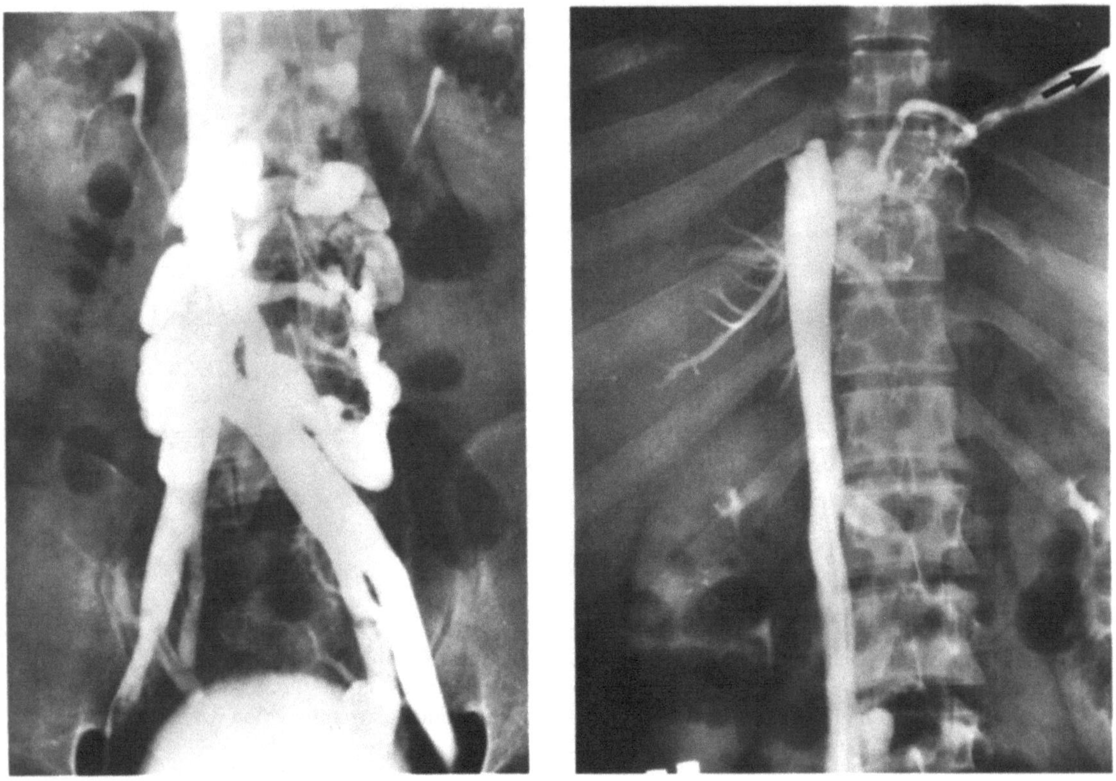

Fig. 4.36a–d. Stenosis of the terminal segment of the inferior vena cava. a Bifemoral percutaneous cavography. Voluminous varices on the inferior hemiazygos system. Patency of both iliac veins and of the inferior vena cava. b Inferior cavography with the catheter positioned in the retrohepatic segment of the inferior vena cava. Complete obstruction of the inferior vena cava caudally to its entry into the right atrium. Collateral circulation via a large left inferior diaphragmatic vein (↗). Note on this case the interest of carrying out systematically the opacification with an intracaval catheter: a would not have lead to the correct diagnosis. c Right auricular injection in order to determine the length of the membrane or of the stenosis. In the present case there was a 1.5-cm-long stenosis and no membranous occlusion. d Postoperative film following pericardiac graft anastomosing the terminal segment of the inferior vena cava with the right atrium

4.36c

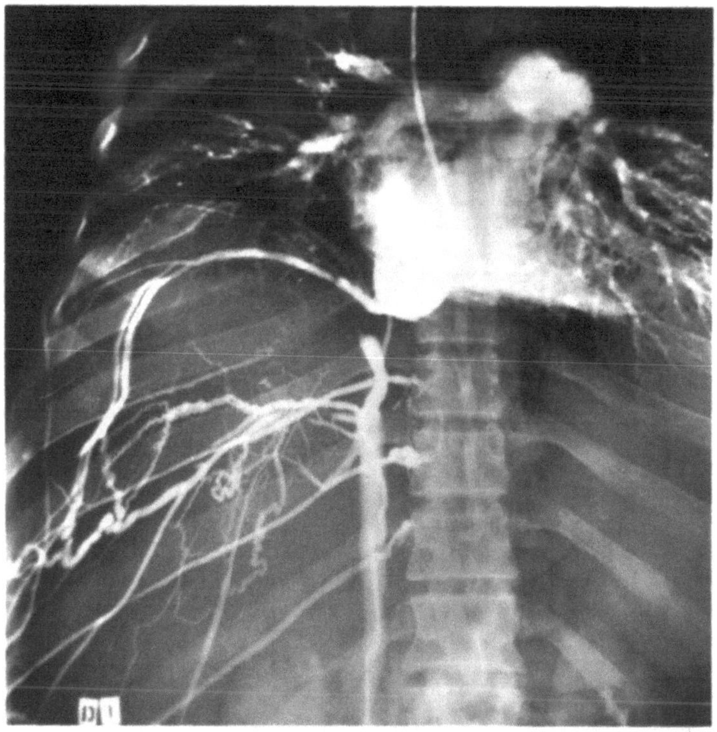

4.36d

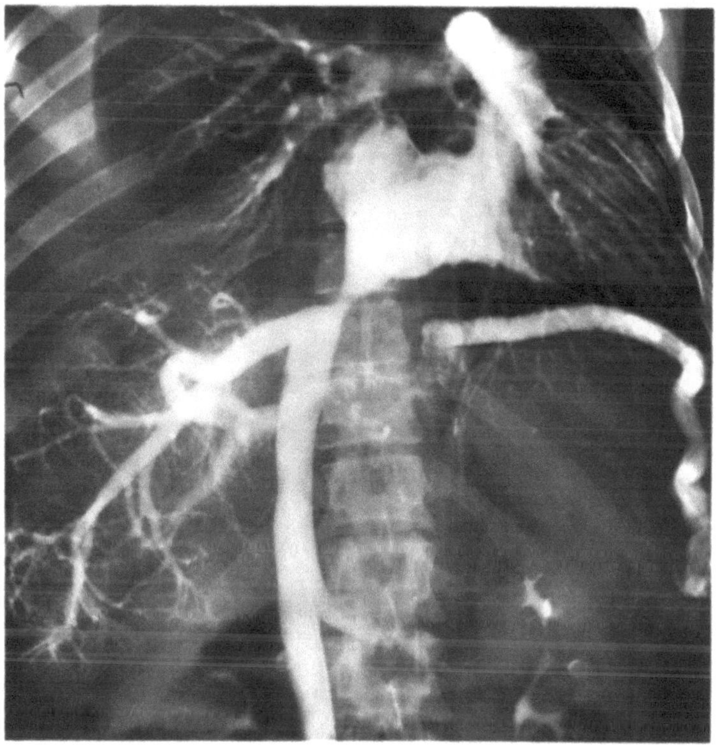

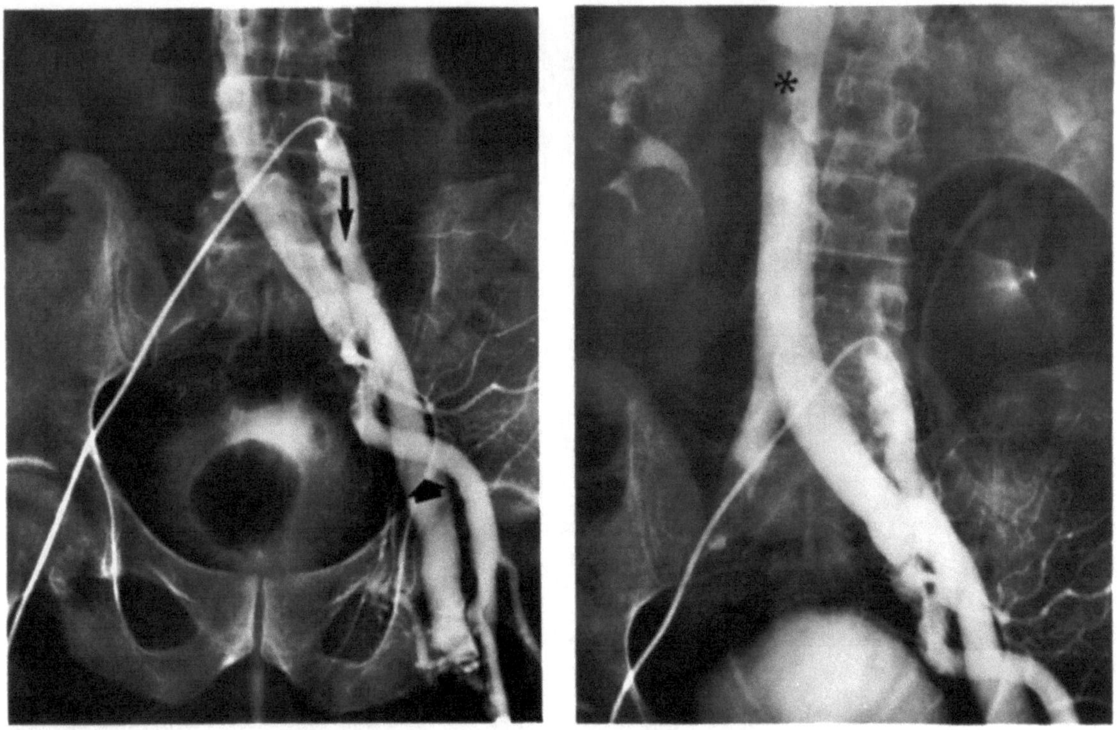

Fig. 4.37. a Left iliac arteriography (right femoral Seldinger) after left iliac thrombectomy associated with arterialization in the Scarpa triangle. Opacification of the left iliac arterial axis (↙), then of the arteriovenous fistula and left iliac venous system (⬅) and finally of the inferior vena cava. b Later phases of the seriogram show opacification of a former filling defect at the level of L2 corresponding to an inferior caval clip (*)

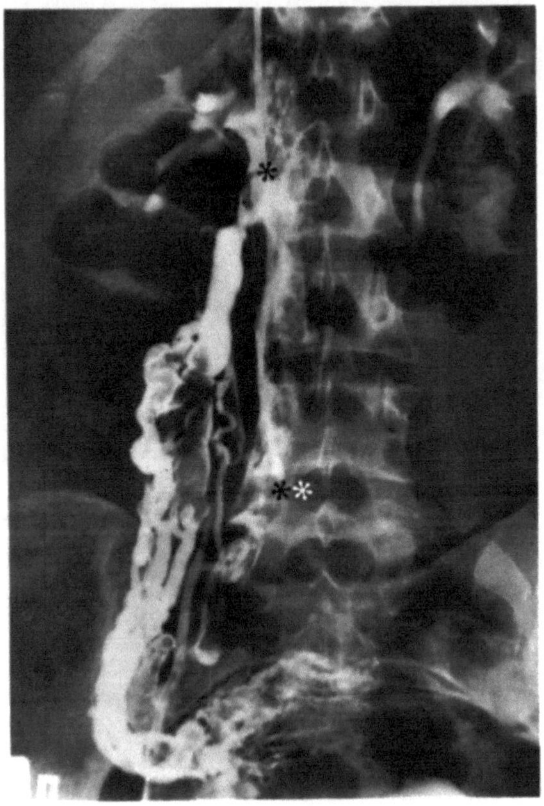

Fig. 4.38. Thrombectomy with arterialization in a case of left iliac phlebitis. Placement of a Teflon clip on the postrenal segment of the inferior vena cava. Postoperative bilateral edema of the legs. Retrograde inferior cavography with brachial approach. The catheter has been pushed through the clip (*) at the L4 level. The clip is located on the postrenal segment of the inferior vena cava (**). Diffuse inferior caval thrombosis below the clip. Downward reflux in the right ovarian vein which shows also a huge thrombus

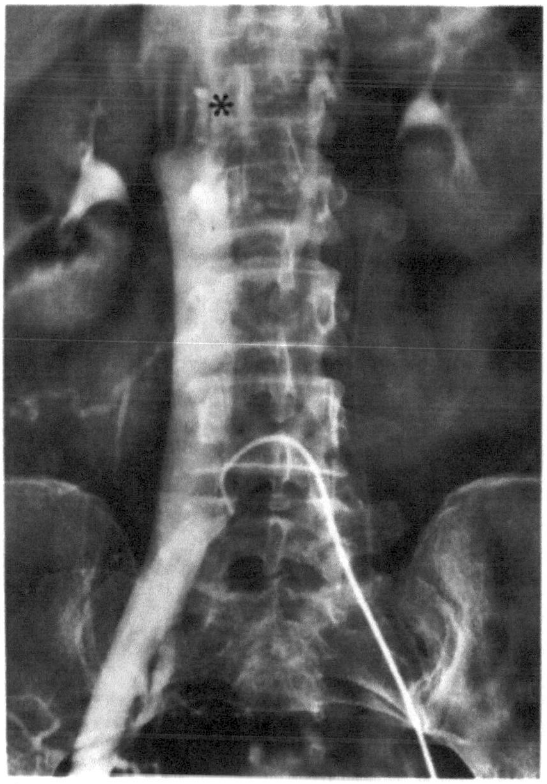

△

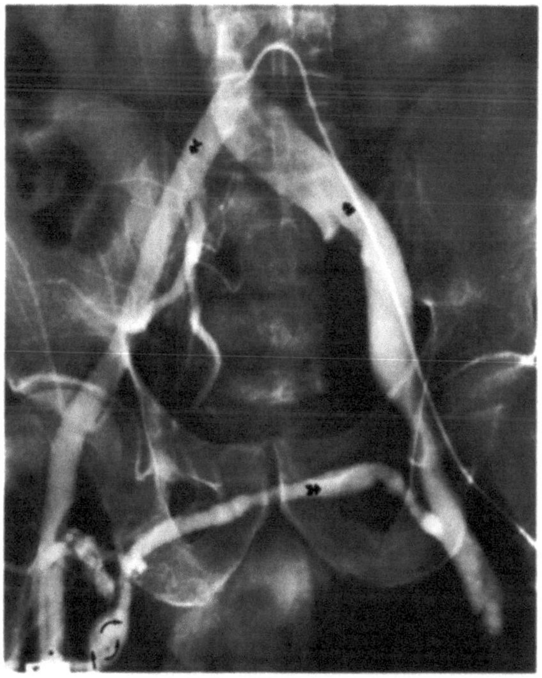

4.40

Fig. 4.39. Right iliac phlebitis. Right iliac venous thrombectomy with arterialization. Postoperative selective right iliac arteriography (left femoral artery Seldinger). Opacification of the arterial axis, later of the right venous axis, and finally of the inferior vena cava. Note the typical appearance of the inferior caval Teflon clip (*)

Fig. 4.40. Right iliac chronic phlebitis. Postoperative arteriogram. Transposition of the saphena with arterialization. Right iliac arteriography with left femoral approach. Successive opacification of the right iliac arterial route (↙) then of the arteriovenous fistula in the right Scarpa triangle (↗) which drains the left internal saphenous vein, placed in a retropubic location (↦). Subsequent opacification of the left iliac system which serves effectively for drainage (↖)

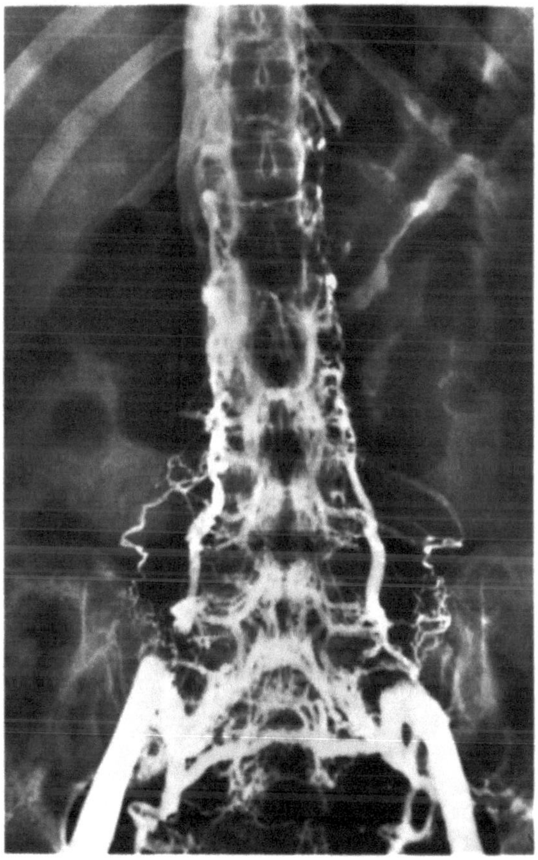

Fig. 4.41. Plication of the inferior vena cava. Thrombosis below. Collateral circulation via the azygos system

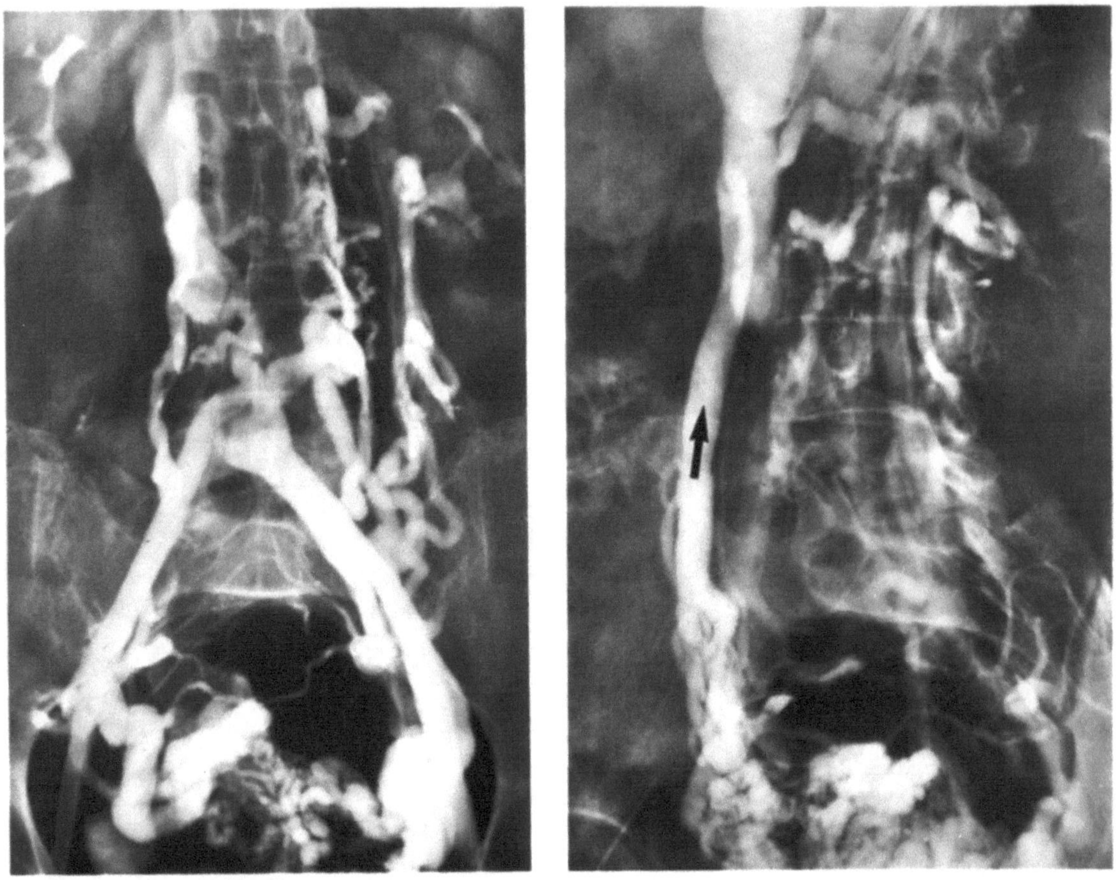

Fig. 4.42 a, b. Ligation of the inferior vena cava. Very marked pelvic collateral circulation, but also lumbar collateral channels draining into the left renal vein via the left ovarian vein which is well displayed on the left anterior oblique projection (↗)

Chapter 5. Collateral Circulation

5.1 General Remarks

The development of angiography has allowed a more precise study of the collateral circulation, based upon the level of obstruction, i.e., whether it is in the iliac veins or the inferior vena cava. The anatomic descriptions, which seemed complete, have been slightly modified, not from the morphological but from the functional point of view. As a matter of fact, some collateral routes which had been described by the anatomists were very rapidly confirmed as existing in vivo.

Before describing these collateral pathways it is necessary to recall the three principles advanced by Edwards to ensure unquestionable authentification of collateral routes:

Course of the collateral vessels: All vessels paralleling the axis of an obstructed vessel are potential collaterals if they are directly or indirectly linked to the venous trunk above or below the level of obstruction.

Presence and orientation of valves: If a vein is valved against the direction of the collateral flow, it cannot act as a collateral channel, at least not immediately. It will have to dilate to twice its diameter in order to render the valves incompetent and allow bidirectional flow.

Size of the collateral vessels: A single large channel is more effective than multiple small collateral channels. According to Poiseuille's law, flow is proportional to the fourth power of the diameter of the vessel.

5.2 Unilateral Iliac Obstruction
(Figs. 5.1–5.3)

In 1967 Mavor and Galloway provided a precise new description of the collateral circulation in obstruction of the deep veins of the lower limb. They distinguished two systems: an inferior system, up to the level where the deep femoral vein joins, and a superior system, above this point. The latter is the one dealt with here.

Several collateral systems could be described, according to the level of their origin on the iliac axis. Participation of this or that collateral system necessitates the patency of the iliac segment from which it originates. We shall consider first the collateral routes of the iliofemoral segment and then those of the common iliac segment.

5.2.1 Collateral System of the Iliofemoral Segment

This consists of two groups: a homolateral and a contralateral group.

Homolateral Group

This comprises, firstly, the hypogastric vein and its tributaries, especially the obturator vein, which is extensively anastomosed with the circumflex veins, branches of the deep femoral vein. This collateral system naturally develops only when there is no thrombosis in the hypogastric system (Fig. 5.4). There is also a second homolateral group, the only one to be visualized when there is a thrombosis of the hypogastric vein. It consists of subcutaneous cavocaval pathways toward the upper caval system via branches of the arch of the internal saphenous vein (subcutaneous abdominal vein and superficial iliac circumflex vein) and via retrocrural branches of the external iliac vein (deep iliac circumflex vein and epigastric vein). Because of the valves in the abdominal wall veins, it takes several weeks before bidirectional flow becomes functional. Subcutaneous cavocaval circulation is a sign of an already rather old, often bilateral, extended iliocaval obstruction (Fig. 5.5). The inferior epigastric vein is anastomosed with the internal mammary vein. Some periumbilical anastomoses may drain into the portal system via the umbilical vein (Fig. 5.6). More rarely, internal mammary and phrenic anastomoses may redirect the blood into the inferior vena cava at the level of the diaphragm. The lateral veins of the abdominal wall (deep and superficial iliac circumflex veins) anastomose with the lateral thoracic veins (external mammary vein, and then axillary vein) (Fig. 5.7). More rarely, the veins of the lateral abdominal wall bypass the inferior caval obstruction and redirect the venous flow toward the lumbar veins and vertebral venous plexus, and from there into the inferior vena cava.

Contralateral Group

The contralateral system implies patency of the opposite iliac venous axis. It comprises superficial veins, i.e., branches of the arch of the internal saphenous vein (pre- and suprasymphysial superficial abdominal ramus, external pudendal veins), which anastomose with their mates on the opposite side and form a spontaneous, functional Palma operation (Figs. 5.8–5.10).

This contralateral system also includes the system of the hypogastric veins, which is very efficient. It is situated at different levels. On the one hand, it functions in the retrosymphysial area, anastomosing branches such as the obturator vein and the internal pudendal vein with their mates on the opposite side. On the other hand, there are deep anastomoses connecting one side to the other: the perigenital and perivesical venous plexuses. The contralateral group is supplemented by the presacral venous plexuses, which anastomose the two hypogastric systems. Moreover, these presacral venous plexuses anastomose with the intravertebral plexuses through the sacral foramina (Figs. 5.11 and 5.12).

A tributary of the external iliac vein, the epigastric vein, may also participate in this contralateral system, partly via a communication, usually large, with the obturator vein, but especially via a constant suprapubic branch that anastomoses with its opposite mate.

Only the presacral venous plexuses are valveless (Fig. 5.13). There are usually one or more competent valves on the origin of the hypogastric system. Because of the vicarious dilatation of the hypogastric vein, bidirectional flow rapidly becomes practical, permitting efficacious collateral circulation from one side of the lesser pelvis to the other.

5.2.2 Collateral System of the Common Iliac Segment

This collateral system is particularly efficacious and is always well displayed on cavograms.

The Azygos System (Fig. 5.14)

This is an extremely important collateral route. It is the ascending lumbar vein which, at the level of the common iliac segment, gives rise to this collateral circulation system. The ascending lumbar vein is one of the origin branches of the azygos system; it communicates with the inferior vena cava through the caval portion of the lumbar veins and also through the peri- and intravertebral plexuses via the intervertebral veins (Fig. 5.15). Chapter 11 deals with the radioanatomy of the intra- and extravertebral plexuses in more detail. When it is patent, the renal vein serves as a pathway toward the inferior caval system via multiple renoazygolumbar anastomoses. In the case of total obstruction of the cava, the azygos system drains all the blood from the lower part of the body toward the superior caval system, via the great azygos vein and the left inferior hemiazygos vein which traverses the diaphragm. This extravertebral collateral azygos drainage is commonly associated with drainage via the intravertebral plexuses, which are connected by multiple anastomoses with the azygos system.

The Sex Vein

The sex vein – spermatic or ovarian – though it is not a branch of the common iliac system, acts as a large collateral pathway in obstruction of the common iliac segment. It may have a very large caliber, and its dilatation serves to carry the additional blood flow, via the hypogastric system, in case of blockage of the common iliac vein.

Middle Sacral Vein

Finally, the middle sacral vein, on the left, may serve as a collateral route in proximal obstruction of the common iliac vein.

5.3 Bilateral Iliac Obstruction (Without Caval Obstruction)

This is a rather infrequent condition. The collateral channels are above all the thoracoabdominal superficial veins, with cavocaval shunt. Involvement of both hypogastric systems usually impedes any contralateral collateral flow within the lesser pelvis. Most often, this type of obstruction is associated with obstruction of the infrarenal segment of the inferior vena cava, described below.

5.4 Postrenal Occlusion of the Inferior Vena Cava

Schematically, two cases may be distinguished, according to whether or not there is recanalization at the level of the renal veins.

5.4.1 With Recanalization

Besides the previously described collateral systems, there may be marked dilatation of the ureteral veins, with extrinsic compression visible on an intravenous urogram. These features are particularly well visualized when cavography is performed with the patient carrying out a Valsalva maneuver or standing upright.

Recanalization occurs especially in the left renal vein, which receives the ureteral veins and the gonadal vein (Figs. 5.16–5.18). The azygos system also communicates extensively with the renal vein system (Figs. 5.19 and 5.20).

The portal system (Fig. 5.21) may serve as collateral channel in cases of infrarenal caval occlusion. Using a large volume of contrast material in cavography succeeds more and more often in demonstrating cavoportal drainage pathways. Filling is via the hemorrhoidal plexus, which anastomoses the hypogastric vein with the superior hemorrhoidal vein and with the inferior mesenteric vein, which drains into the portal system (Fig. 5.22). Much more rarely, filling occurs via the abdominal wall veins, which drain toward the epiploic veins or toward a patent umbilical vein. This portal system (Fig. 5.23) tends especially to develop when the usual pathways, especially the central routes (azygos system) are affected; this is not, however, an absolute rule.

Other collateral routes may also develop, but they are only rarely visualized cavographically. They connect the portal system with retroperitoneal structures. Thus there may be communications between the posterior parietal veins, depending on the inferior caval system, and portal veins of the ascending colon and distal terminal ileum, which both derive embryologically from the subcardinal veins. Also there may be a communication between the right ovarian vein and the superior mesenteric vein, producing cavoportal drainage (the gonadal vein being a branch with the same embryologic origin). The descending colon and sigmoid may also communicate with branches derived from the subcardinal system. Much more rarely, there are portocaval communications with greater flow and larger caliber, e.g., the splenorenal anastomosis and the mesentericogonadal anastomosis, which are more often encountered in portal hypertension than in inferior caval thrombosis.

5.4.2 Without Recanalization

The tributaries of the renal veins, mainly the renoazygolumbar venous arch, but also the left gonadal vein, are thus suppressed, and the collateral circulation is via the azygos system, which carries it as far as the thorax (Fig. 5.24), and via the parietal collateral channels. This type of obstruction causes functional cavoportal shunts more frequently than the previous type.

5.5 Obstruction of the Middle Portion of the Inferior Vena Cava

Obstruction of the inferior vena cava between the renal and the hepatic veins is rather rare, at least when there is no subjacent inferior caval obstruction. Most often there is complete obstruction of the ilio-inferior caval system. Collateral circulation is partly via the azygos system and the vertebral venous plexus (Fig. 5.25) and mainly via the superficial collateral routes and the portal system. The gonadal and ureteric venous systems as well as the renoazygolumbar arch do not usually serve as collateral routes.

The venous drainage of the kidney is via suprarenal-phrenic anastomoses into the azygos system. There are in fact at this level very important posterior drainage pathways, which establish communication between the suprarenal veins, the azygos system, the phrenic veins, and also the internal mammary veins and even the veins of the esophagus.

5.6 Obstruction of the Upper Portion of the Inferior Vena Cava

This is a very rare level for obstruction of the inferior vena cava. As in the middle segment, when obstruction occurs it tends to be complete and accompanied by obstruction of the subjacent caval segment. All previously described collateral routes play a role. It is important to see whether there is obstruction of the hepatic veins (Fig. 5.26). With partial obstruction of the hepatic veins the portal system may still serve as a collateral route. Contrariwise, with thrombosis of the hepatic veins the portal system cannot serve as a collateral channel, and reversal of flow in the portal system will occur. This is well displayed by selective hepatic arteriography. Thus, the problems are the same as for the Budd-Chiari syndrome (see also Chap. 12).

References

Berlin L, Waldam I, Fong JK (1965) Occlusion of the inferior vena cava. A major roentgenographic abnormality with minor clinical manifestations. JAMA 194:984–986

Bramwit DN, Hummel WC (1969) The superior and inferior mesenteric veins as collateral channels in inferior vena cava obstruction. Radiology 92:90–92

Chermet J, Tubiana JM, Monnier JP, Rouanet JP, Wesley C, Chalut J (1977) Les phlébites iliaques. A propos de 100 observations. Valeur de l'angiographie pré- et post-opératoire. Ann Radiol (Paris) 20/7:649–666

Ferris EJ, Vittimberga FJ, Byrne JJ, Nabseth DC, Shapiro JH (1967) The inferior vena cava after ligation and plication. Radiology 89:1–10

Ferris EJ, Hipona FA, Kahn PC, Phillps E, Shapiro JH (1969) Venography of the inferior vena cava and its branches, Vol. 1. Williams & Wilkins, Baltimore p 229

Filler RM, Edwards EA (1962) Collaterals of the lower inferior vena cava in man revealed by venography. Arch Surg 84:10–16

Fletcher EWL, Lea Thomas M (1968) Chronic post-thrombotic obstruction of the inferior vena cava investigated by cavography. A report of 11 cases. Am J Roentgenol Radium Therapy Nucl Med 102/2:363–369

Hipona FA, Gabriele O (1967) Portal venous system as a major collateral in iliac and inferior vena caval obstruction. Radiology 89:1077–1079

Lea Thomas M, Fletcher E, Cockett FB, Negus D (1967) Collaterals in external common iliac vein obstruction. Clin Radiol 18:403–409

Mavor GE, Galloway JM (1967) Collaterals of the deep venous circulation of the lower limb. Surg Gynecol Obstet 185:561–571

Pacalon D (1974) Etude radiologique des suppléances portales dans les thromboses de la veine cave inférieure. Thèse Med, Besançon

Sakaguchi S, Ischitobi K, Baba S, Kameda T (1970) Dynamic phlebography of the lower extremities with special reference to our new approach to the classification of findings. Angiology 21:283–294

Serradimigni A, Mercier C (1973) Les thromboses veineuses profondes des membres. Actualités diagnostiques et thérapeutiques. Masson, Paris

Stein S, Blumsohn D (1962) Clinical and radiological observations of inferior vena caval obstruction. Br J Radiol 35:159–164

Weese JA de, Rogoff SM (1963) Phlebographic patterns of acute deep venous thrombosis of the leg. Surgery 53:99–108

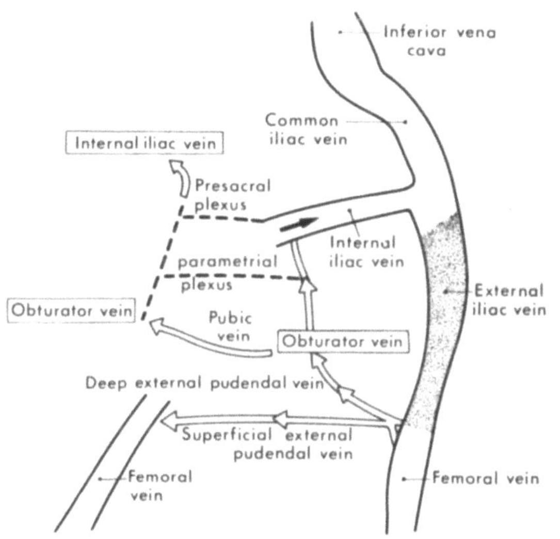

Fig. 5.1. Obstruction of the left external iliac vein

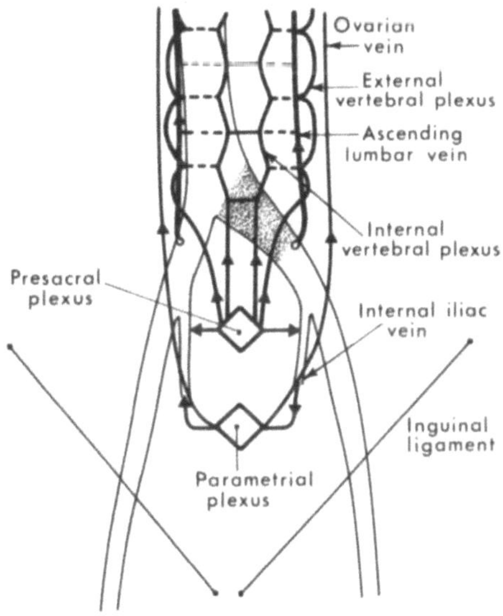

Fig. 5.2. Obstruction of the left common iliac vein

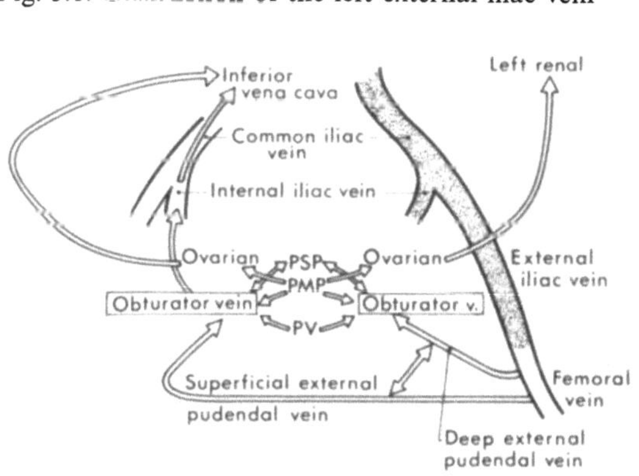

Fig. 5.3. Complete iliac obstruction (common iliac, external iliac and left internal iliac vein)
PSP Presacral plexus
PMP Parametrial plexus
PV Pubic vein

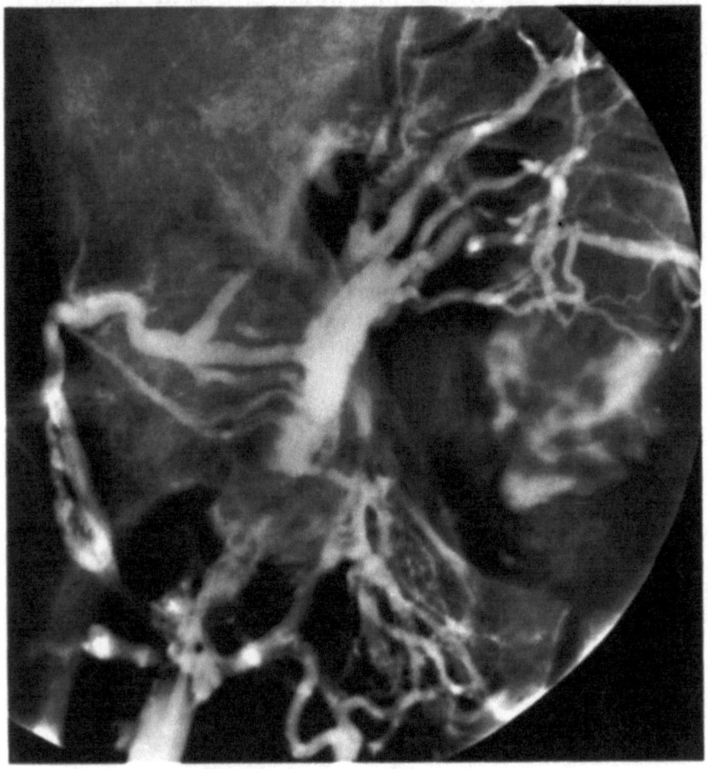

Fig. 5.4. Iliofemoral obstruction. The obstruction involves the common femoral vein, where a thrombus has been punctured, and the right external iliac vein. Collateral circulation via branches of the deep femoral vein (circumflex vein, inferior gluteal vein and obturator vein) draining into the right hypogastric system which is opacified. Right-to-left communication via the presacral venous plexuses

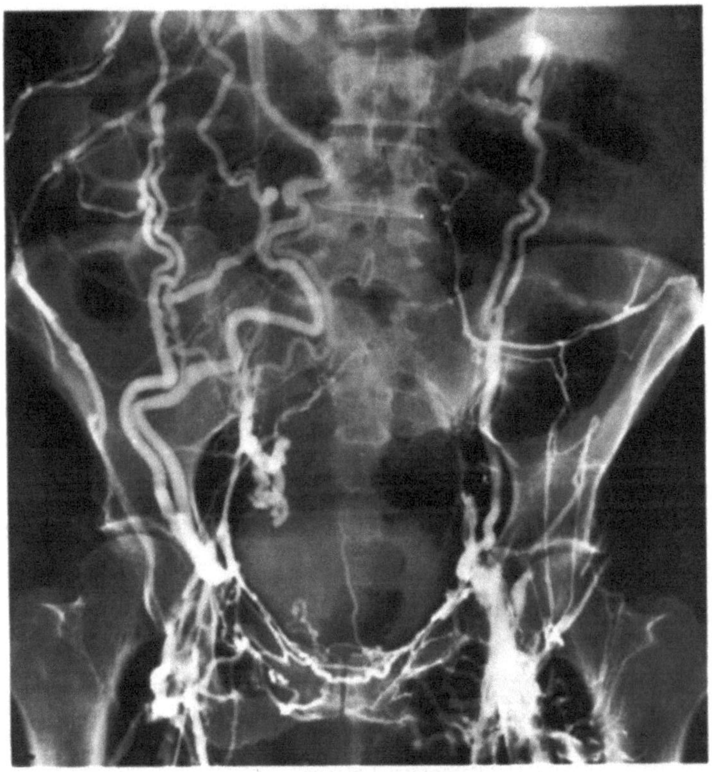

Fig. 5.5. Iliocaval thrombosis. Very long-standing thrombosis with superficial parietal circulation via the epigastric, circumflex iliac, and superficial abdominal veins

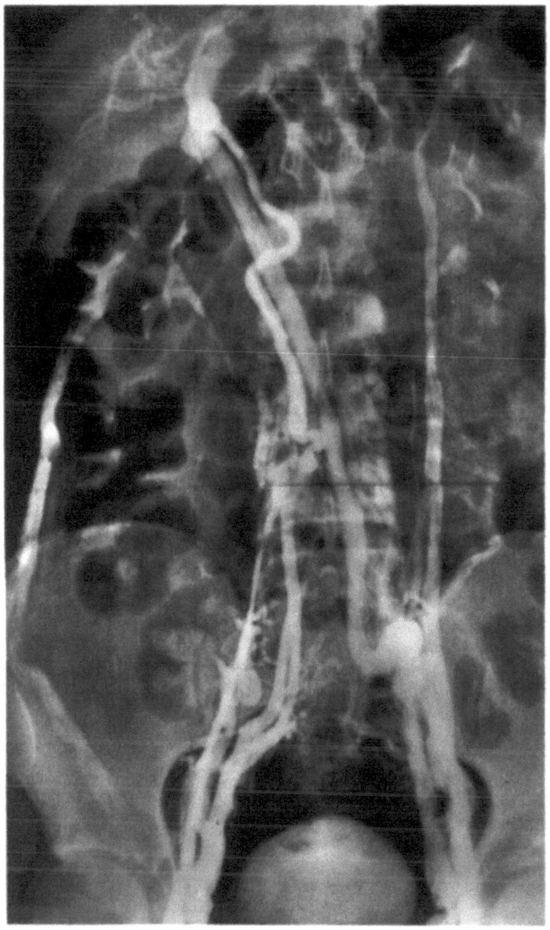

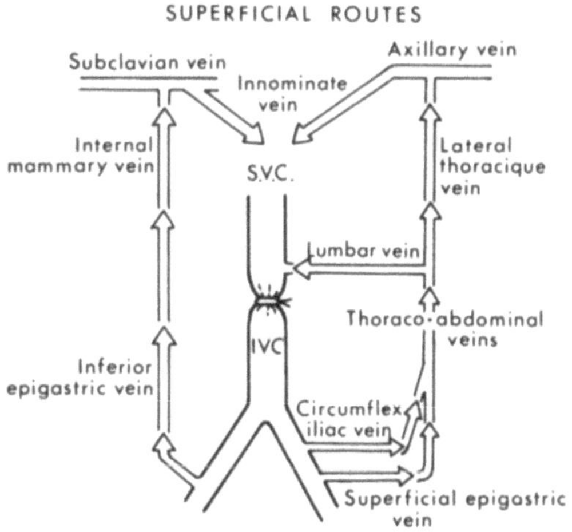

Fig. 5.7. Collateral drainage via the superficial veins of the thoraco-abdominal wall

◁
Fig. 5.6. Complete iliocaval thrombosis. Collateral circulation via two epigastric veins which drain over umbilical anastomoses into an umbilical vein and a vein of the round ligament of the liver. (By courtesy of Prof. Ag. J. Tongio)

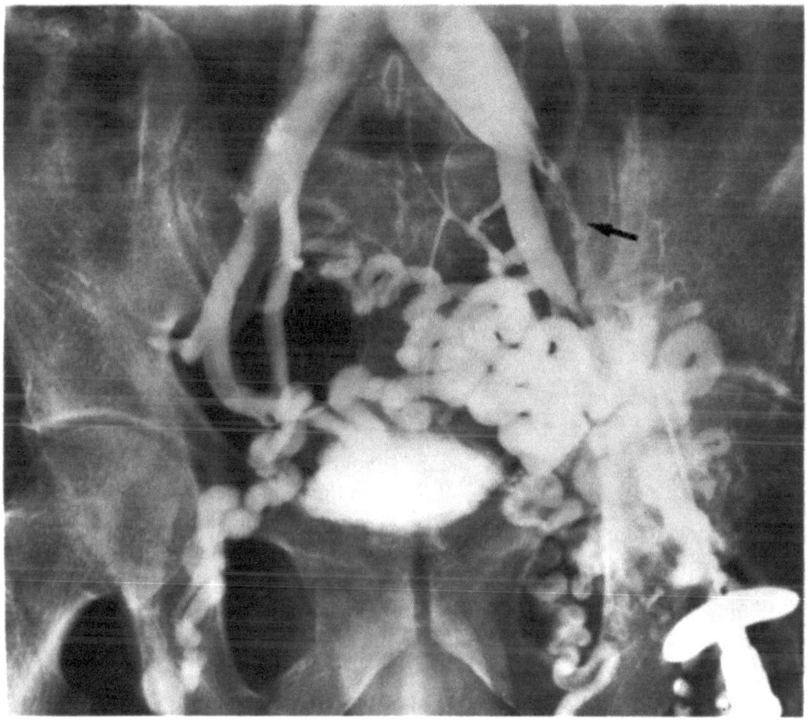

Fig. 5.8. Post-traumatic stenosis of the left external iliac vein (injury caused by a Fogarty's catheter with balloon); grid-like appearance of the external iliac vein (←). Huge supra- and retropubic inguinal varices diverting the blood flow towards the right side

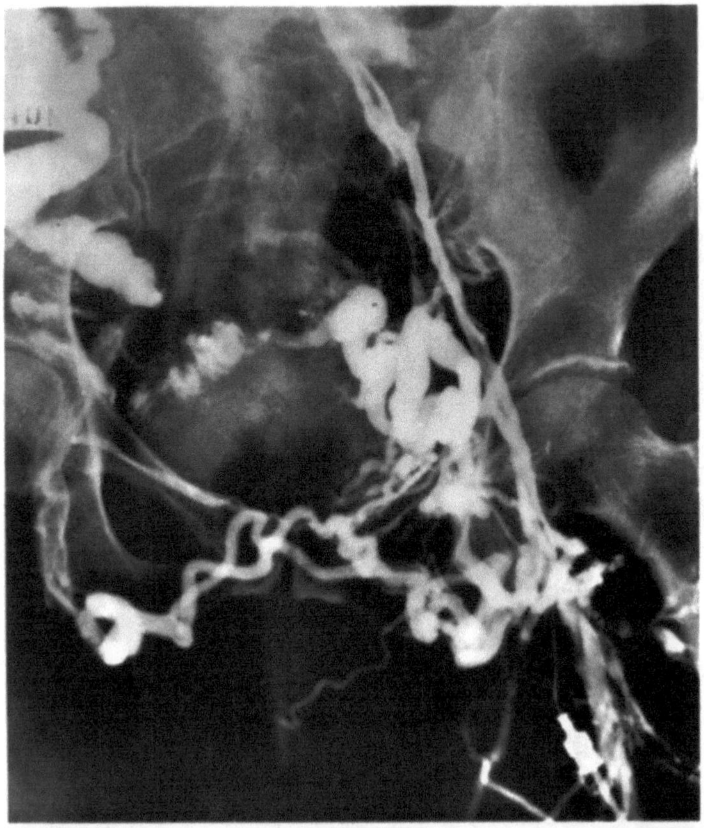

Fig. 5.9. Left iliofemoral chronic phlebitis. Puncture with the catheter-needle into the thrombus on the left. Collateral circulation via the obturator and the inferior gluteal vein, and mainly supra- and retropubic toward the right side. Residual barium in the ascending colon

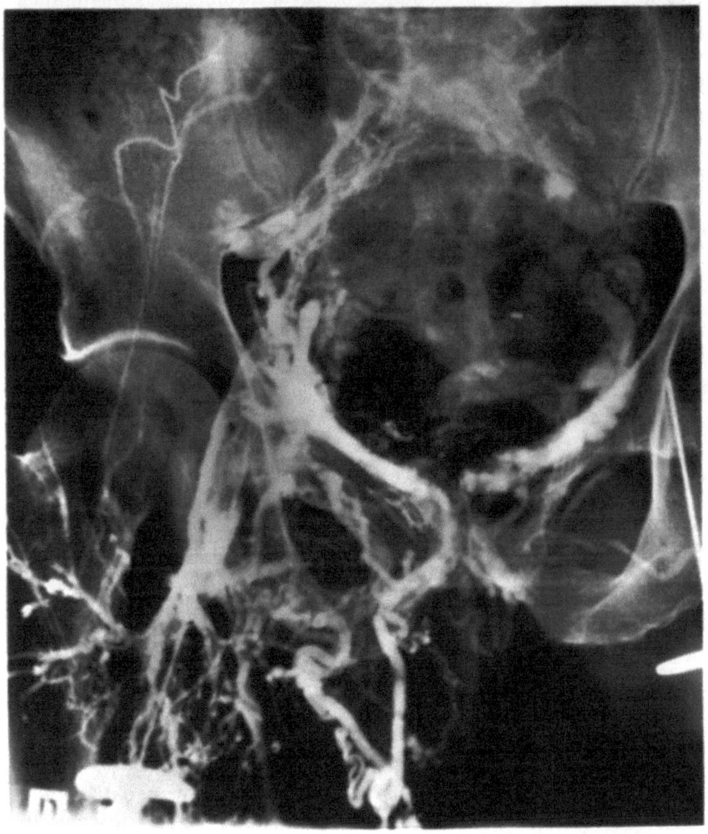

Fig. 5.10. Percutaneous bifemoral cavography. Puncture into a thrombus on the right side. Opacification of the external pudendal veins, of a right varicocele and of the parietal (Retzius space) and deep (internal pudendal vein) branches of the right hypogastric system. Note also the opacification of the veins of the Retzius space on the left side of the pelvis. Absence of parietal collateral circulation

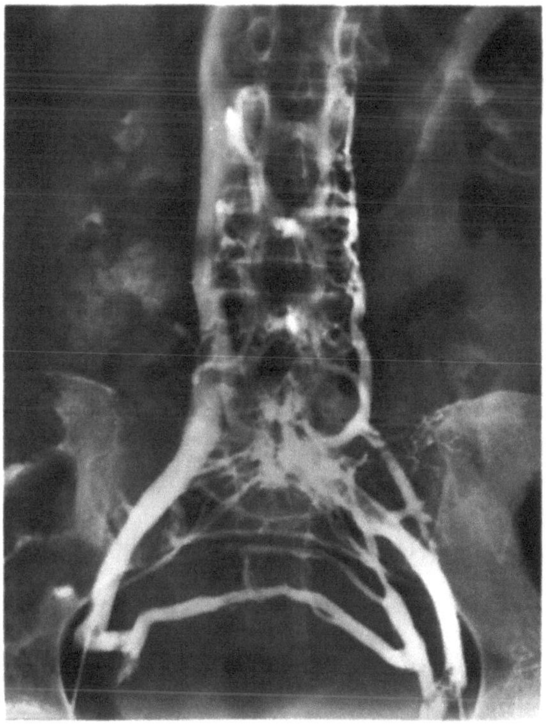

Fig. 5.11. Obstruction of the left common iliac vein by a paraganglioma of the organ of Zuckerkandl. Left to right opacification via the presacral venous plexuses

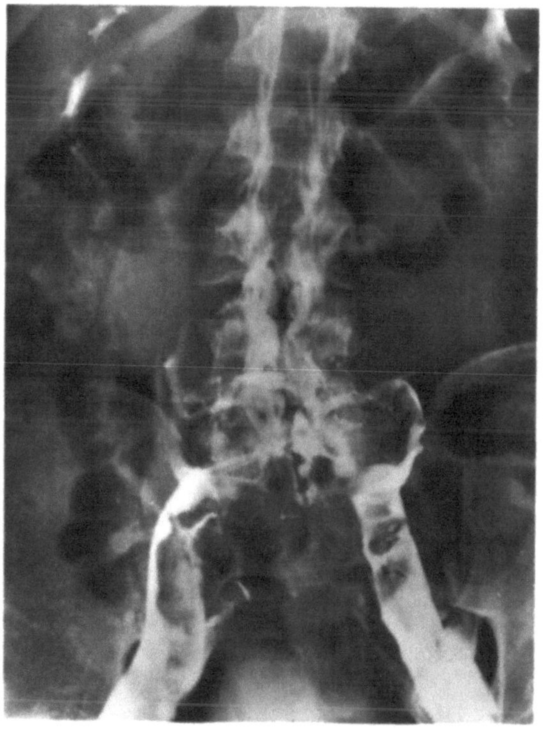

Fig. 5.12. Percutaneous bifemoral cavography in a 29-year-old male who presented a sudden, hard and cyanotic edema of both lower limbs. Complete functional impotence. Appearance of free thrombus in both iliac veins. The inferior vena cava is not opacified. This is a later sequence showing nothing but collateral circulation via the intervertebral venous plexuses outlining the medullary cavity. Collateral circulation is unusually moderate. This patient had in fact had phlebitis of the iliocaval confluence during his childhood. The actual symptoms are due to obstruction in the collateral circulation which had probably been more marked before

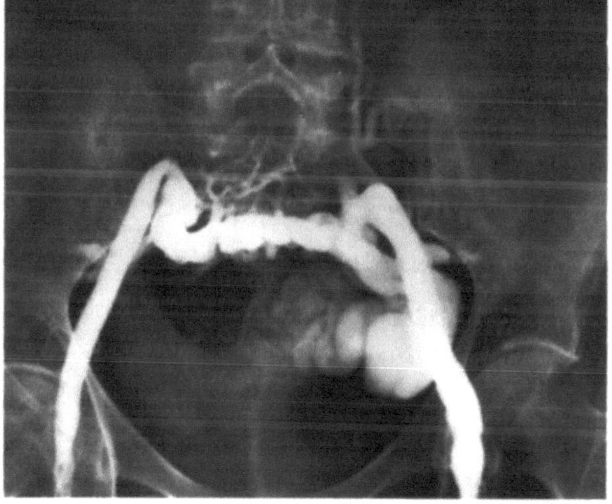

Fig. 5.13. Obstruction of both common iliac veins and of the infrarenal segment of the inferior vena cava. Opacification of the dilated presacral plexuses. Faint visualization of large pelvic varices which drain into a double right ovarian vein depicted in Fig. 5.18

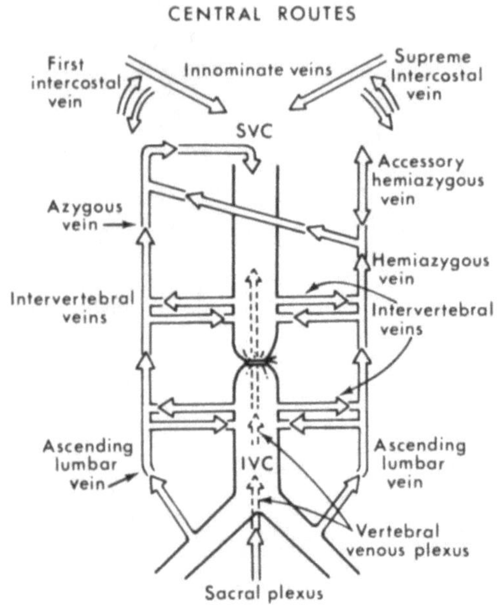

Fig. 5.14. Collateral circulation via the azygos system

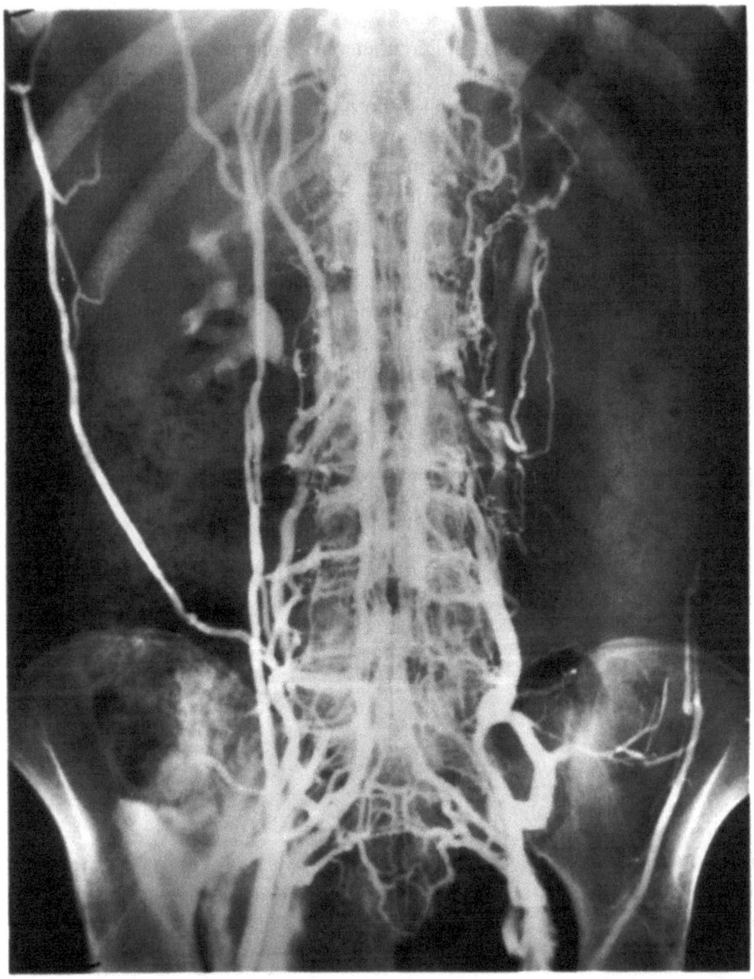

Fig. 5.15. Iliocaval obstruction and collateral circulation via parietal veins, mainly via the intravertebral azygos system. Budd-Chiari disease with caval thrombosis

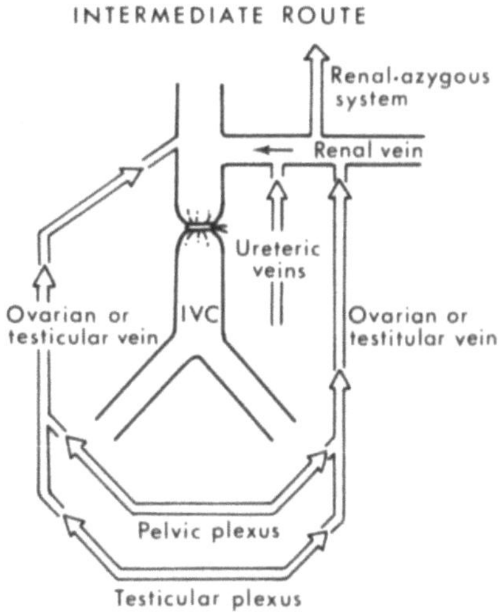

Fig. 5.16. Collateral circulation via the sex veins

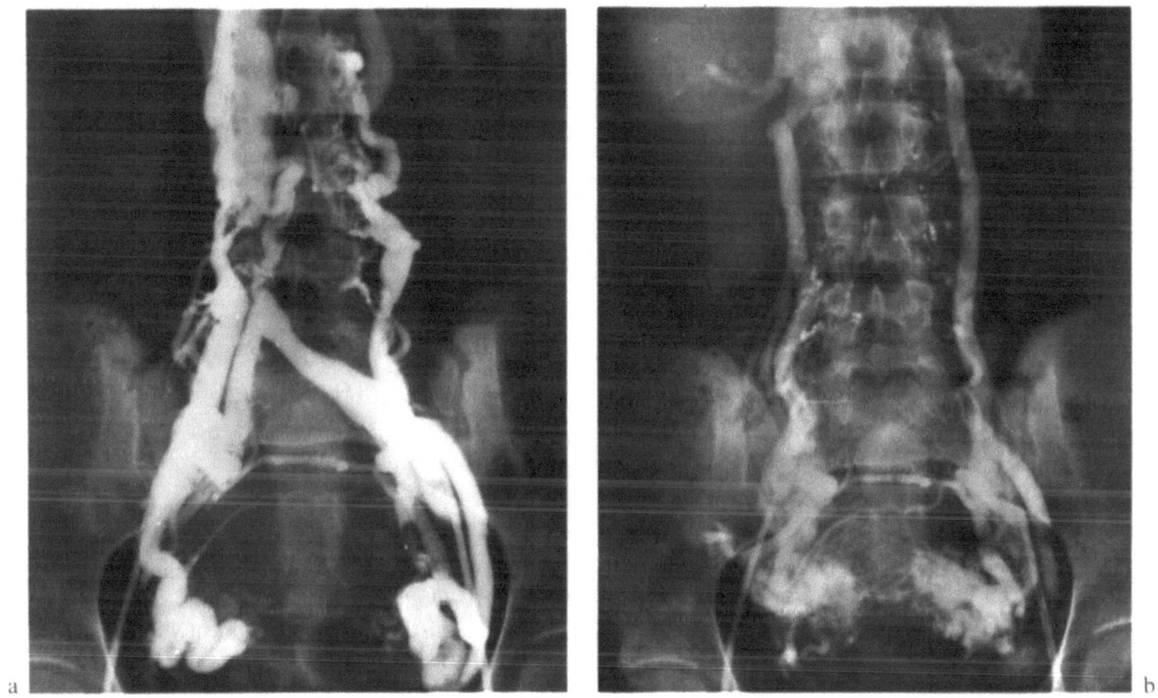

Fig. 5.17. a Obstruction of the infrarenal segment of the inferior vena cava secondary to ligation of the cava. b There is marked collateral circulation via the pelvic plexuses draining into the right and left sex veins and reopacifying the inferior vena cava and the left renal vein

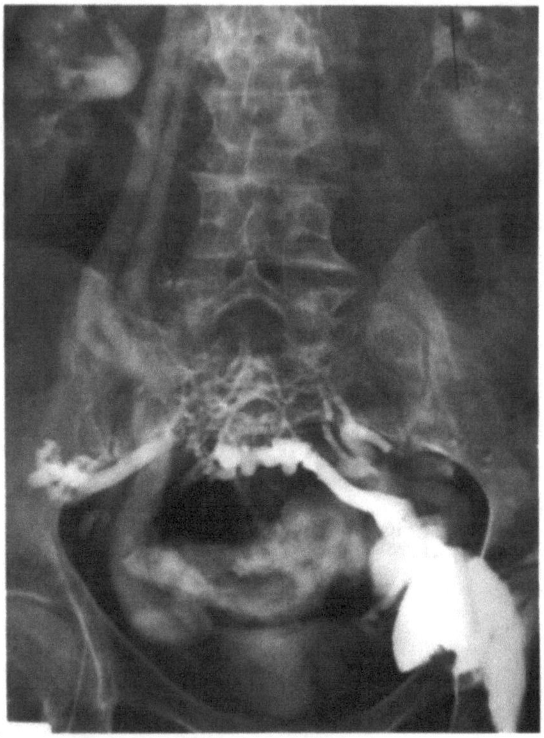

a

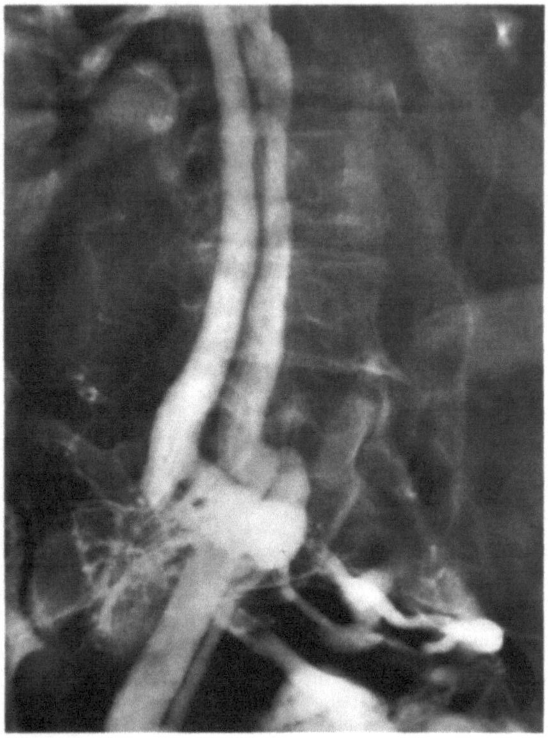

b

Fig. 5.18. a Late phase of percutaneous bifemoral iliocavography showing obstruction of both common iliac veins and of the infrarenal segment of the inferior vena cava. Mild extravasation of contrast material on the left. Filling of a double right ovarian vein via the parametrial venous plexus. b Left posterior oblique projection providing a good visualization of the double right ovarian vein which serves as collateral route for the recanalization at the level of the right renal vein and of the adjacent part of the inferior vena cava

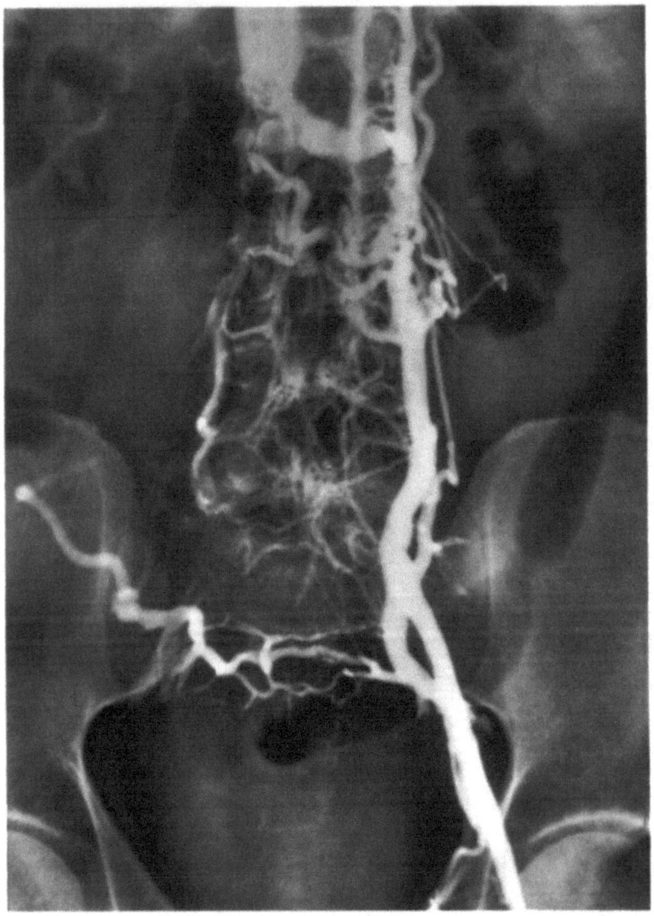

Fig. 5.19. Left unifemoral iliocavography. Occlusion of the left common iliac vein and of the infrarenal segment of the inferior vena cava. Opacification of a large ascending lumbar vein and reopacification of the infrarenal segment of the inferior vena cava via a direct anastomotic arch, corresponding very likely to a dilated large lumbar vein

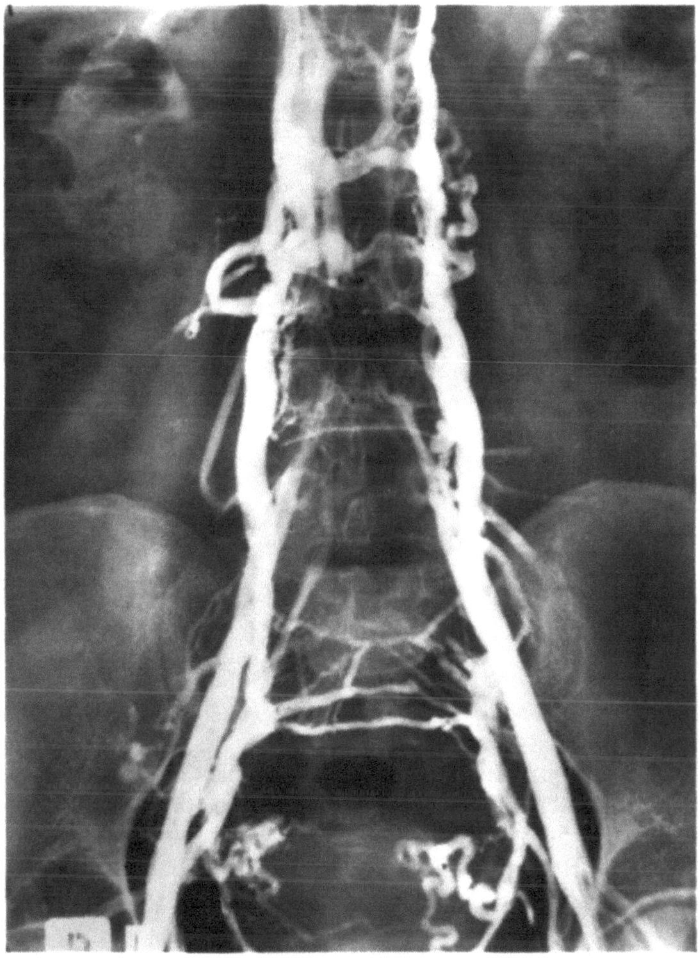

Fig. 5.20. Common iliac and infrarenal caval obstruction. Opacification of a large left ascending lumbar vein. Reopacification of the inferior vena cava via lumbar veins. Opacification of an ascending iliolumbar vein on the right, which communicates with the azygos system and with the right sex vein

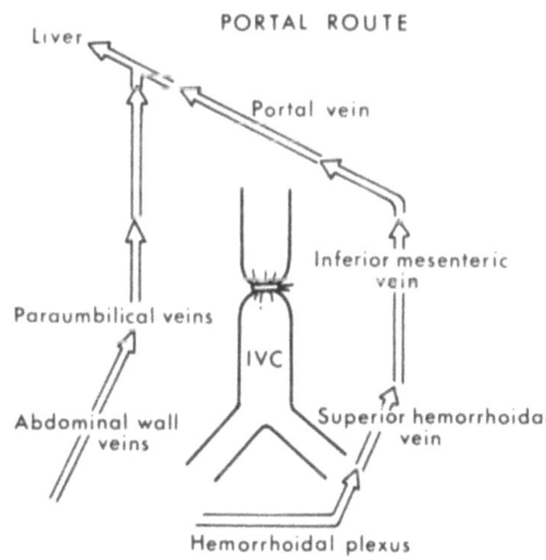

Fig. 5.21. Collateral drainage via the portal system

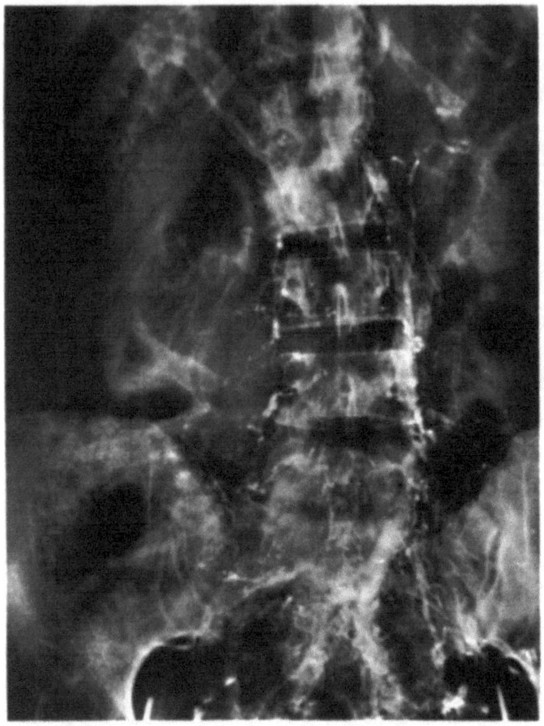

Fig. 5.22. Late phase of percutaneous bifemoral iliocavography showing diffuse iliocaval thrombosis. Opacification of the inferior mesenteric vein via the superior hemorrhoidal plexus and the plexus of the portal system

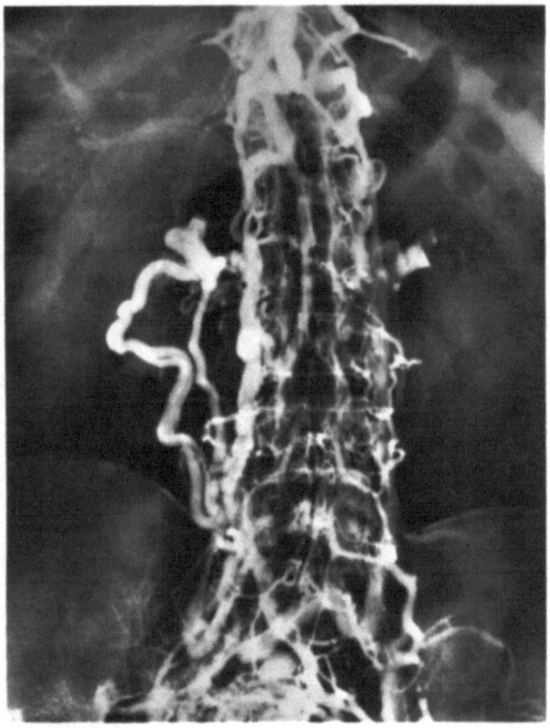

Fig. 5.23. Diffuse iliocaval thrombosis following venous catheterization in a patient with Hodgkin's disease. Thrombosis of the inferior vena cava and of both renal veins confirmed by surgery. Associated nephrotic syndrome. Percutaneous bifemoral inferior vena cavography: a late sequence shows diffuse iliocaval thrombosis. Opacification of the portal vein is very likely via the inferior mesenteric vein and via hemorrhoidal plexuses arising from the lesser pelvis

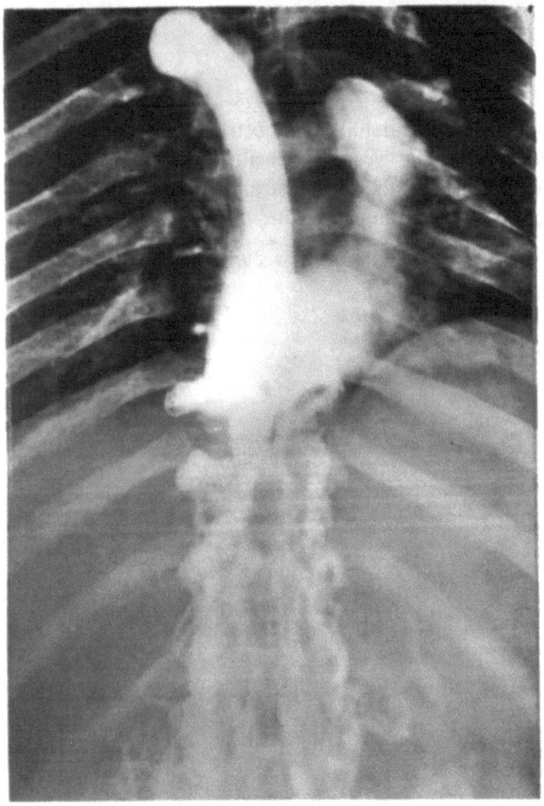

◁ Fig. 5.24. Diffuse iliocaval thrombosis in a case of Budd-Chiari syndrome. Collateral circulation via the azygos system reopacifies the great azygos vein at the level of its arch in T4 (Projection centered onto the chest)

Fig. 5.25a, b. Obstruction of the middle portion of the inferior vena cava, comprised between the renal and the hepatic veins. The infrarenal segment of the inferior vena cava is patent (a). Huge lumbar varices and drainage via the azygos system (b). No portal collateral circulation ▷

Fig. 5.26. a Obstruction of the retrohepatic portion of the inferior vena cava. The collateral circulation is via the left renoazygolumbar arch, draining into the inferior hemiazygos vein which empties directly into the great azygos vein. Filling of accessory hepatic veins and then of the right main hepatic vein. b The suprahepatic venous system serves as collateral route to circumvent the obstacle situated in the retrohepatic portion of the inferior vena cava. The infra- and interrenal portions are patent ▷

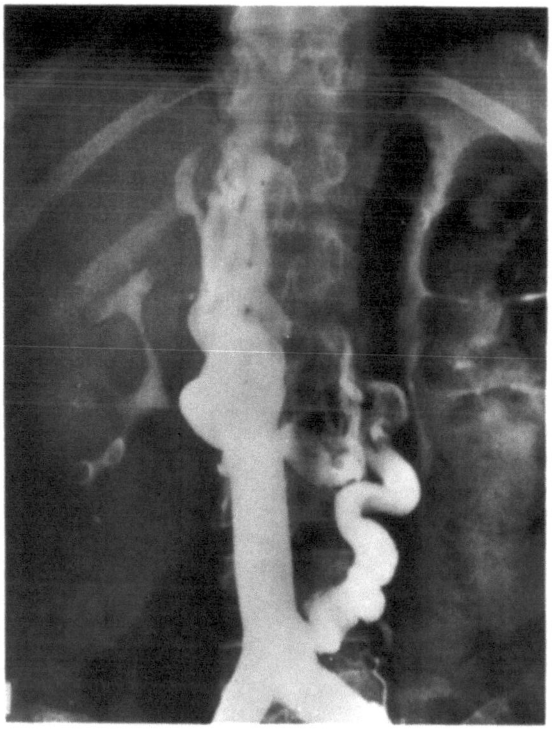

5.25a

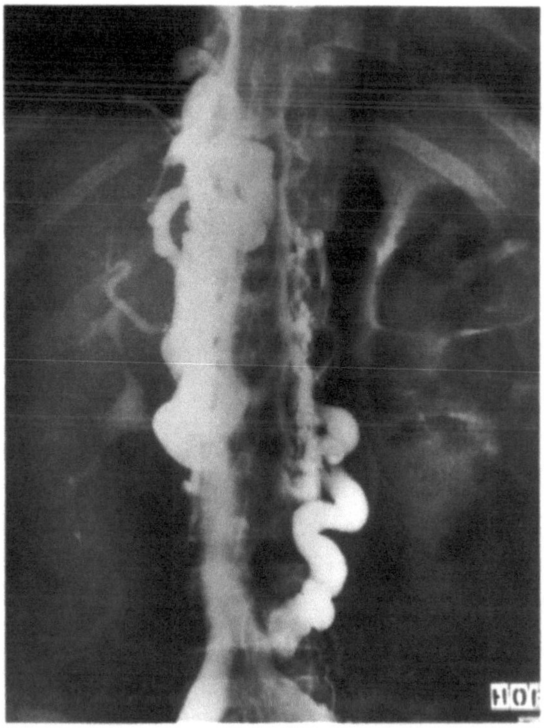

5.25b

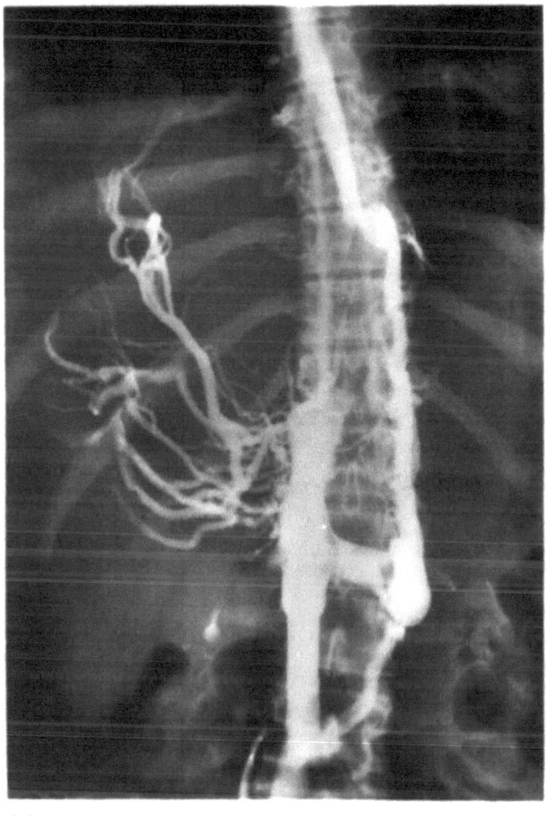

5.26a

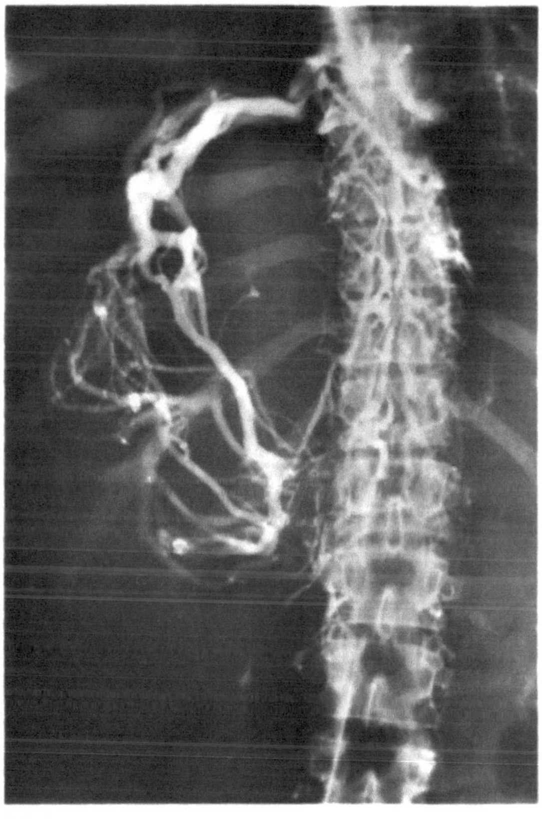

5.26b

Chapter 6. Retroperitoneal Compressions of the Inferior Vena Cava

In the retroperitoneal space the inferior vena cava is situated to the right of the spine. Due to its thin wall and low pressure, and to its close relations with the retroperitoneal anatomic structures, the inferior vena cava is precociously affected by any pathologic process developing in the retroperitoneal space.

6.1 The Retroperitoneal Space

6.1.1 Limits

It is anatomically defined by following limits:

Cranially by the inferior aspect of the diaphragm at the level of the posterior phrenicocostal sinus.

Caudally, by the lesser pelvic rim (promontory and innominate lines. At this level the retroperitoneal space is continuous with the pelvic subperitoneal tissue.

Posteriorly by the muscular masses of the psoas, of the quadrature lumborum and of the transverse muscle of the abdomen covered by their fascia.

Anteriorly, by the areas of the viscera devoid of peritoneum (duodeno-pancreas, colon and liver) and by the other viscera through the posterior parietal peritoneum.

Laterally, the limits may be defined with regard to the transverse processes of the lumbar vertebrae, or with regard to the external edge of the quadrature lumborum muscle, or with regard to the urinary system. In fact, it is continuous with the lateral extraperitoneal space.

6.1.2 Contents

The retroperitoneal space contains:

1) The great vessels: aorta, inferior vena cava, and their branches.
2) Nervous structures: splanchnic nerves, colic plexus, the lumbar sympathetic trunk, the roots of the presacral nerve.
3) Structures of the lymphatic system.
4) The kidney, the adrenals, and the ureters.

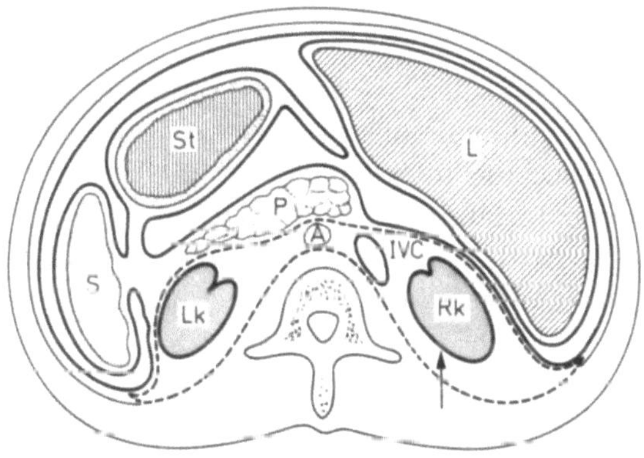

Scheme 6.1. Transverse section of the retroperitoneal space at the level of the renal hilus

S	Spleen	*P*	Pancreas
L	Liver	*S*	Stomach
LK	Left kidney	*A*	Aorta
RK	Right kidney	*IVC*	Inferior vena cava

6.2 Kidney

The right kidney is closer to the inferior vena cava than the left and causes thus more often compressions of this vessel. Renal masses may affect the inferior vena cava in three different manners:

The tumor produces extrinsic compression.

Hilar lymph nodes may be involved with tumor and compress the inferior vena cava.

Invasion of the lumen from the renal vein.

The renal mass produces lateral compression of the infrarenal segment in tumors developing from the inferior pole of the kidney, and of the suprarenal segment in tumors of the superior pole. The exploration of the inferior vena cava is part of the preoperative investigations of renal tumors, especially of right renal tumors, when the renal veins fail to be opacified in a later phase of arteriography (Figs. 6.1–6.3).

Other renal anomalies may affect the inferior vena cava, e.g., malformations (horse-shoe kidney...) ptosis, or huge hydronephrosis (Fig. 6.4).

6.3 Adrenals

Right adrenal masses may compress and displace the inferior vena cava. The right adrenal gland is attached to the inferior vena cava by the suprarenal vein, and is thus in close contact with it (Fig. 6.5). Left adrenal tumors affect the inferior vena cava only when they are of large volume. Adrenal masses cause usually lateral compression, but they may also affect the posterior wall of the inferior vena cava and even the right hepatic veins (Fig. 6.6).

Cases have even been reported of endocaval adrenal tumors, but these are most often recurrences of operated on normotopic tumors.

6.4 Arterial Anomalies

Tortuous arteries and, a fortiori, aneurysms may cause compression of the inferior vena cava. In the case of the right renal artery it ensues posterior compression due to aneurysmal dilatation. Anomalies of the iliac arteries may affect the common iliac veins or the onset of the inferior vena cava.

The aorta causes a smooth pressure defect on the left lateral wall of the inferior vena cava and displaces this vessel to the right. Aneurysms of the aorta may rupture into the inferior vena cava and cause caval hypertension and cardiac insufficiency of rapid evolution.

In very old patients cavography may be a method for demonstrating aneurysms of the aorta below the level of origin of the renal arteries; an early film will show the right border of the aneurysm and a later sequence the aneurysmal lumen (Fig. 6.7).

6.5 Retroperitoneal Tumors

Due to their particularly deep anatomic location, the diagnosis of retroperitoneal tumors is difficult, clinically as well as radiologically. They are very rare tumors; their frequency is reported to be of about 0.2% (Pack). They seem to be more frequent in females (61%) and may also be seen in children (14%). Most often they are malignant (70 to 91% according to the different authors).

They are defined as tumors developing in the retroperitoneal space, excepted tumors of the kidney, of the adrenals or of aortic aneurysms. Patel and Tubiana define them more precisely as "primary tumors located in the retroperitoneal space which do not arise from an organ normally developing in this space, as far as a histologic examination could prove this." It is thus a matter of tumors developing from mesenchymatous, nervous, embryonic and lymphatic elements.

6.5.1 Histologic Classification

Schematization is difficult because of the number of different tissues to be involved. Patel and Tubiana propose following classification:

Mesodermal Tumors (60%)

These arise from the following structures:

Adipous tissue: lipoma and liposarcoma.

Connective tissue: fibroma and fibrosarcoma (relatively frequent and particularly voluminous).

Muscular tissue: leiomyoma, leiomyosarcoma, rhabdomyosarcoma.

Mesenchymal tissue: myxoma, myxosarcoma.

Lymphoid tissue: lymphangioma and lymphangiosarcoma.

Vascular tissue: hemangioma and hemangiosarcoma.

Mesenchymatous and sarcomatous tumors which are difficult to classify from the histologic point of view.

These tumors are most often malignant and tend to disseminate to the liver and to the lungs.

Tumors Originating in the Nervous Structures (20%)

These arise from:

The peripheral nerves: neurinoma, Schwannoma.

The sympathetic system: ganglioneuroma, sympathoblastoma, sympathoma, usually seen in children.

Embryonal Tumors (10%)

They are either dermoid cysts, or teratomas which contain often organoid-type calcifications. Chordomas are also seen.

Unclassifiable Tumors (10%)

These are either tumors of hemorrhagic appearance which cannot be classified histologically, or parasitic cysts.

All these retroperitoneal tumors are close to vascular or lymphatic structures which are easy to opacify (lumbar lymphatic chain, aorta and its branches, inferior vena cava).

Of all these structures the inferior vena cava is doubtless the most easily affected by the tumor so that cavography will provide the most significant data.

6.5.2 Technique

Inferior vena cavography is performed with simultaneous injection of both femoral veins. It is very important to visualize a possible associated deformation of the common iliac veins.

Precise localization of the compression requires a frontal and a lateral projection. Selective catheterization might be useful to improve the images.

6.5.3 Cavographic Radiosemiology in Retroperitoneal Tumors

Retroperitoneal tumors may affect the inferior vena cava according to two fashions: either extrinsically or intrinsically.

There may be, moreover, association of collateral circulation.

Extrinsic Compression

Signs of extrinsic compression are the following: either displacement (Fig. 6.8), or unilateral impression (Fig. 6.9), or bilateral impression producing more or less complete stenosis. The displacement is particularly clear in the postero-anterior direction, the inferior vena cava being displaced more or less far from the spine. Appreciation of stenosis should take into account eventual arterial compressions; impressions are usually associated to displacement of the inferior vena cava axis.

In the practice, displacement of the axis of the inferior vena cava is considered the most tangible sign with retroperitoneal tumors (Hayt) (Fig. 6.10).

Thrombosis

Retroperitoneal tumors may cause thrombosis of the inferior vena cava, i.e., fibrinocruoric thrombosis close to the narrowing, or tumoral thrombosis due to parietal invasion and neoplastic extension into the caval lumen (Figs. 6.11 and 6.12).

Collateral Circulation

The development of collateral circulation is the more marked that the flow rate is diminished. Since compression occurs most often below the level of the origin of the renal veins, the collateral circulation is either via the deep veins (vertebral, paravertebral and lumbar ascending systems), or via intermedian routes (gonadal veins) or via superficial routes (parietal veins) or, finally, via portal derivation routes.

6.5.4 Value of Cavography in the Diagnosis of Retroperitoneal Tumors

Indirect methods by opacification of neighboring structures (stomach, colon and kidney) provide valuable data only with large tumors (Kemp, Lowman, Bismuth, North). Diagnostic retropneumoperitoneum is not an easy method and its results are far from being reliable (Davidson). Thus vascular opacification plays an important role in the diagnosis of retroperitoneal tumors. Arteriography, associated if need be, with selective opacification of the lumbar arteries, may demonstrate direct signs of tumoral development (vascular disorganization), though indirect signs, for instance displacement of the aorta, are seen much later than displacement of the cava. Besides its interest for the diagnosis, inferior vena cavography provides two types of data:

It shows the relations of the retroperitoneal tumor with the inferior vena cava, a most important precision in view of the surgical technique to be utilized. Extension of the tumor to the suprarenal segment of the inferior vena cava requires restorative surgery whereas involvement of the infrarenal segment can be treated by simple resection.

Moreover it may provide the diagnosis of malignity when there is an intracaval tumoral invasion.

6.6 Retroperitoneal Lymph Node Involvements

The radiologic investigation of retroperitoneal lymph node involvements may present in two fashions: either it is a matter of an isolated abdominal mass and the investigations will show its ganglionic nature when its origin is unknown; or it is a matter of lymph node involvements looked for in a case of lymphoma or of a neoplasm of known lymphophilic type.

Without reviewing the anatomic distribution of the lymphatic chains in the retroperitoneal space, it should be recalled that the right lateral location of the inferior vena cava causes it to have closer relations to the right lateral and to the median chains, and also that the retroperitoneal lymphatic chains are continuous with the chains of the abdomen and of the lesser pelvis.

The most frequent histologic type of retroperitoneal lymph node involvements are: hodgkinian and non-hodgkinian lymphomas, genital neoplasms (testicles, ovaries, body and cervix of the uterus), urinary carcinoma, rectal carcinoma. Lymph node metastases of a retroperitoneal tumor (sympathoblastoma) are much more rare (Ferris).

6.6.1 Technique

Catheterization is performed bilaterally so as to obtain a good opacification of the common iliac venous system. Several projections, both frontal and lateral, are required to demonstrate small lesions that are only visible with a tangential beam. A right posterior oblique projection seems the most useful to demonstrate lateral and posterior compressions of the inferior vena cava (Pradel). Some authors have proposed to perform the radiographs in the upright position to obtain a better filling of the inferior vena cava and closer relations with lateral lymph node involvements (Hayt). The Valsalva maneuver gives similar results with less discomfort.

6.6.2 Radiosemiology

As with retroperitoneal tumors, signs of *extrinsic compression* are seen; this compression may produce fibrinocruoric thrombosis and collateral circulation.

Exceptionally there may be invasion of the inferior vena cava by contiguity of metastatic lymph nodes.

Since the lymph node involvement is usually multiple each hypertrophied node will leave its impression on the inferior vena cava. Thus there are multiple, polycyclic impressions that may be very marked, involve several segments and several aspects of the inferior vena cava, which allows to differentiate easily this condition from a unilaterally developing tumor. These multiple impressions may be faintly visible on a frontal projection and much more clear on right posterior oblique projections (Figs. 6.13 and 6.14). They may be associated with similar images on the iliac venous axes, hence the interest of performing an iliocavography by bifemoral venous approach.

Severe compression by enlarged lymph nodes may be responsible for *stenosis* or even *thrombosis* of the infrarenal segment of the inferior vena cava. Marked collateral venous circulation may develop.

Sometimes the contact with metastatic lymph nodes may produce direct *invasion* of the inferior vena cava (Fig. 6.19).

When, in the presence of an abdominal mass of unknown origin, there is a marked displacement to the right of the inferior vena cava and a lesser degree of displacement of the aorta in the opposite direction at the level of the renal hilus, one must consider the possibility of involvement of the right lateral aortic lymph nodes due to an undetected seminoma (Fig. 6.18).

6.6.3 Place of Cavography in Investigation of Retroperitoneal Lymph Node Involvements

The presence of retroperitoneal lymph node involvements having a therapeutic repercussion in numerous neoplastic conditions, justifies the utilization of a more or less agressive investigation method. Thus inferior vena cavography has been proposed for the detection of retroperitoneal lymph node involvements in hodgkinian and in non-hodgkinian lymphomas (Allen, Filler, Lee, Schwarz, Baum, Hops, Brower, Laurin), and in involvements of the lymph nodes with genital cancers, especially of the testicles (Hillman, Kolstad, Baum, Hops, Lee, Masselot).

There is actually a general agreement that the diagnosis of retroperitoneal lymph node involvements, whatever their origin, requires the combined use of three investigations: intravenous urography, lymphangiography and inferior vena cavography. The comparative value of these investigations has been studied by numerous authors (see Table 6.1).

For lymphomas in general, lymphangiography appears as the most sensitive investigation (between 34 and 73% of positive results in the reported series).

The average for Hodgkin's disease is about 50% of positive results.

Cavography is second best. Its sensitivity ranges according to the different authors, between 21% and 47%. The average is by 37% in Hodgkin's disease (Figs. 6.14–6.16).

Table 6.1. Value of the investigations in the diagnosis of retroperitoneal lymph node involvements in lymphomas in general

Reference	Number of patients in the series	Cavography % of abnormal results	Lymphography % of abnormal results	IVU % abnormal results
Baum et al., 1963	34	43%	65%	20%
Lee et al., 1964	104	47%	65%	13%
Schwarz et al., 1965	100	38%	73%	14%
Hopf and Fuchs, 1970	58	36%	62%	10%
Brower and Seale 1974	98	25%	37%	5%
Laurin, 1975	98	21%	34%	17%

Modified from Laurin et al.

Table 6.2. Value of the investigations in the diagnosis of retroperitoneal lymph node involvements secondary to genital neoplasms

Reference	Number of patients	% results of cavography	% results of lymphangiography	% results of urography
Baum et al., 1963	40	30%	70%	30%
Hopf and Fuchs, 1960	136	17%	30%	26%
Lee et al., 1971	24	83%	75%	
Masselot et al., 1971	60	31%	55%	38%
Lien et al., 1977	120	23%	28%	16%

Modified from Laurin et al.

Intravenous urography appears to be less interesting with between 10 and 15% of positive results (Table 6.1).

Thus lymphography appears to be the investigation of choice. Cavography permits however to demonstrate anomalies in cases where the lymphangiography was normal (4 to 5% of cases) (Laurin). In practice, as concerns diagnosis, cavography is reserved for the cases with lymphomas for which lymphangiography has not been technically satisfactory.

In genital cancers (see Table 6.2) lymphangiography appears usually to be the best diagnostic procedure for retroperitoneal lymph node metastases. The results seem however to be quite dispersed (30 to 75%). Cavography provides somewhat lower results, safe for Lee's series (neoplasms of the uterine cervix). However, cavography detected anomalies of the inferior vena cava in 11% of the patients in whom lymphangiography was normal. Its diagnostic value in genital tumors appears thus clearly more reliable than in lymphomas (Lee, Hops) (Figs. 6.13, 6.18, and 6.19).

The value of cavography varies for the different lymphatic chains:

In the right lumbar region the sensitivity of cavography depends on the pre- or retrocaval location of the lymph nodes. When the lymph node enlargement is retrocaval, the sensitivity of cavography, especially with lateral projections, is at least equal to that of lymphangiography; If it is precaval, lymphangiography is clearly more sensitive and to be visible on a cavogram the nodes have to reach a considerable size.

In the left lumbar region, cavography provides only later data than lymphangiography, because the inferior vena cava is too distant.

In the area of the hilus of the right kidney, cavography provides more interesting data than lymphangiography.

In the region of the common iliac vein, the lateral and posterior location of the nodes with regard to the common iliac vein accounts for the fact that only huge nodes are visible. The external iliac nodes are separated from the vein by a considerable distance.

The limits of cavography with regard to lymphangiography are as follows:

Iliac veins involvement is a late indicator of pelvic lymph node enlargement.

Left paravertebral lymph node masses can only be detected when they are huge.

Anterior preaortic lymph nodes are only detected late.

Right lumbar nodes anterior to the inferior vena cava are visible only when they are very large.

6.6.4 Conclusion

The diagnosis of retroperitoneal lymph node enlargement with inferior vena cavography requires multiple incidences, the most informative being the right posterior oblique projection. The most typical feature consists of multiple indentations of the margins, without invasion of the inferior vena cava and most of the time, without hemodynamic changes.

6.7 Tumors of the Inferior Vena Cava

Tumors of the inferior vena cava are rare. They derive from the caval walls and are most often leiomyosarcomas and more seldomly endotheliomas. The first case of caval wall tumor has been described in 1871 by Perl. In 1976 Bailey reports about 46 cases collected in the literature.

The leiomyosarcoma is a tumor occurring in females in their sixties. It is most often located in the median part of the inferior vena cava but may have a large extension involving the superior hepatic veins, the renal vein and even the right atrium. There are occasionally distant metastases in the liver or in the lungs. Sometimes there are also leiomyomas located elsewhere (uterus and esophagus).

Very exceptionally the inferior vena cava is the site of endoluminal tumoral processes: ectopic site of a nearby located tumor (pheochromocytoma) (Rote).

Inferior vena cavography is the method of choice for demonstrating caval wall tumors. Initially the tumor develops within the lumen. On an X-ray it is visualized as a rounded defect, often voluminous, more or less polycyclic with craniocaudal extension. Usually blood flow is not disturbed and all projections show relative distension of the inferior vena cava caused by the tumor (Figs. 6.21–6.23). These features are quite similar to those seen with leiomyomas of the esophagus (Hivet, Maillet, Tegtmeyer).

In a more advanced stage, especially when the tumor has reached the right atrium, the renal and superior hepatic veins, the radiologic features change. There is now more or less complete obstruction of the afferent vessels and of the inferior vena cava lumen.

Most often these tumors are only found at surgery or even at postmortem examinations. Very rarely (in 6% of cases) cavographic data lead to consider this diagnosis before surgery, in case of an abdominal mass of unknown origin. This points out the importance of inferior vena cavography in such circumstances.

References

Allen, JE, Morse TS, Frye TR, Clatworthy HW (1964) Vena cavograms in infants and children. Ann Surg 160:568–570

Bailey RV, Stribling J, Weitzner S, Haroy JD (1976) Leiomyosarcoma of the inferior vena cava. Ann Surg 184:169–173

Baum S, Bron K, Wexler L, Abrams H (1963) Lymphangiography, cavography and urography. Comparative accuracy in the diagnosis of pelvic and abdominal metastases. Radiology 81:207–218

Bismuth V, Blery M, Gaux JC, Guenin P (1971) Le diagnostic radiologique des tumeurs rétropéritonéales primitives de l'adulte. Ann Radiol 14:419–436

Brower AC, Seale DL (1974) A cortical appraisal of radiographic studies employed in the staging of patients with Hodgkin's disease. Radiology 110:97–101

Davidson JK, Havard CW, Scott RB (1959) Radiological demonstration of enlarged retroperitoneal lymph nodes. Lancet 1.1008–1012

Ferris EJ, Hipona FA, Kahn PC, Philipps E, Shapiro JH (1969) Venography of the inferior vena cava and its branches. Williams & Wilkins, Baltimore

Filler, RM, Harris SH, Edwards EA (1962) Characteristics of the inferior cava venogram in retroperitoneal cancer. N Engl J Med 266:1194–1201

Hayt DB (1966) Upright inferior vena cavography. Radiology 86:865–870

Hietala SO, Kan Garloo H, Ranninger K (1977) Cavography in the management of malignant abdominal tumors. Acta Radiol 18:217–224

Hilleman DC, Tristan TA (1963) Inferior vena cavography with detection of abdominal extension of pelvic cancer. Radiology 82:416–422

Hivet M, Poilleux J, Gastard J, Hernandez (1973) Sarcome de la veine cave inférieure. Nouv Presse Med 2:569–572

Hopf MA, Fuchs WA (1970) Die Lymphographie, Cavographie und Urographie als Kombination. Radiologe. 10:280–288

Kemp A, Harder RA (1960) Radiology in the diagnosis of retroperitoneal tumors. Clin Radiol 11:69–73

Kolstad P (1963) The relation between stage, pain, roentgenological and operative findings in cancer of the cervix. Acta Obstet Gynecol Scand [Suppl 6] 42:35–38

Laurin S (1975) Cavography and lymphography in Hodgkin's disease. Acta Radiol 16:98–106

Lee BJ, Nelson JH, Schwartz G (1964) Evaluation of lymphography, inferior venocavography and intravenous pyelography in the clinical staging and management of Hodgkin's disease and lymphosarcoma. N Engl J Med 271:327–330

Lee F, Greening R, Kramer S, Mahn G, Kuroda K, Lin SR, Koslow S (1971) The value of pelvic venography and lymphography in the clinical staging of carcinoma of the uterine cervix. AJR 111:284–296

Lien HH, Kolbenstvedt A (1977) Phlebography, urography and lymphography in the diagnosis of metastases from testicular tumors. Acta Radiol 18:177–186

Lowman R (1965) Retroperitoneal tumors. A survey and assessment of roentgen techniques. Radiol Clin North Am 3:543–549

Maillet P (1976) Leiomyosarcome de la veine cave inférieure. Chirurgie 102:658–664

Masselot J, Bergiron C, Markovits P (1971) Valeurs comparées de la lymphographie, de la cavographie, et de l'urographie intra-veineuse dans l'étude des métastases ganglionnaries (rétropéritonéales) des cancers du testicule. J Radiol Electrol Med Nucl 52:653–662

Mc Coy RM, Klatte EC, Thamy RK (1969) Use of inferior vena cavography in evaluation of renal neoplasms. J Urol 102:556–562

Missal ME, Robinson JA, Tatum RW (1965) Inferior vena cava obstruction; clinical manifestations, diagnostic methods and related problems. Ann. Intern. Med 62:133–138

North JP (1960) Primary tumors of the retroperitoneum. Ann Surg 151

Pack GT, Tabam E (1954) Primary retro-peritoneal tumors. A study of 120 cases. Surg Gynecol Obstet 99:209–213

Patel J, Tubiana R (1947) Les tumeurs rétropéritonéales. Ann Anat Pathol (Paris) 17:329–334

Perl L (1871) Ein Fall von Sarkom der vena cava inferior. Virchows Archiv 53:378

Pleasants JH (1911) Obstruction of the inferior vena cava, with a report of 18 cases. Johns Hopkins Hosp Rept 16

Pradel J, Bigot JM, Monnier JP (1970) Tumeurs et adénopathies rétro-péritonéales. Encycl. Med. Chir. Radiodiagnostic IV. 33660, A10.

Rote AR, Flint LD, Ellis FH (1977) Intracaval recurrence of pheochromocytoma extending into right atrium. N Engl J Med 296:1269–1271

Schwartz G, Lee BJ, Nelson JH (1965) Lymphography, cavography and urography in the evaluation of malignant lymphomas. Acta Radiol., 3:138–144

Tegtmeyer CJ, Buschi A (1977) The angiographic diagnosis of leiomyosarcoma of the inferior vena cava. Radiology 122:683–686

Tucker AS (1965) The roentgen diagnosis of abdominal masses in children: intravenous urography vs inferior venacavography. AJR 95:76–79

Wright FW (1965) Cavography in the assessment of renal tumors. Br J Urol 37:380–382

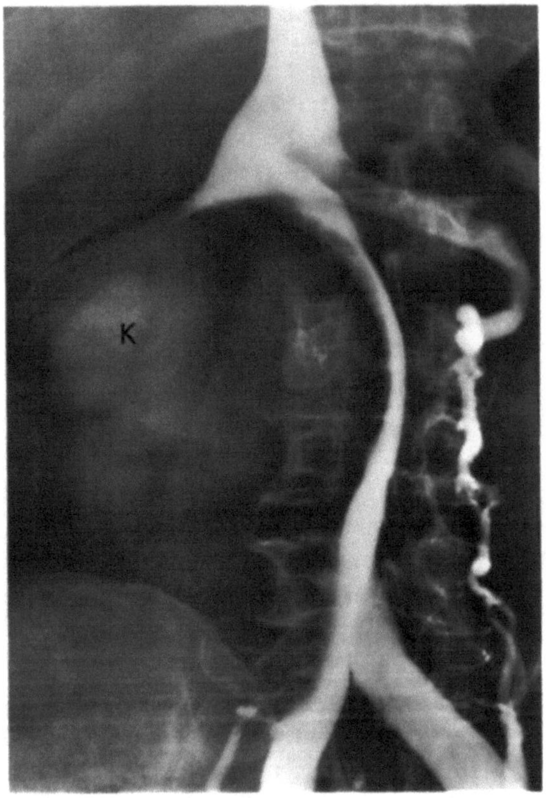

Fig. 6.1. Extrinsic compression of the postrenal segment of the inferior vena cava due to carcinoma of the right kidney (K). The postrenal segment of the inferior vena cava is deviated to the left by a huge carcinoma of the right kidney. The pressure deformity is smooth and graceful, along the right aspect of the vena cava

a

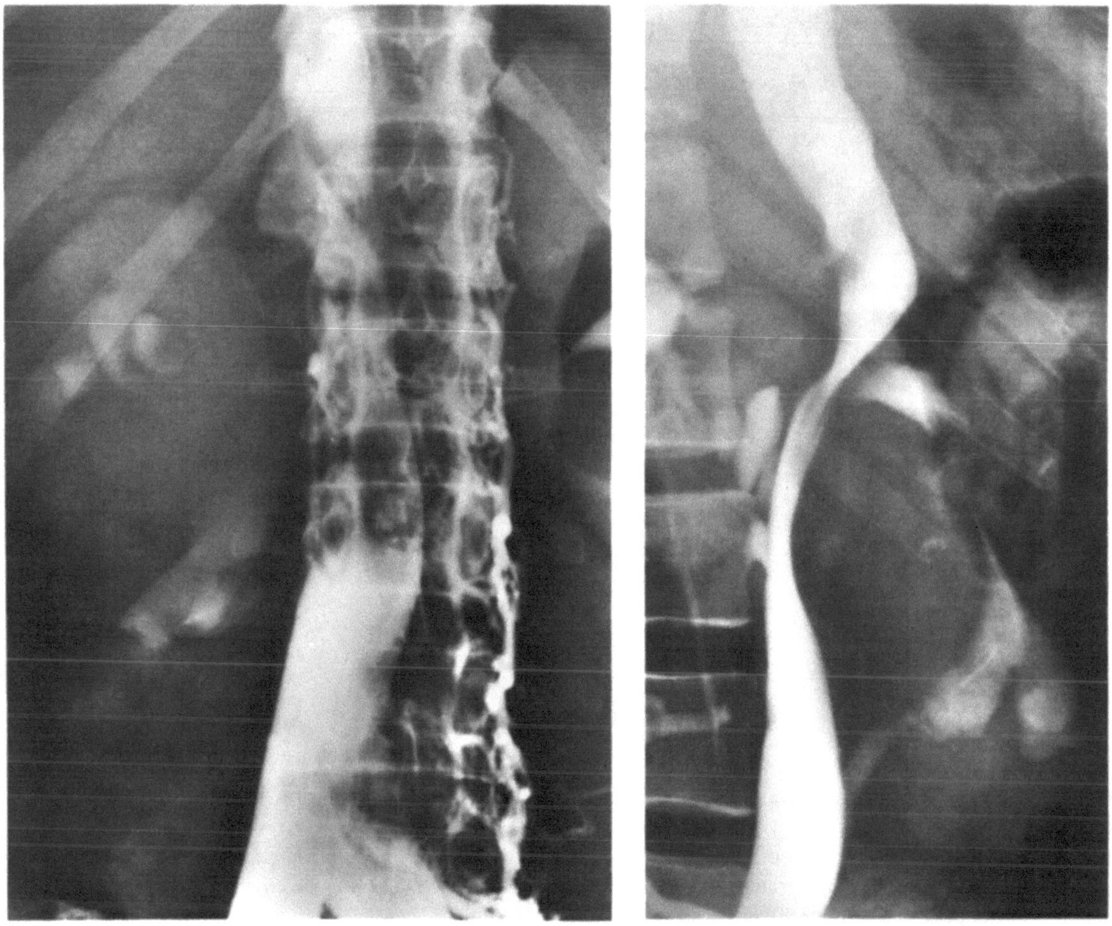

b

c

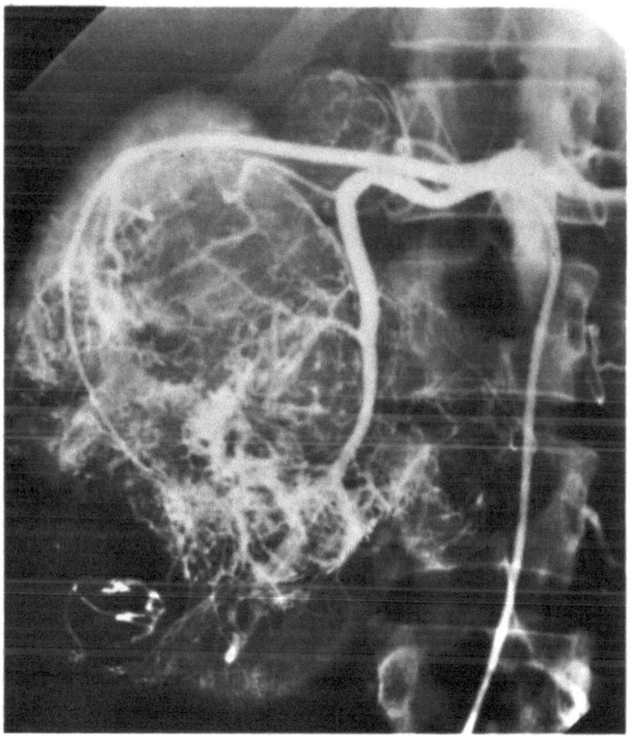

Fig. 6.2a–c. Extrinsic compression caused by a right renal mass and secondary adenopathy. a Frontal view. b Lateral view. Note the anterior extrinsic compression caused by the tumor itself. There is also an extrinsic compression of the posterior wall of the vena cava above the superior pole of the kidney secondary to adenopathy. c Selective right renal arteriography confirms the presence of suprahilar adenopathies. The adrenal is spared

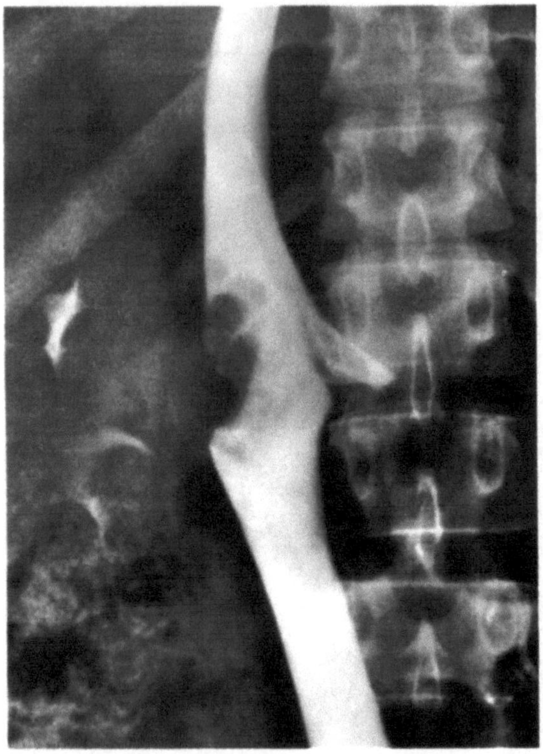

Fig. 6.3. Extrinsic compression by satellite adenopathies of a right renal mass. Small polycyclic impressions along the right lateral wall of the inferior vena cava. Surgery confirms the right renal vein to be free and shows the presence of hilar adenopathies

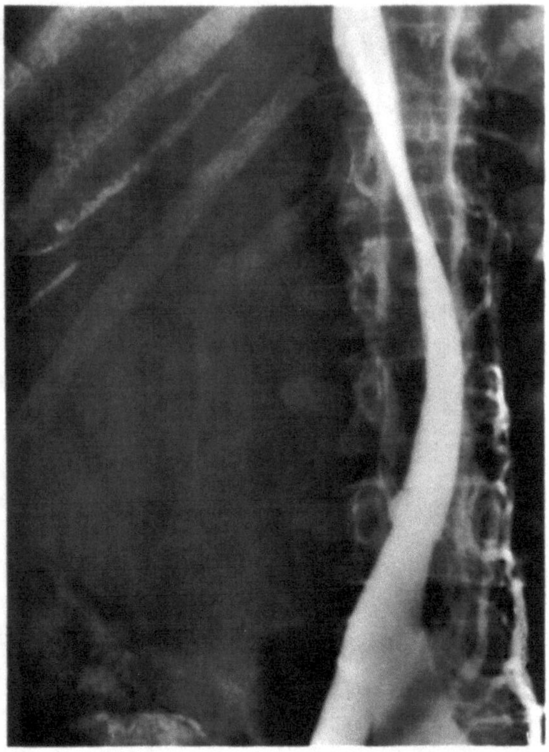

Fig. 6.4. Extrinsic compression secondary to right hydronephrosis. The inferior vena cava is displaced toward the left and the impression involves mainly the right aspect. The displacement is quite regular and graceful

Fig. 6.5. a Frontal view. b Lateral view. Tumor of the right adrenal gland (pheochromocytoma). There is a simple extrinsic compression of the right posterior aspect of the inferior vena cava ▷

Fig. 6.6a, b. Adrenal tumor (pheochromocytoma). a Frontal view. b Lateral view. The adrenal tumor causes extrinsic compression of the posterior and right lateral wall of the inferior vena cava. It mainly produces a pseudo-syndrome of Budd-Chiari: note on the frontal view the arciform displacement of the right large suprahepatic vein (*) with pooling of the contrast medium in this vein during the late phase of the study

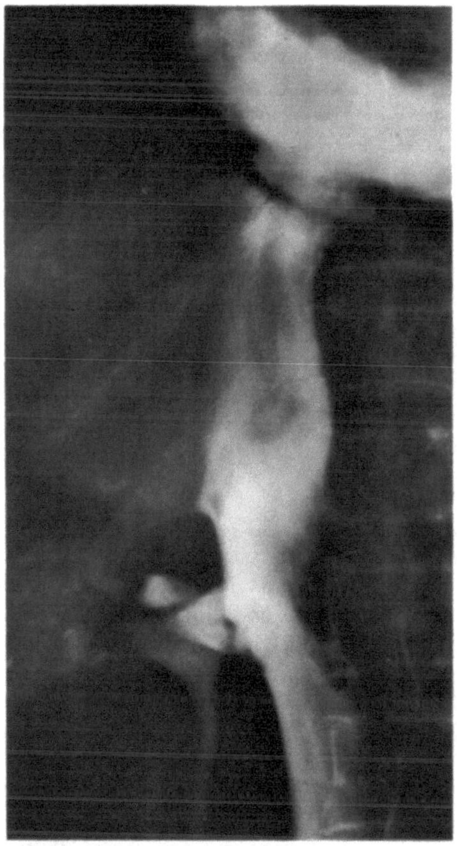

6.5a

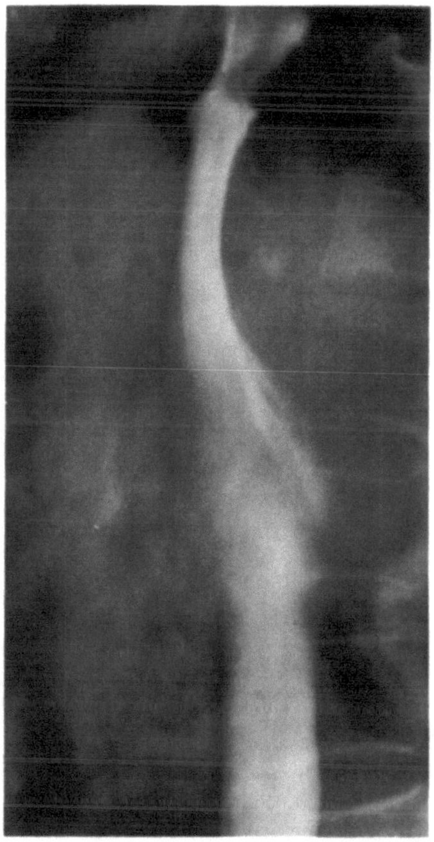

6.5b

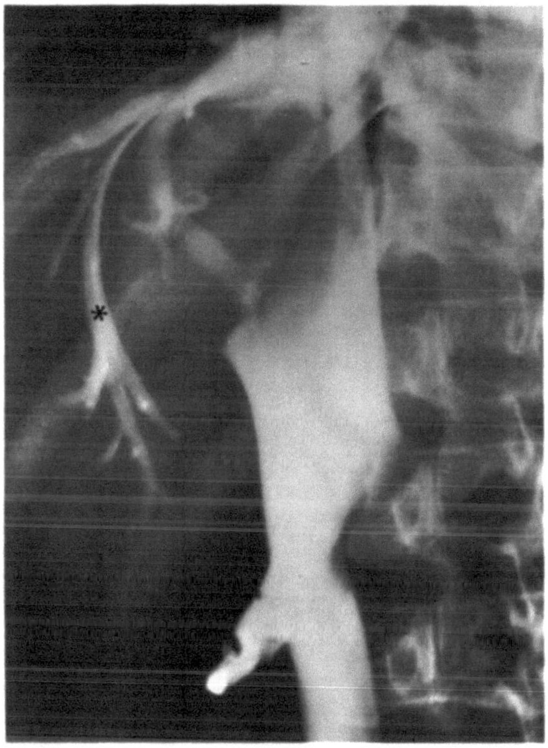

6.6a

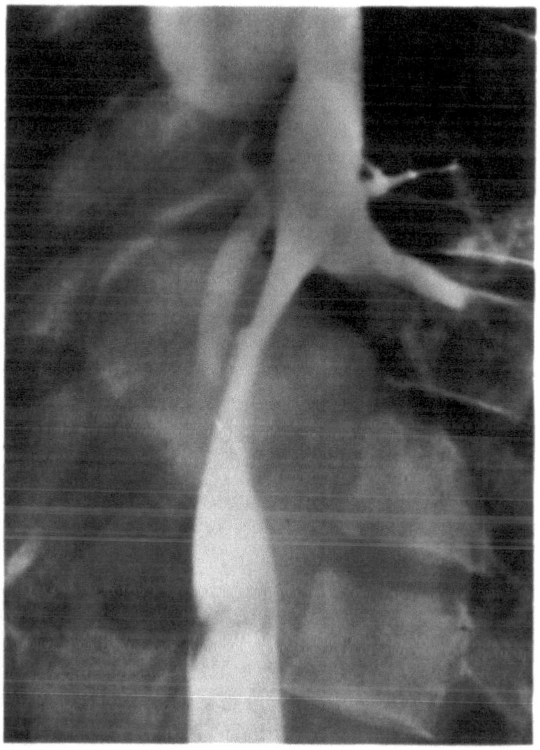

6.6b

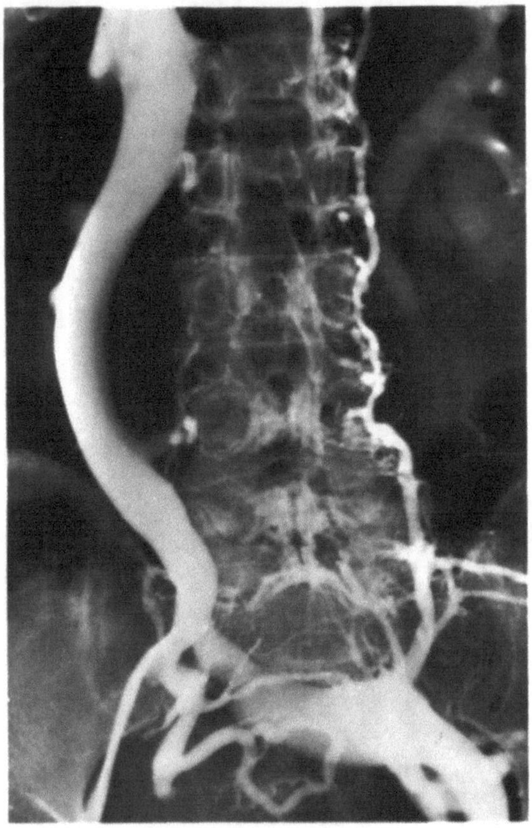

Fig. 6.7. Extrinsic compression of the inferior vena cava secondary to aortic aneurysm. Fusiform aneurysm causing a graceful displacement of the inferior vena cava toward the right. Note a similar impression with displacement of the left common iliac vein. Cavography with additional late phases may be a method for studying aortic aneurysms

Fig. 6.8. Retroperitoneal tumor (mesenchymoma). Ptosis and tilting of the right kidney. Marked opacity in the right hypochondrium and flank. Graceful displacement toward the left of the suprarenal segment of the inferior vena cava

Fig. 6.9. Retroperitoneal tumor (reticulum cell sarcoma). Note the ptosis and displacement toward the right of the kidney and the posterior compression of the inferior vena cava which is flattened anteroposteriorly

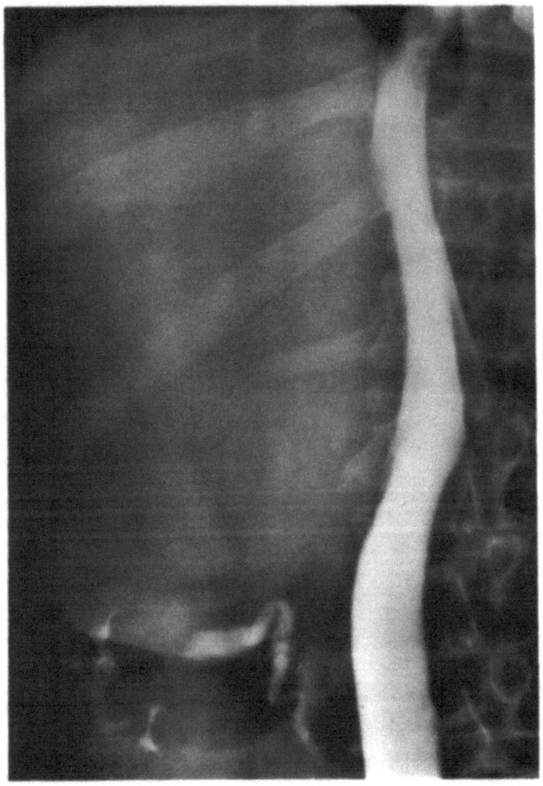

Fig. 6.8

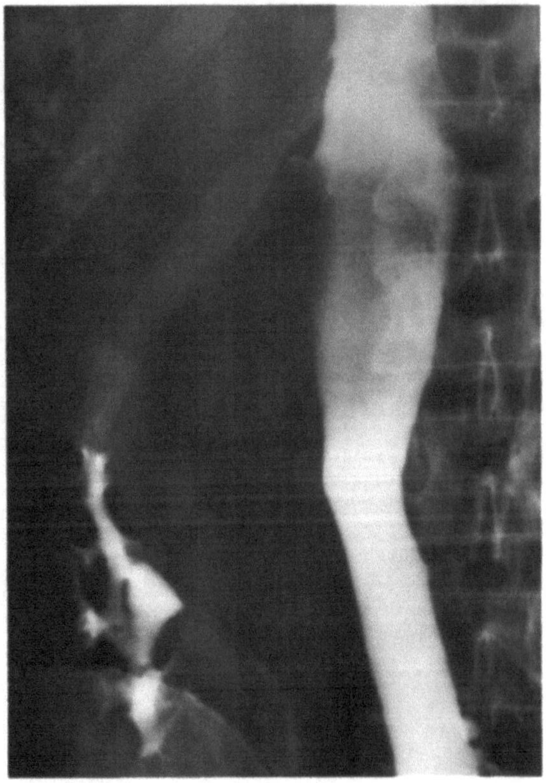

Fig. 6.9

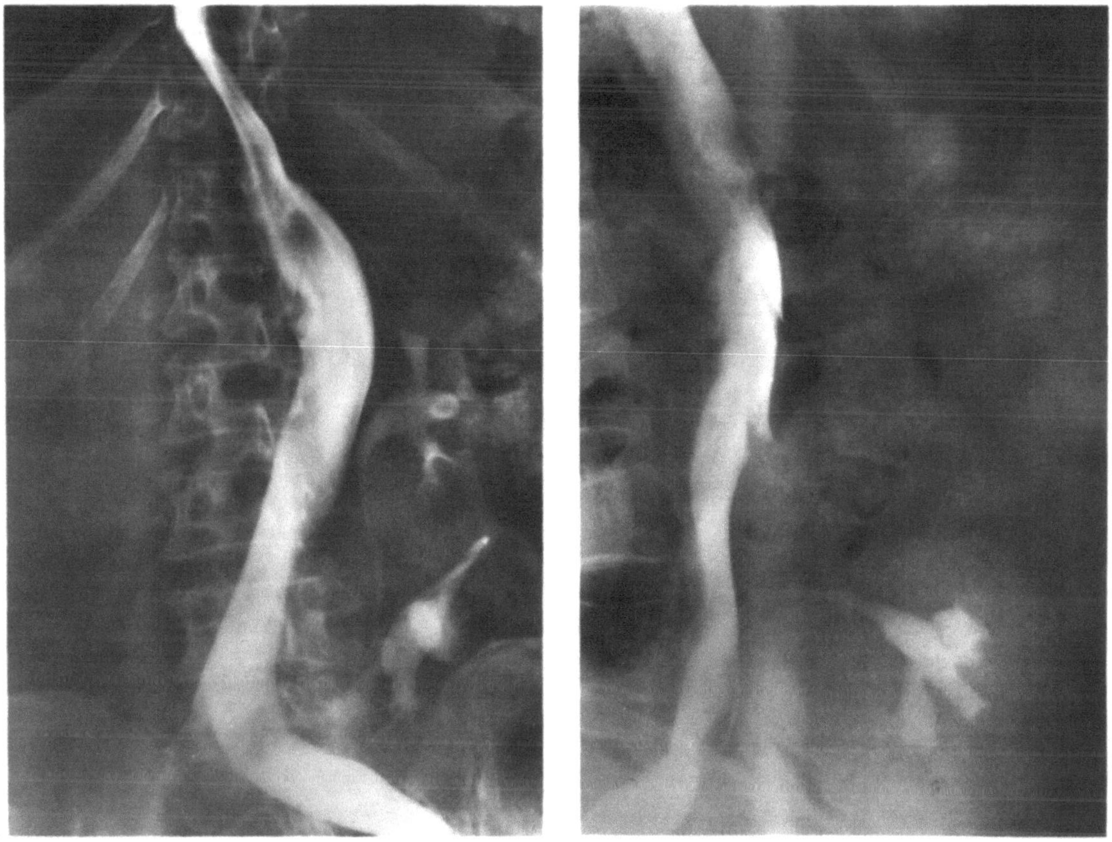

a b

Fig. 6.10a, b. Retroperitoneal tumor (fibrosarcoma). a Frontal view. b Lateral view. Note that the inferior vena cava is markedly displaced toward the left and also anteriorly. The right kidney is entirely tilted anteriorly and is visualized on the left side of the spine. The inferior vena cava is normal. There are no collateral channels: the retroperitoneal mass causes displacement of the inferior vena cava without narrowing of its lumen nor invasion

---

Figs. 6.11–6.14 see pages 110 and 111

Fig. 6.11. Retroperitoneal tumor (mesenchymoma). The inferior vena cava is displaced anteriorly by a retroperitoneal mass. The inferior vena cava is almost entirely involved and is opacified cranially to the compression by important collateral channels in the lumbar region

Fig. 6.12. Invasion of the inferior vena cava by a retroperitoneal mass (reticulum cell sarcoma). The tumor has partly destroyed L3 and L4 and invades by contiguity the vena cava. Intraluminal tumoral bud

Fig. 6.13a, b. Retroperitoneal adenopathy (seminoma). a Frontal view. b Lateral view. On the frontal view the inferior vena cava is not displaced but its borders show regular small indentations suggesting the presence of adenopathies. The lateral view shows a marked anterior displacement of the inferior vena cava, unsuspected on the frontal view. Numerous polycyclic indentations corresponding to adenopathies

Fig. 6.14a, b. Retroperitoneal adenopathies (Hodgkin's lymphoma). a Frontal view. b Right posterior oblique projection. Note the numerous bilateral small indentations, perfectly regular on the different aspects of the inferior vena cava very well visualized on the right posterior oblique projection

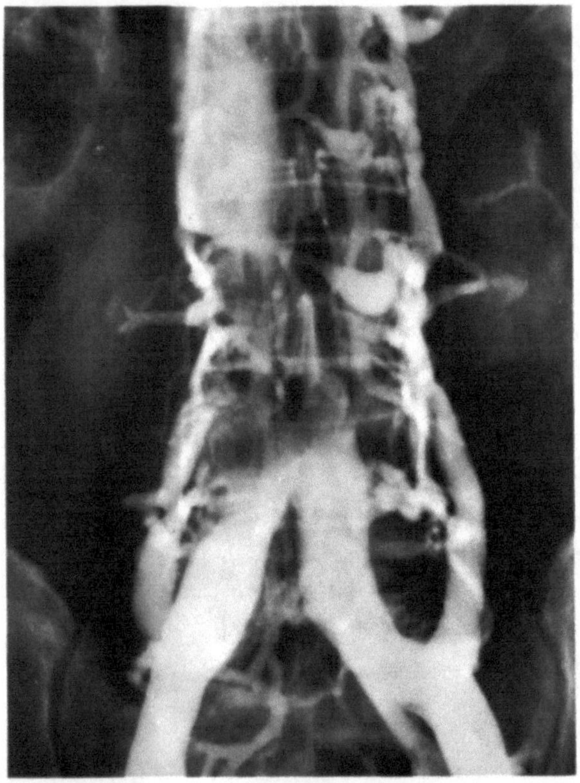
6.11 a

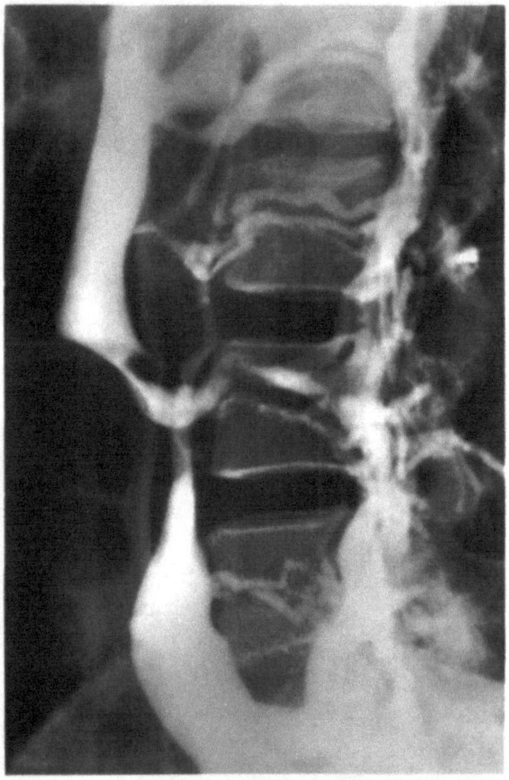
6.11 b

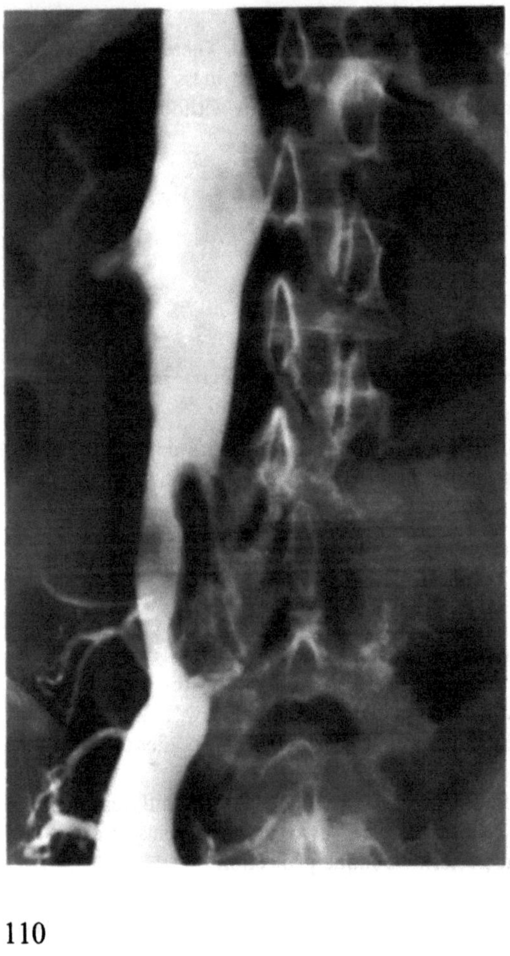
6.12 a

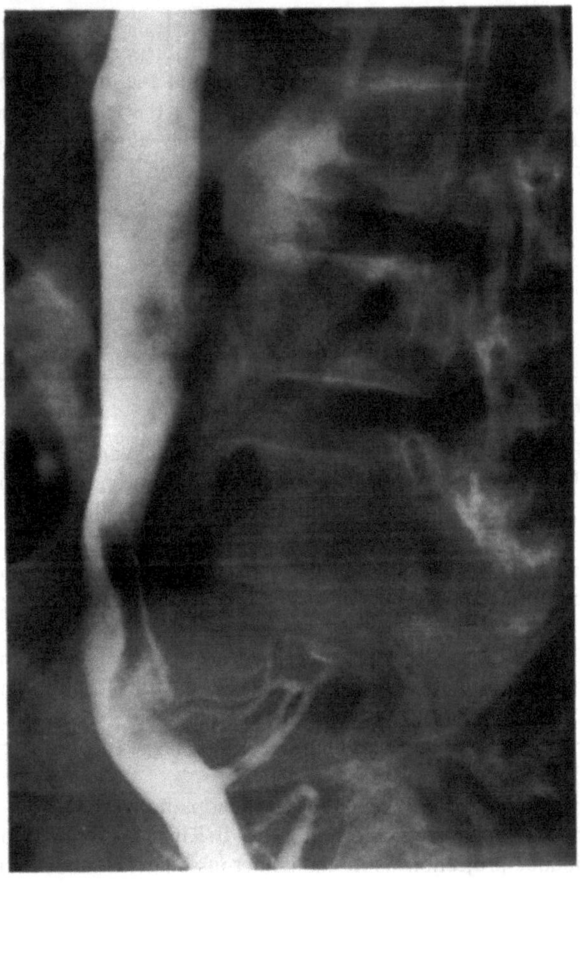
6.12 b

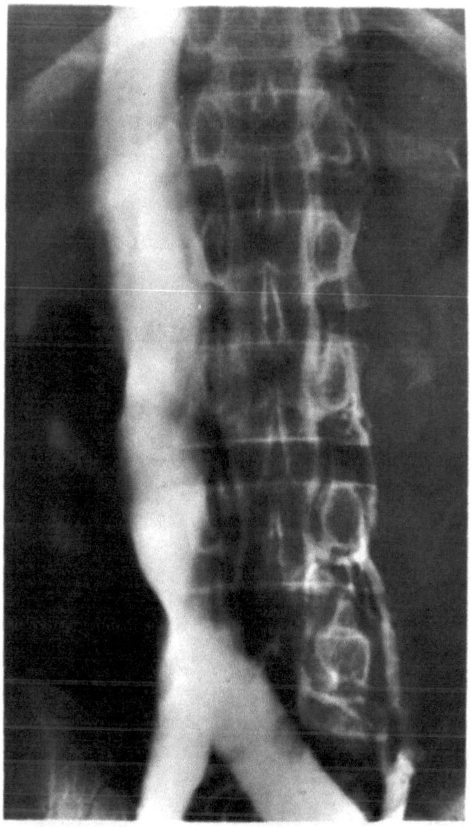
6.13a

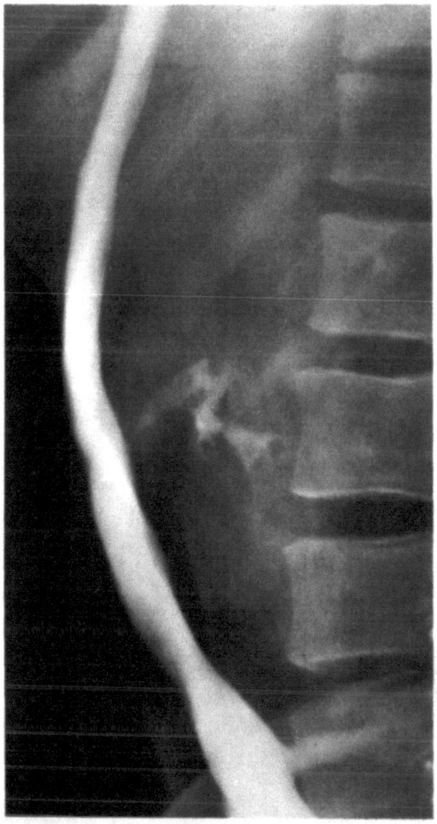
6.13b

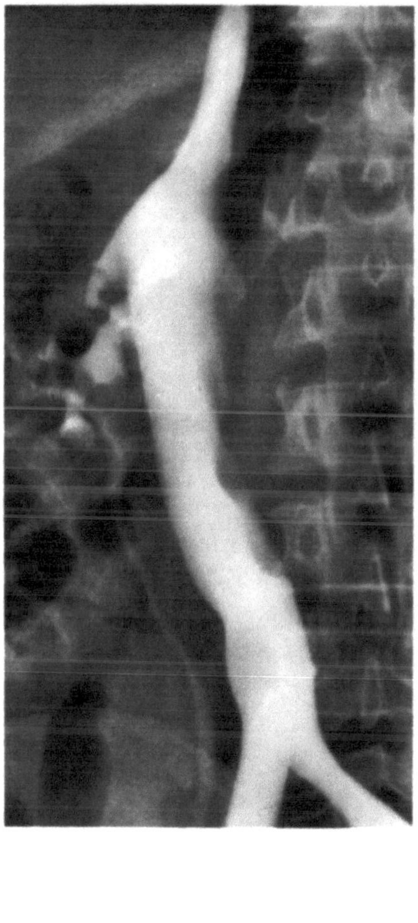
6.14a

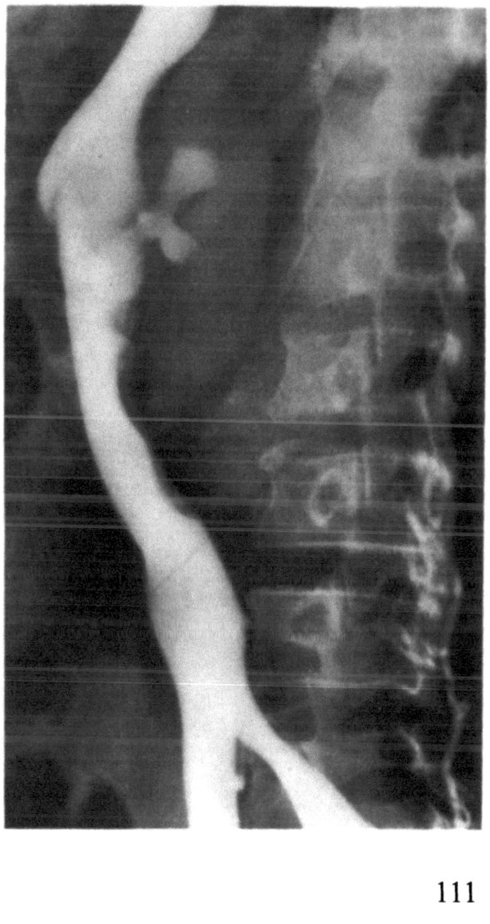
6.14b

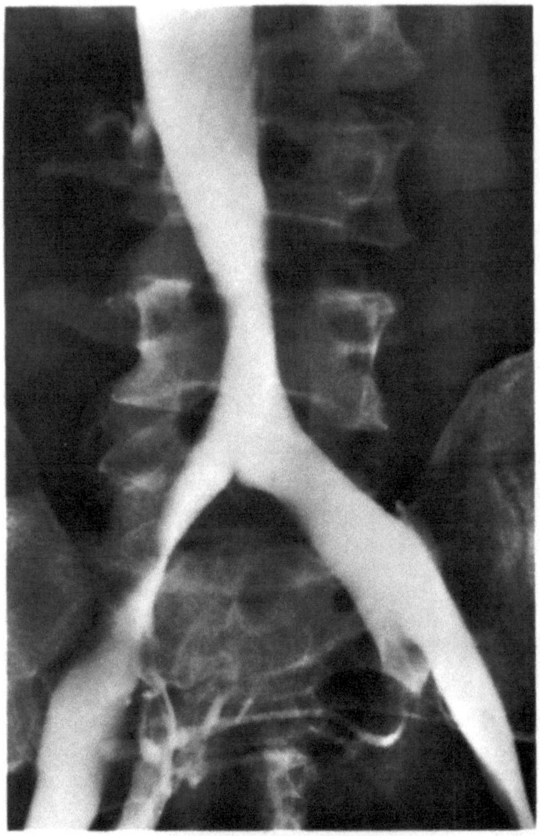

6.15a

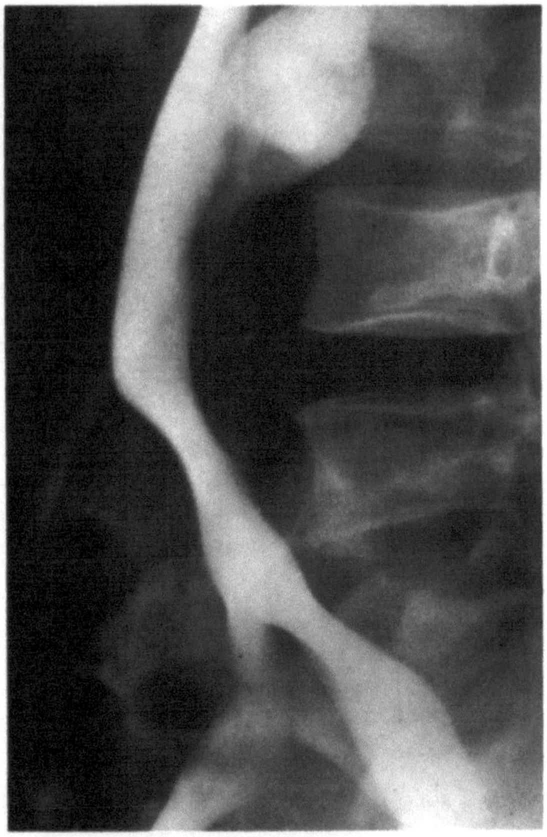

△6.15b

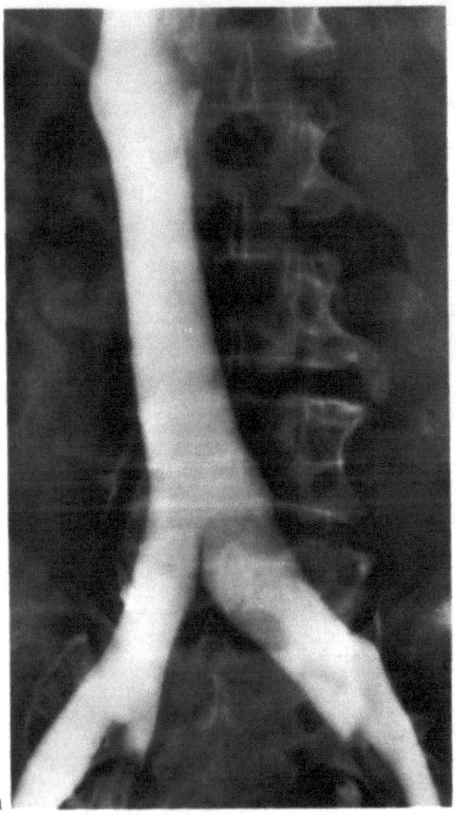

6.16a

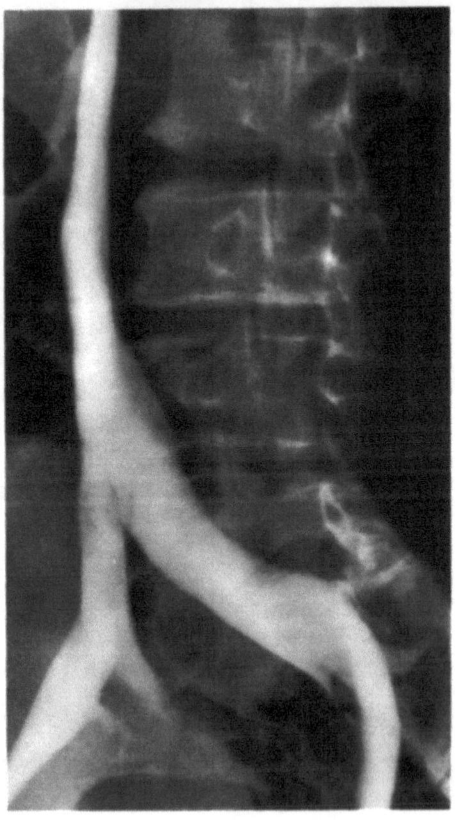

6.16b

Fig. 6.17. Retroperitoneal adenopathies (lymphosarcoma). Cavography is a complementary method for the study of retroperitoneal adenopathies, especially as concerns the upper lumbar lymph nodes. In this patient lymphography had shown some clearly hypertrophic left lumbar nodes but the right lumbar lymph nodes were not opacified. There exists a smooth extrinsic compression at the level of L1–L2 consistent with the extension of the sarcomatous process

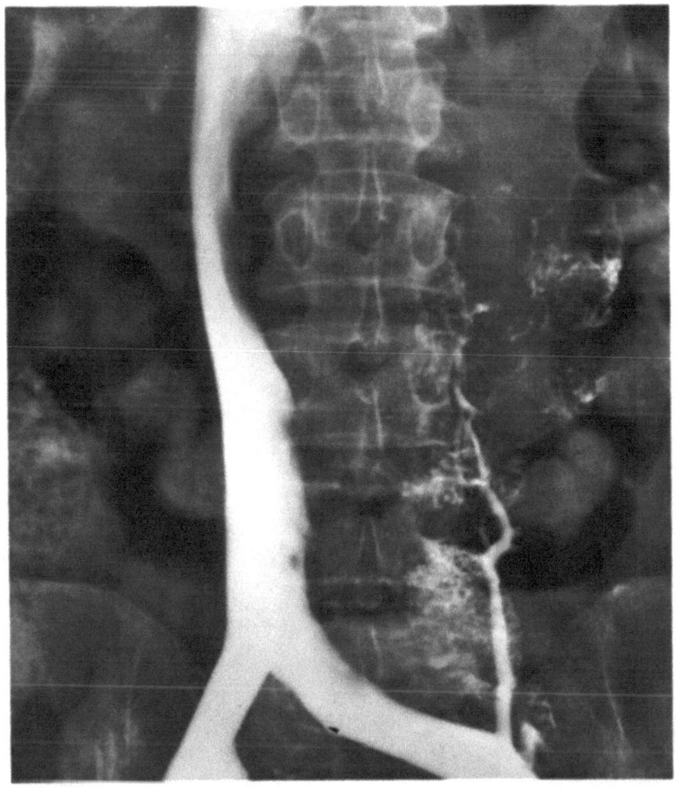

6.17

◁ Fig. 6.15a, b. Retroperitoneal adenopathies (Hodgkin's lymphoma). a Frontal view. b Left anterior oblique projection. Regular stenosis of the right common iliac vein and of the initial segment of the inferior vena cava. The left anterior oblique projection shows regular small indentations along the different walls of the inferior cava. These features probably correspond to adenopathies. Moreover, there is anterior displacement of the vena cava

◁ Fig. 6.16a, b. Retroperitoneal adenopathies (Hodgkin's lymphoma). a Frontal view. b Right posterior oblique projection. The frontal view shows merely an extrinsic impression along the left wall of the common iliac vein. The oblique projection shows several indentations on the aspects of the inferior vena cava suggesting adenopathies

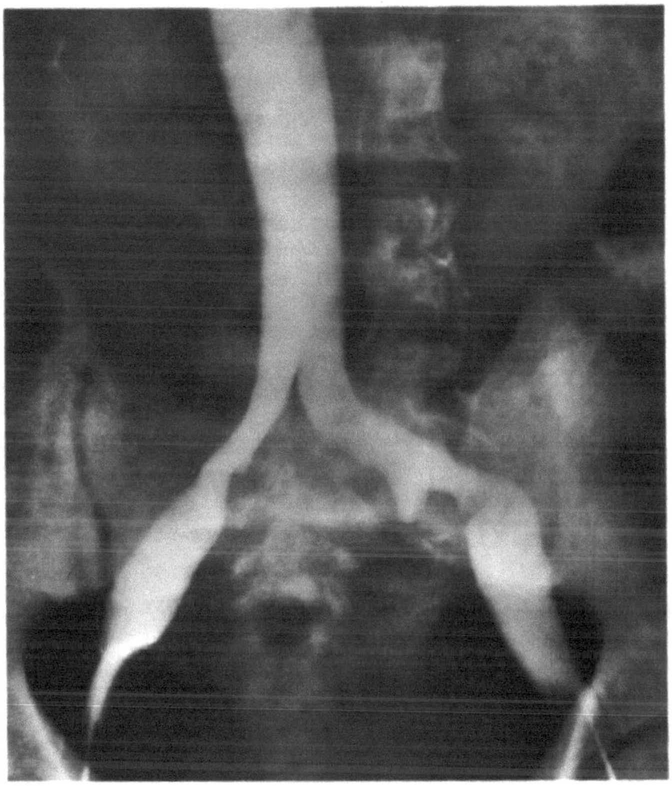

6.18

Fig. 6.18. Bone mastocytosis with huge pelvic and lumboaortic lymph nodes (confirmed by a lymphography which is not shown here). Stenosis and extensive ensheathing of both iliac veins. Extrinsic pressure upon a vein may be visualized as an elongated stenosis and not as an indentation

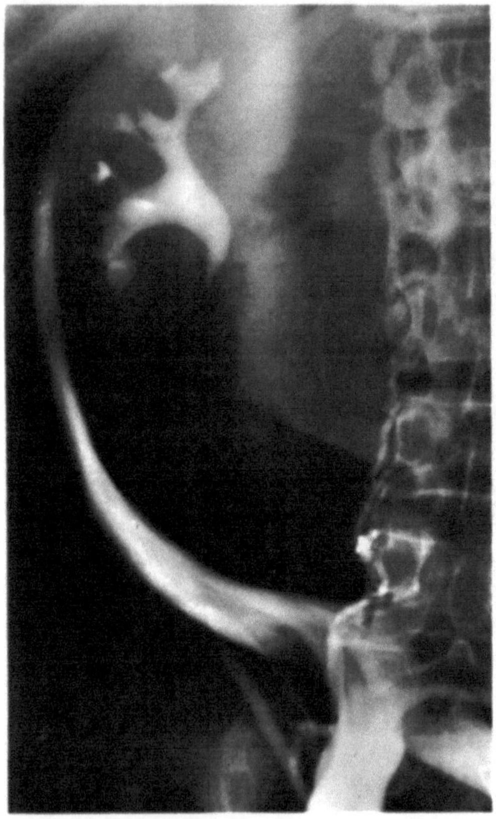
6.19a

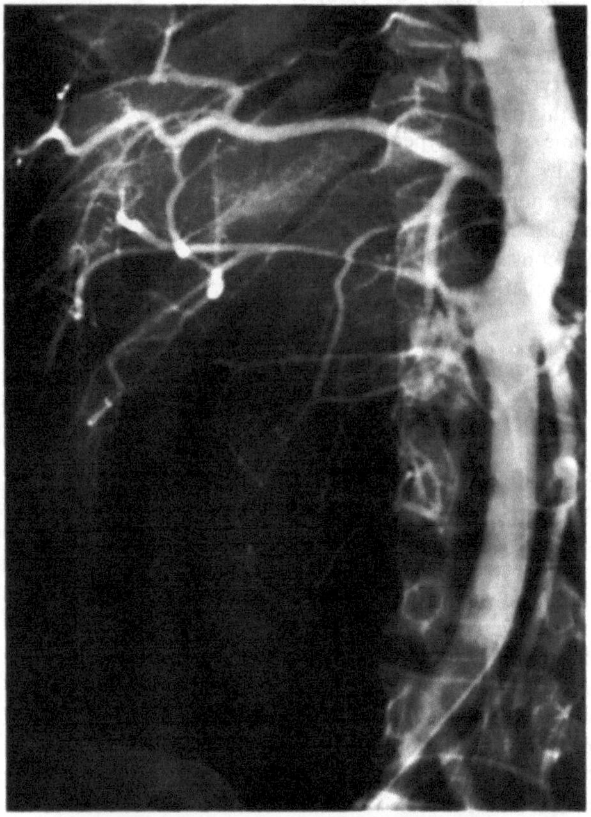
6.19b

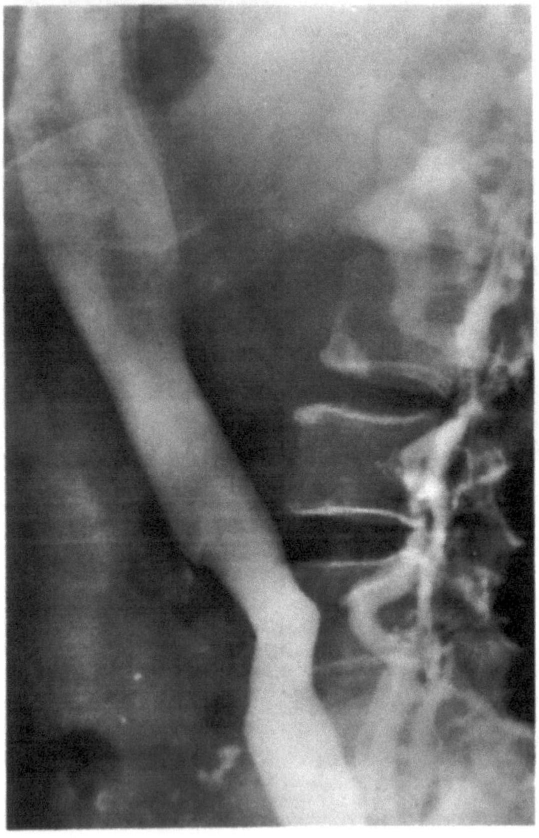
6.19c

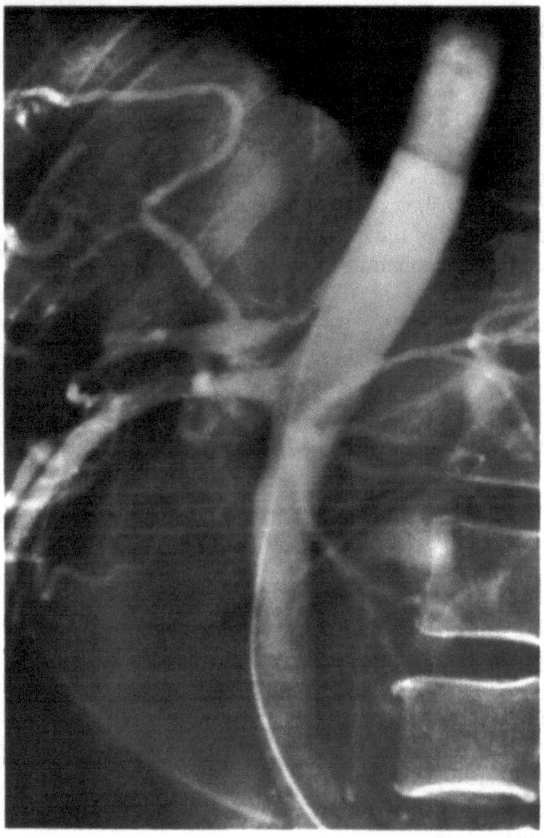
6.19d

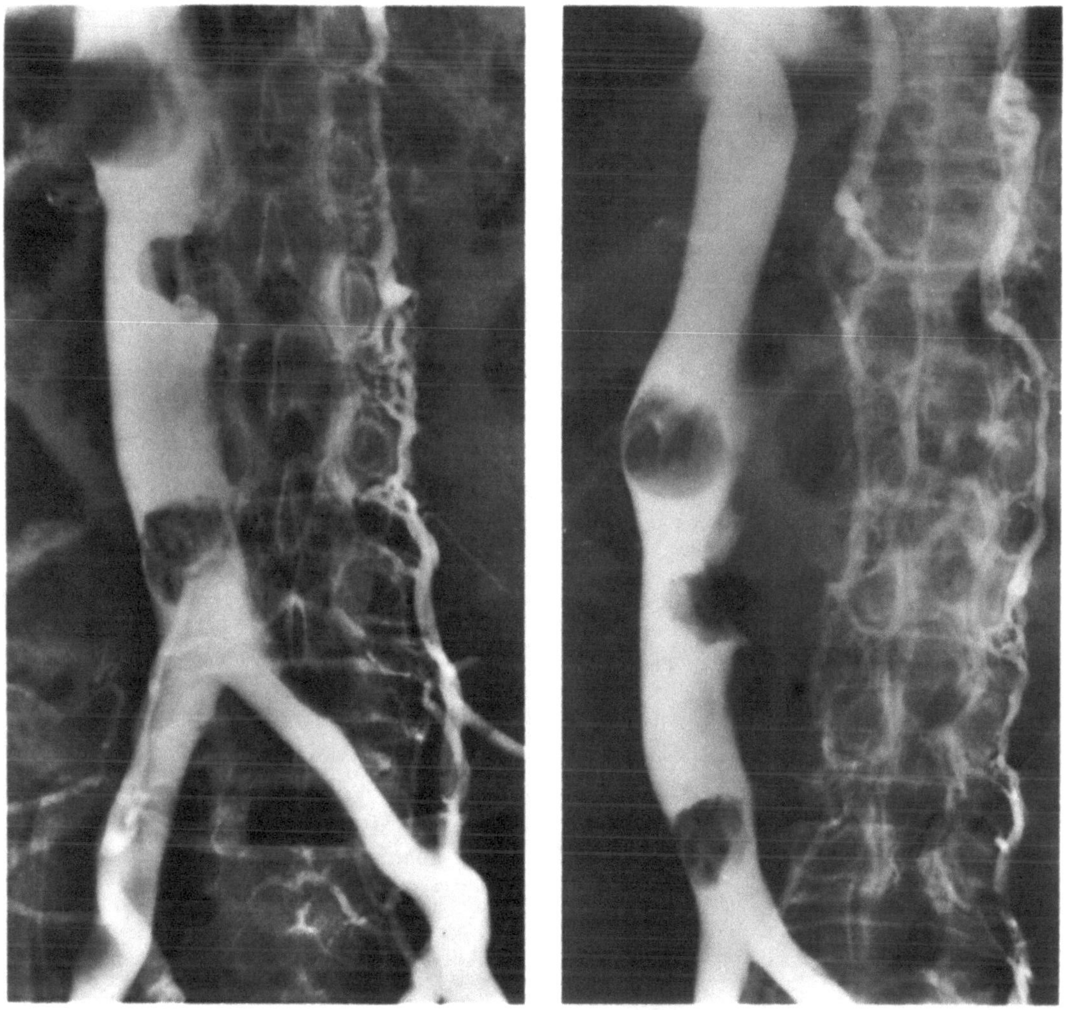

a b

Fig. 6.20a, b. Invasion by contiguity of the inferior vena cava by malignant adenopathies (cancer of the prostata). Numerous indentations, some of them forming real intracaval defects. Note on the right posterior oblique projection (b) the tumoral invasion, well visible on the left posterior aspect of the inferior vena cava at the level of L3. The invasion of the inferior vena cava by contiguity of a malignant adenopathy is an uncommon occurrence

◁ Fig. 6.19a–d. Retroperitoneal adenopathies (seminoma). a Frontal cavogram: The inferior vena cava is markedly displaced toward the right in a graceful and arciform fashion. The kidney is also displaced to the right; no changes of its cavities. b Frontal aortogram: It shows a very marked arciform displacement of the aorta toward the left and a major elongation of the renal artery. c Lateral cavogram: the inferior vena cava is free, displaced anteriorly on its entire course and laminated from right to left. d Lateral aortogram: the aorta is displaced anteriorly with regard to the spine. The right renal artery and the lumbar arteries are stretched. Note the important displacement of the digestive arteries to the left and anteriorly

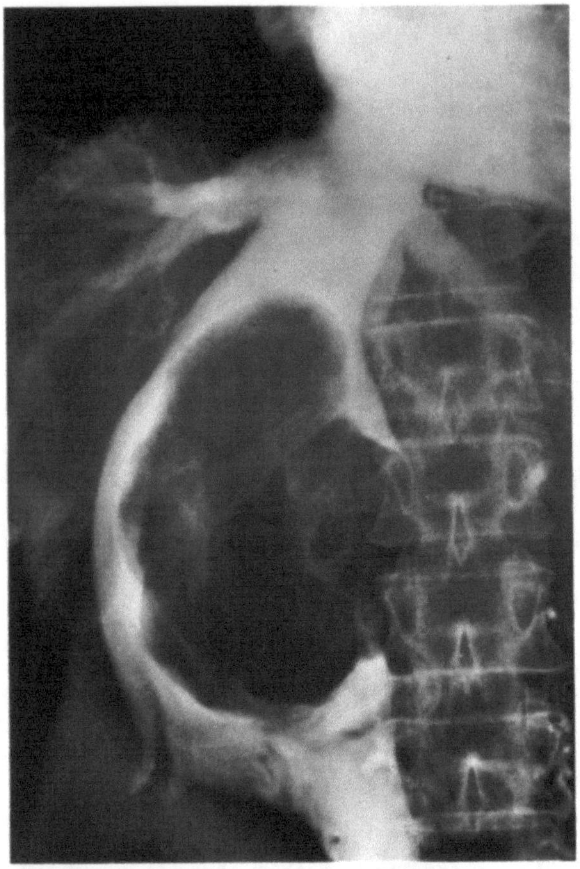

6.21

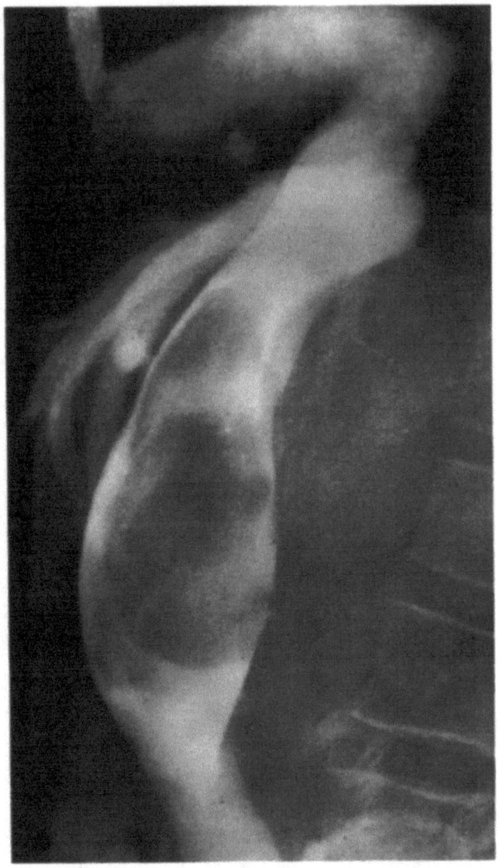

6.22

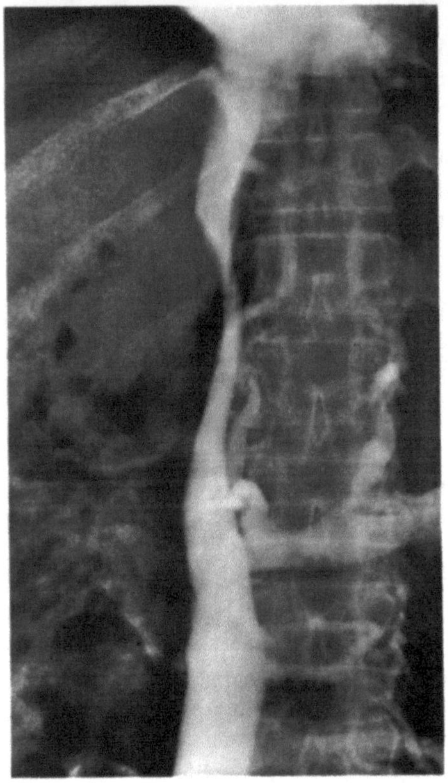

◁ 6.23

Fig. 6.21–6.23. Primary leiomyosarcoma of the inferior vena cava. 21, 22 Frontal and lateral views of an inferior vena cavogram show a huge intrinsic defect on the left wall of the inferior vena cava and widening of this vein in all its diameters. In this case there was a dilatation of the whole inferior vena cava without interruption of the flow. A more advanced tumor would cause thrombosis of the inferior vena cava. 23 Postoperative control. Total resection of the tumor necessitated removal of the right kidney (invasion of the renal hilum). The continuity of the inferior vena cava could be restituted. There persists however a marked diminution of the inferior vena cava caliber at the level of L1–L2 with reflux toward the renal and lumbar system. (By courtesy of Dr. Hernandez)

Chapter 7. Retroperitoneal Fibrosis

This condition was known at the beginning of the century (Albarran 1905) but it was individualized as an entity only in 1948 by Ormond. Retroperitoneal fibrosis is a clinical and radiological entity involving the ureters, the inferior vena cava, the iliac veins and the rectosigmoid. It is a fibroblastic proliferation with polymorphic inflammatory infiltrations of the retroperitoneal region. Different mechanisms have been considered to produce this extensive fibrosis and among them mainly urinary diseases, systemic diseases, neoplasms of the small pelvis, and drugs. These iatrogenic retroperitoneal fibroses deserve to be individualized since they regress as soon as the treatment is stopped; they are secondary to Methysergide, Ergotamine, Hydralazine (Arger et al. 1973; Morrison 1968). Retroperitoneal fibrosis may be isolated or form a part of a multifocal fibrosis involving the lungs, mediastinum, peritoneum, etc. (Kittredge 1974).

Among the radiological signs the most precocious is the effect on the inferior vena cava, whence the interest of inferior vena cavography when this condition is clinically suspected.

7.1 Clinical Data

The age of occurrence is very variable (from 8 to 80 years) but most often situated in the fourth or fifth decade of life.

The incidence is three times higher in males than in females. The frequency in treatments for migraine is of about 1/10,000 (Gelford and Cronwell 1968).

The involvement is most often rightaway bilateral but frequently asymmetrical (Richet and Meyrier 1970). The clinical symptoms are rather polymorphic, the most important being renal insufficiency (21 among Michel's 25 cases).

Renal insufficiency may develop without major distention of the cavities (Lalli 1977). There may also be abdominal pains of different types but quite often there is nephritic colic. The other clinical signs consist of nausea, vomiting, wasting, arterial hypertension and headache. More rarely there may be venous signs, i.e., edema of the lower limbs or phlebitis (20% of the patients, according to Richet), or gastrointestinal symptoms, i.e., constipation secondary to sigmoid flexure involvement. There is very often a long delay between the appearance of the first signs and the diagnosis; this may reach in certain cases more than 25 years (Reboul and Manigand 1974).

7.2 Radiologic Investigations

The diagnosis of retroperitoneal fibrosis is generally founded on conventional X-raying, i.e., intravenous urography and inferior vena cavography.

7.2.1 Intravenous Urography

Intravenous urography is an easy investigation but brings to light only late signs, i.e., more or less marked, usually bilateral and asymmetrical obstruction of the ureter. Medial deviation of the ureters which has been considered up to now as a characteristic sign, seems in fact questionable (Arger, Michel 1978). As a matter of fact, hypertrophic psoas muscles may cause a similar displacement of the ureters (Bree et al. 1976).

7.2.2 Inferior Vena Cavography

Inferior vena cavography is the method of choice for demonstrating this condition (Helander and Lindbom 1956; Manigand et al. 1972; Lien and Kolbenstvedt 1977; Virtama and Helela 1967; Michel et al. 1971).

Development of collateral circulation arising from the lumbar ascending vessels (Fig. 7.3) though the stenosis is rather mild.

At a later stage the signs are obvious, the stenosis is very tight with marked collateral circulation (Figs. 7.3 and 7.5–7.7). The termination of the iliac veins may be involved (Figs. 7.3, 7.4, and 7.7)

The ultimate stage causes complete obstruction (Fig. 7.6a); the whole blood is drained via collateral channels, which are mainly intraspinal. Inferior vena cavography with approach from above allows to localize the upper level of the obstruction (Fig. 7.6b).

The cavographic appearance is the same with primary and with secondary retroperitoneal fibrosis (Figs. 7.2 and 7.7).

7.2.3 Other Radiologic Investigations

Opacification with barium, retrograde ureteropyelography, lymphography, and arteriography are only of interest in some peculiar cases. But inferior vena cavography provides the earliest and most significant data.

7.3 Treatment

As concerns retroperitoneal fibrosis, the treatment is actually double. Early applied corticotherapy gives excellent results (Kearney 1976). Of course, interruption of the causal anti-migraine treatment prevents extension of the fibrosis (Morrison, Gelford 1968). In more advanced stages surgery consisting in decompression and intraperitonealisation of the ureter is always undertaken (Declercq, Dufour, Auvert). This suppresses the risk of mechanic complications in the urinary tract but does not restore the renal function in very advanced cases.

The technique is the following: bifemoral puncture and free flow injection which allows to demonstrate not only the state of the inferior vena cava but also the eventual invasion of the iliac veins. In some cases (Fig. 7.6b) when the lower segment of the inferior vena cava is completely obstructed, it may be necessary to utilize the approach from above so as to verify the patency of the renal veins. Frontal and lateral projections are systematically performed so as to demonstrate displacements in the frontal as well as in the sagittal plane. Early venographic films and later arteriographic films are necessary to appreciate the state of the inferior caval venous axis as well as that of the aorta. It is also possible to carry out at the same time a cavography and an intravenous urography when there is a strong clinical doubt (Michel et al. 1978).

The cavographic signs are the earliest. The venous walls are very flexible and thus easily deformed.

The site of the lesions is always the same, i.e., the postrenal segment of the inferior vena cava.

At the onset the radiologic appearance is as follows: (Michel et al.).

More or less extended, regular, well centered and symmetrical stenosis (Figs. 7.1 and 7.2).

Medial displacement of the inferior vena cava which projects on the spine on a frontal projection (Fig. 7.1).

Marked anterior displacement on the lateral projection; the inferior vena cava is displaced anteriorly and is visible in front of the anterior margin of the spine (Figs. 7.1 and 7.3).

Inferior vena cavography is of great importance for the diagnosis of retroperitoneal fibrosis since it is the only method which provides early diagnosis and thus the possibility for a medical therapy at a time when it is still efficacious.

References

Albarran J (1905) Rétention rénale par périurétérite: Libération externe de l'uretère. AFV 511–517

Arger PH, Stollz JL, Miller WJ (1973) Retroperitoneal fibrosis: An analysis of the clinical spectrum and roentgenographic signs. AJR 119:812–821

Auvert J, Xerri A (1970) Fibrose rétropéritonéale idiopathique extensive. J Urol Nephrol (Paris) 76:274–276

Bar-Ziv J (1972) Injury to the inferior vena cava. Br J Radiol 45:307–310

Bree RL, Green B, Keiller OL, Genet EF (1976) Medial deviation of the ureters secondary to psoas muscle hypertrophy. Radiology 118:691–695

Bricker DL (1970) Successful management on an injury to the suprarenal inferior vena cava. Surg Clin North Am 50:999–1002

Declercq M, Mazeman E, Wemeau L (1974) Les fibroses rétropéritonéales. Diagnostic, évolution et conduite thérapeutique à propos de 15 observations. Ann Urol 8:53–60

Dufour B (1973) Les obstructions de l'uretère lombo-iliaque à l'exclusion des tumeurs urétérales. J Urol Nephrol (Paris) 79:107–139

Gelford GJ, Cronwell DK (1968) Methysergide, retroperitoneal fibrosis and retrosigmoid stricture. AJR 104:566–570

Gelford GJ, Wilets AJ, Nelson D, Kroll LL (1967) Retroperitoneal fibrosis and methysergide. Report of 3 cases. Radiology 88:976–982

Graham JM (1978) Traumatic injuries of the inferior vena cava. Arch Surg 113:413–418

Helander CG, Lindbom A (1956) Roentgen examination of the inferior vena cava in retroperitoneal expanding processes. Acta Radiol 45:289–297

Kairaluoma MI (1976) Prolonged recovery after extended right hepatic lobectomy in a patient with severe blunt liver injury and laceration of the vena cava. A report of case with special references to autotransfusion and complications of biliary decompression. Acta Chir Scand 142:345–349

Kearney GP (1976) Venacavography, corticosteroids and surgery in the management of idiopathic retroperitoneal fibrosis. J Urol 115:32–35

Kittredge RD (1974) The many facets of sclerosing fibrosis. AJR 122:288–298

Lalli AF (1977) Retroperitoneal fibrosis and inapparent obstructive uropathy. Radiology 122:339–342

Lien HH, Kolbenstvedt A (1977) Non malignant venographic abnormalities of the inferior vena cava. Radiology 122:105–110

Madding GF (1977) Hepatic and vena caval injuries. Surg Clin North Am 57:275–289

Manigand G, De Lara C, Benchetrit J, Reboul M, Deparis M (1972) Fibrose rétropéritonéale. Remarques cliniques à propos d'une observation avec cavographie. Ann Med Interne (Paris) 123:497–502

Mc Master P (1976) Hepatic trauma involving the hepatic veins and vena cava. Injury, 7:299–305

Michel JR, Masselot J, Chung KH (1971) Intérêt de la radiologie dans la fibrose rétropéritonéale avec accent mis sur la phlébographie cave inférieure en flux libre. Ann Radiol (Paris) 14:409–417

Michel JR, Moreau JF, Deltour F, Affre J, Lyonnet D (1978) Fibrose rétropéritonéale (FRP). Apport des méthodes de radiologie conventionnelle. Journ Cult Lat (Paris)

Morrison G (1968) Retroperitoneal fibrosis associated with methysergide therapy. J Can Assoc Radiol 19:61–63

Ormond JK (1948) Bilateral ureteral obstruction due to enveloppement and compression by an inflammatory retroperitoneal process. J Urol 59:1072–1079

Reboul M, Manigand G (1974) Intérêt d'un diagnostic précoce dans la fibrose rétropéritonéale idiopathique. Place de la cavographie. Phlebologie 27:167–174

Richet G, Meyrier A (1970) Liposclérose rétropéritonéale. Thrombose des veines rénales. Masson, Paris

Turpin I (1977) Injuries to the inferior vena cava and their management. Am J Surg 134:25–32

Virtama P, Helela T (1967) Lymphography and cavography in retroperitoneal fibrosis. Br J Radiol 40:231–232

Weichert RF (1971) Blunt injury to intrahepatic vena cava and hepatic veins with survival. Am J Surg 121:322–325

Weichert RF (1970) Injuries to the inferior vena cava: report of 35 cases. J. Trauma, 10:649–657

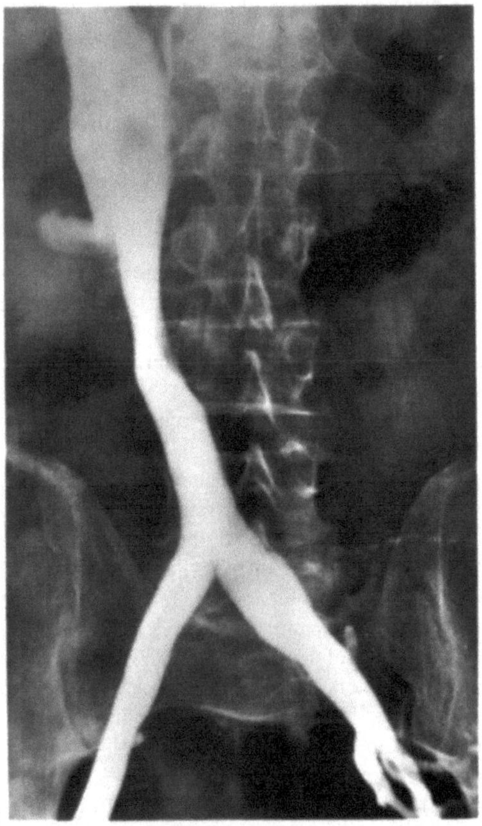
7.1 a

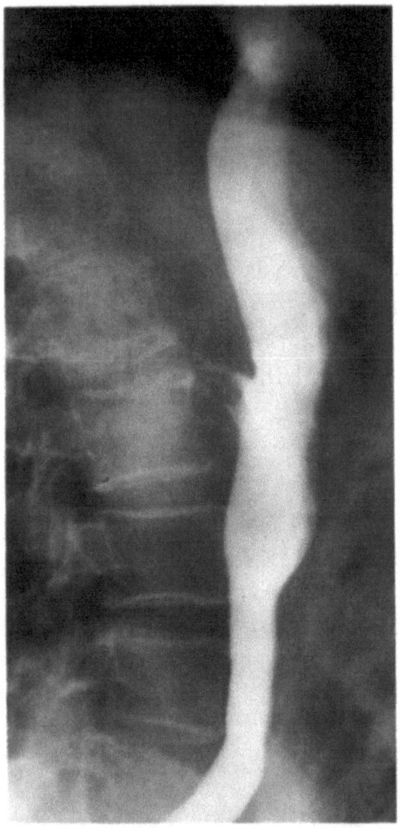
7.1 b

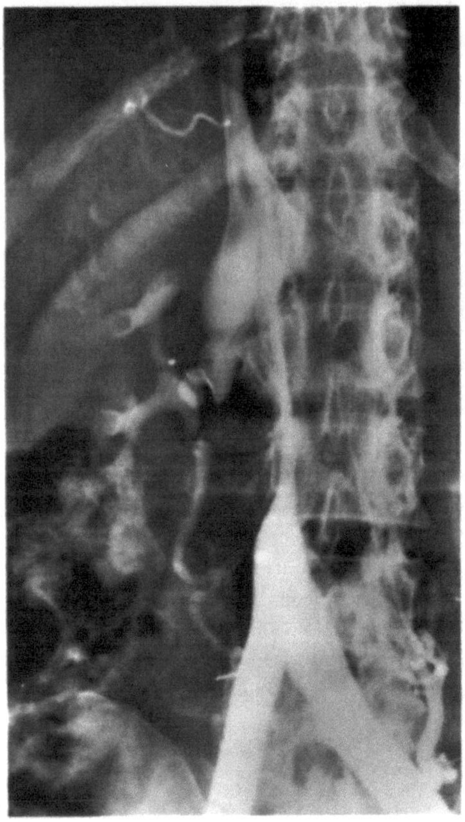
7.2 a

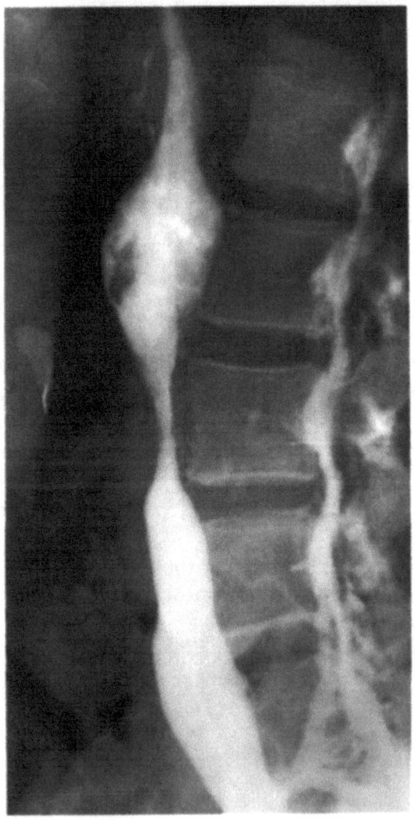
7.2 b

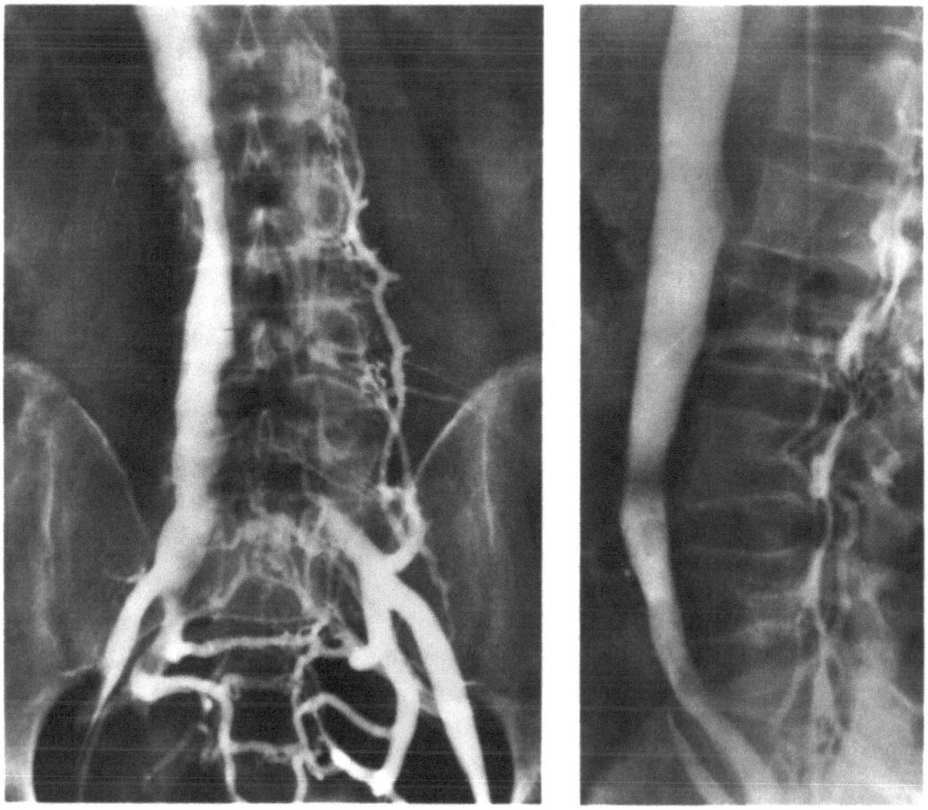

a b

Fig. 7.3a, b. Retroperitoneal fibrosis. a Frontal view. b Lateral view. Regular extended stenosis of the inferior vena cava at the level of the three lower lumbar vertebrae. There is a marked narrowing of the right common iliac vein with marked lumbar ascending and presacral collateral circulation. Note the clear forward displacement of the inferior vena cava at the level of the lower lumbar vertebrae

◁ Fig. 7.1a, b. Retroperitoneal fibrosis. a Frontal view. b Lateral view. Long, regular, symmetrical concentric stenosis of the inferior vena cava at the level of L2, L3, and L4. In its inferior part the stenosis is concentric and narrows globally the caliber of the inferior vena cava; in the superior part the narrowing occurs mainly in the lateral direction as it is well visible on a frontal view. Moreover, fibrosis causes a displacement of the inferior vena cava which is now visible anteriorly to the spine (on the lateral view) whereas it is normally projected onto the spine at this level

Fig. 7.2a, b. Retroperitoneal fibrosis. Very regular, 3-cm-long stenosis of the infrarenal segment of the inferior vena cava. Appearance of extrinsic compression with onset of peri- and intraspinal collateral circulation. Surgery suggests the presence of peritoneal carcinosis of undetermined etiology. The histologic examination proved it to be retroperitoneal fibrosis of sarcoidosic origin. A liver puncture confirms this diagnosis

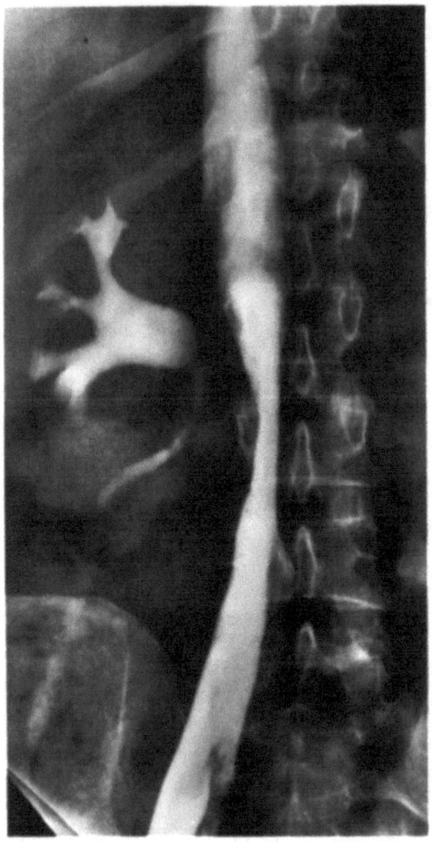

Fig. 7.4. Retroperitoneal fibrosis. This patient had already undergone surgery for intraperitonealization of the right ureter which accounts for the position of the ureters. Edema of the left leg leads to perform cavography. Thrombosis of the left iliac axis. There is a thrombus issuing from the right hypogastric artery. Extended, regular and concentric stenosis of the infrarenal segment of the inferior vena cava at the level of L3 and L4

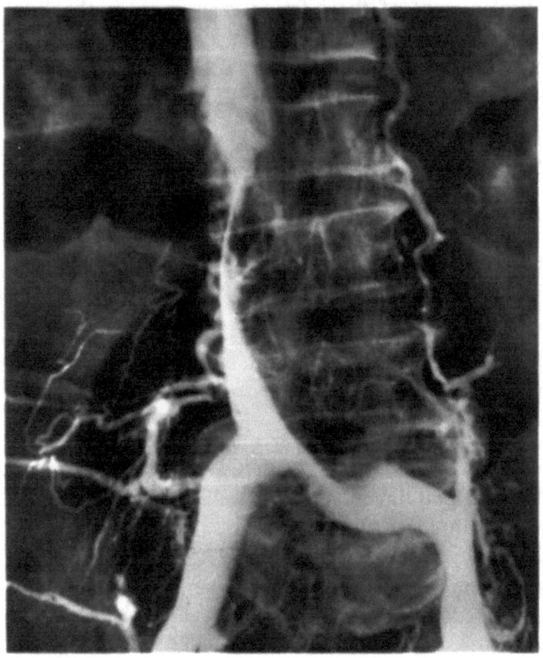

a

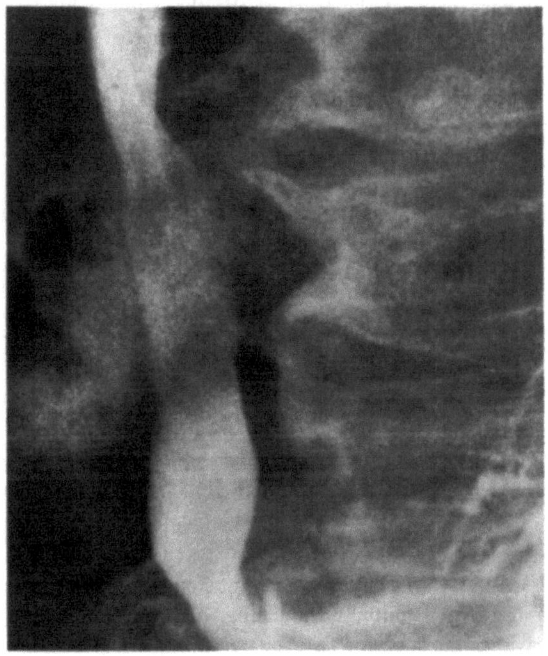

b

Fig. 7.5a, b. Retroperitoneal fibrosis. a Frontal view. b Lateral view. Very tight stenosis of the inferior vena cava, especially in the lateral direction. The inferior vena cava resembles a thin thread at the level of L3. The lateral view shows the flattened appearance of the vena cava at this level, and its image clearly projected in front of the spine

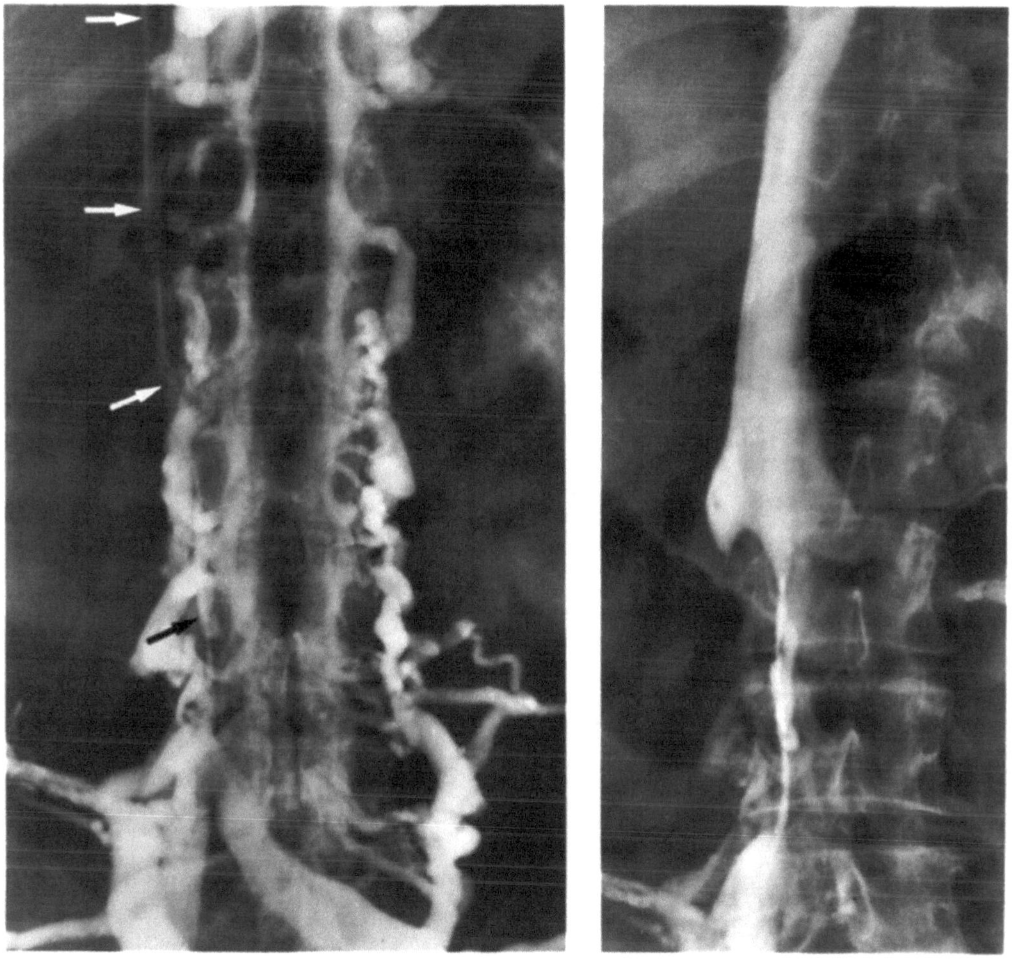

7.6a 7.6b

Fig. 7.6a, b. Retroperitoneal fibrosis. a Frontal view showing the very tight stenosis of the inferior vena cava at the level of L2–L3 (↗). The inferior vena cava is reduced to a thin thread (↗) and there is marked collateral circulation via the subcutaneous abdominal and lumbar system and via the lumbar ascending and the intraspinal system. b Retrograde cavography to verify the patency of the renal veins and of the prerenal segment of the inferior vena cava. This shows also the markedly reduced caliber of the inferior vena cava at the L2 and L3 level

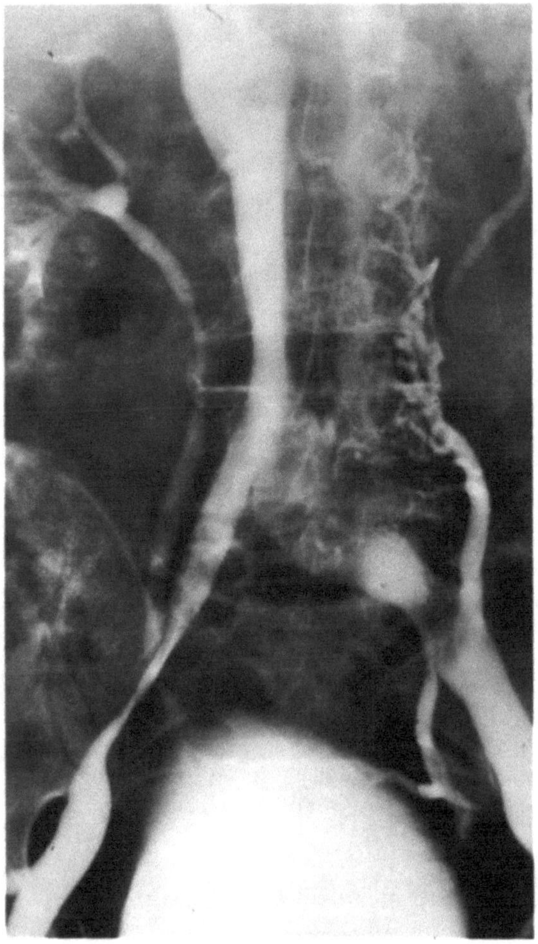

Fig. 7.7. Retroperitoneal stenosis due to cancer of the bladder. Note on this film the defect in the inferior aspect of the bladder. Resulting retroperitoneal fibrosis causes extended and concentric stenosis not only of the postrenal segment of the inferior vena cava but also of the right common iliac axis

Chapter 8. Inferior Vena Cavography in Hepatic and Intraperitoneal Diseases

This chapter deals with the changes in the inferior vena cava due to pathologic conditions involving the intraperitoneal organs, e.g., liver, pancreas, digestive tract, and peritoneum. Tumors of the lesser pelvis with intra-abdominal development are dealt with concomitantly, since they raise similar diagnostic problems.

Intraperitoneal tumors are separated from the inferior vena cava by the posterior parietal peritoneum, but they nevertheless affect this vessel when they reach a certain volume: the inferior vena cava has very supple walls and low pressure so that it is easily modified by hypertrophic neighboring structures. The caval caliber and hence the blood flow are reduced, which increases the risk of inferior vena cava thrombosis. In some cases it is the pulmonary embolism, secondary to this thrombosis, which draws attention on involvement of the inferior vena cava, especially after surgical treatment for voluminous abdominal tumors.

The posterior parietal peritoneum hinders direct parietal invasion of the inferior vena cava by intraperitoneal malignant tumors. Invasion is thus only seen in the hepatic region.

8.1 Anatomical Considerations

Anteriorly and laterally the inferior vena cava is related to the intraperitoneal anatomic structures. The relations are distributed on two levels:

The upper segment corresponds to the hepatic area and shows two peculiarities: there is no peritoneal covering and the hepatic veins join here.

The lower segment: at this level the inferior vena cava is covered with the posterior parietal peritoneum through which it is related with the intraperitoneal organs.

8.1.1 Upper Segment (Hepatic Segment)

There are major relations between the inferior vena cava and the liver since it is contained within a vertical groove over a distance of about 2 to 3 cm. This groove is occasionally converted into a tunnel between the right lobe and the caudate lobe. The adherence is such that the inferior vena cava plays a role in the fixation of the liver. At some centimeters below its atrial opening, the inferior vena cava receives the left and the right hepatic veins.

Large pelvic tumors may extend to the abdominal cavity, raise the peritoneum of the lesser pelvis which thus protrudes into the cavity and may exert pressure upon the inferior vena cava through the posterior parietal peritoneum. Of course this compression may be direct in the lesser pelvis at the level of the iliac veins and of the commencement of the inferior vena cava.

8.1.2 Lower Segment

Anteriorly to the posterior peritoneum the relations are, from caudal to cranial: the root of the mesentery and hence, the small intestine, the longitudinal part of the duodenum, the head of the pancreas, Winslow's foramen and, through this, the portal vessels. The portal vein, major relation of the inferior vena cava from the surgical point of view, is in fact at some distance caudally and to the right, especially when the junction of the superior mesenteric vein with the spleno-mesareic trunk is situated very cranially; hence, the portal vein is short, so that eventual portocaval anastomosis becomes very difficult.

8.2 Technique

The technical conditions are not the same with hepatic pathology as with nonhepatic pathology.

8.2.1 Hepatic Pathology

Venographic exploration of the liver comprises two steps: first inferior vena cavography and second, hepatic venography (see also Chapter 9). Inferior vena cavography permits to demonstrate the effect of the hepatic disease upon the inferior vena cava and to localize and examine the confluence with the hepatic veins. In case of thrombosis or other obstruction, it may be necessary to utilize brachial approach for opacifying the distal part of the inferior vena cava and, eventually, catheterizing the hepatic veins. Frontal and lateral projections are indispensable since compression may be either only lateral or only frontal. It may also be necessary to change the position of the patient. Indeed, a hepatic mass may compress the inferior vena cava when the patient is in the lateral decubitus position and it suffices to position the patient in the reverse lateral decubitus (Fig. 3.12) to see the compression diminish or even disappear.

Finally, we would like to point out the importance of displaying not only the upper segment of the inferior vena cava, but also the right atrium – especially in case of neoplastic invasion of the hepatic veins – in order to appreciate its integrity.

When the presence of a membranous obstruction in the inferior vena cava is suspected, it may be necessary to perform cavography by introducing a catheter with multiple side-holes above the level of the renal veins so as to obtain a good opacification of the retrohepatic segment.

8.2.2 Nonhepatic Abdominal Pathology

The problem is quite different since there are no venous tributaries draining blood from the peritoneal cavity. Orthogonal projections are also indispensable for a correct appreciation of the narrowing of the inferior vena cava. The position of the patient influences the compression and it is useful to perform a series in the position which produces minimal compression, i.e., right lateral decubitus for a tumor on the right side, and left lateral decubitus for a tumor on the left.

Lateral decubitus with horizontal beam permits to appreciate the exact status of the inferior vena cava in ascites of hepatic or other origin.

8.3 Radiologic Features

8.3.1 Hepatic Diseases

Several hepatic diseases (cirrhosis, Budd-Chiari, tumors) may cause changes in the inferior vena cava. The roentgenographic findings are of two types: either more or less marked compression which may cause thrombosis, or direct invasion by contiguity from the hepatic veins.

Cirrhoses

Three types of features may be encountered:

1) *Stenosis* is the most frequent manifestation. It is a rather extended stenosis occurring on the intrahepatic course of the inferior vena cava; it is symmetrical and regular and the vein resumes its normal diameter above the liver and is, in some cases, even dilated. The stenosis corresponds to the hypertrophic liver tissue exerting pressure upon the inferior vena cava (Figs. 8.1 and 8.2). This stenosis is not concentric but often more marked in the frontal plane, so that the inferior vena cava is markedly narrowed on a frontal projection, and has a normal diameter on a lateral view.

2) *Dilatations* of the inferior vena cava on this level are much more rare. They correspond to atrophy of the liver tissue which causes dilatation of the retrohepatic segment of the inferior vena cava (Fig. 8.3).

3) *Ascites* is responsible for the third type of images (Figs. 8.4 and 8.5). Increased intraperitoneal pressure due to the ascites causes changes in the inferior vena cava which are maximal at the lowest, i.e., most dorsal, point, the patient being supine. The hydrostatic hyperpressure phenomena on a thin-walled supple pipe, with low pressure inside, is well explained by the physics of fluids (Poiseuille's law). Ascites causes a very extended and progressive stenosis beginning at the level of the renal veins and becoming more and more marked toward the right atrium.

This stenosis is perfectly symmetrical and varies with the changes in the patient's position and with the volume of ascites. Roentgenograms performed in the lateral decubitus and with a horizontal beam show that ascites is displaced and hence hydrostatic compression upon the inferior vena cava partly released. These projections allow to differentiate direct hepatic compression from compression by ascites secondary to the hepatic disease. Finally, the compression varies along with the evolution of ascites: when this is punctured, the caliber of the inferior vena cava is again entirely normal.

Catheterization of the inferior vena cava permits moreover *to measure pressures*. Not only the infra- and suprahepatic caval pressure – it is indeed well known that there exists a correlation between caval hypertension, portal hypertension and evolution of the cirrhosis (functional renal insufficiency) but also the measurement of wedge and free pressure in the hepatic veins permitting to appreciate the portal hypertension, and hence providing major data in view of a surgical treatment (portocaval shunt).

Budd-Chiari Syndrome

This corresponds most often to obstruction of the hepatic veins; but it may also be due to obstruction of the suprahepatic inferior vena cava (membranous occlusion, thrombosis, tumor, especially of the kidney). Inferior vena cavography is therefore the first step in the exploration of such patients (see also chapter 11).

There are four types of data provided by inferior vena cavography: normal or abnormal appearance of the cava, appearance of the hepatic veins, compression of the inferior vena cava by the caudate lobe, presence of ascites.

The upper segment of the inferior vena cava may be the site of obstruction. This may be due to a *congenital membrane* which may be either incomplete, so as to permit the passage of a reduced blood flow, or complete of congenital origin, or, finally, rendered complete by a recent thrombosis. Cavography shows then incomplete, or more often complete obstruction of the inferior vena cava with marked collateral channels constituted by the perivertebral and ascending lumbar systems and drainage via the azygos veins.

The second main cause of upper caval obstruction is the extension of tumors, especially renal tumors (these may invade the renal veins and then the inferior vena cava, obstructing its upper segment so as to produce a Budd-Chiari syndrome).

But most often the Budd-Chiari syndrome is not secondary to obstruction of the upper caval segment but to *direct obstruction of the hepatic veins*. When the ostia of the hepatic veins are involved, inferior vena cavography, possibly with Valsalva maneuver, may demonstrate obstruction of the hepatic veins and show a cone-shaped (or beak-like) image corresponding to the non-opacified segment of the hepatic veins. Moreover, the dilution flow which comes normally from the hepatic veins, may be absent. But the Budd-Chiari syndrome may involve only one lobe so that the dilution flow of the still spared hepatic veins persists.

As a rule, obstruction occurs only in the main hepatic veins. The accessory veins, especially those of the caudate lobe are spared, and there is hypertrophy of this segment. This compensating hypertrophy causes compression of the anterior aspect of the inferior vena cava (Fig. 8.6 and 8.7) which is visualized as a regular arciform pressure deformity of the anterior wall.

The fourth type of image seen in a Budd-Chiari syndrome is due to the presence of ascites. It is then useful to perform projections with a horizontal beam and in the lateral decubitus so as to individualize more easily the different features.

Hepatic Tumors

Benign tumors affect the inferior vena cava only if they are voluminous or if they are located in the proximity of the cava. They produce extrinsic compressions which may be responsible for thrombosis. Cysts (Fig. 8.10) especially hydatid cysts (Figs. 8.8 and 8.9) have similar roentgenographic features and imply the same risks, when they are huge. These types of tumors produce perfectly regular extrinsic compressions and some displacement of the inferior vena cava. Contrariwise, primary or secondary malignant tumors may produce compression of the vena cava (Figs. 8.11–8.13) and are moreover, sometimes responsible for invasion of the cava (Figs. 8.14 and 8.15). This invasion may be direct and produces multiple irregular defects within the caval lumen in the retro or suprahepatic segment. It may also be indirect, corresponding to a neoplastic plug originating from the hepatic veins and extending into the inferior vena cava.

Pediculate hepatic tumors have the same effects as intraperitoneal tumors and may produce compressions of the infrahepatic segment of the inferior vena cava (Figs. 8.16 and 8.17).

Intraperitoneal Tumors and Tumors of the Lesser Pelvis Extending to the Abdomen

They produce more or less marked compression, i.e., lateral or frontal regular arciform defects which narrow the inferior vena cava lumen.

These tumors being relatively mobile, their effect upon the inferior vena cava depends on the patient's position. The more they are voluminous, the more marked is the compression. The compression produces a reduction of the flow which may give rise to a sometimes quite marked and rapidly developing collateral circulation. Reduction of the flow risks to cause secondary thrombosis.

These abdominal tumors may be benign but are in fact mostly malignant and of diverse origins: pancreas, mesentery, uterus, ovary. Malignant abdominal tumors may involve the inferior vena cava by other mechanisms then direct compression, i.e. either posterior parietal invasion (rarely) or neoplastic involvement of retroperitoneal lymph nodes, hepatic metastases or neoplastic ascites.

The importance of inferior vena cavography for the investigation of hepatic diseases is no longer to be demonstrated. It belongs indeed to the screening methods utilized for the examination of such patients. But, as concerns abdominal tumors, the inferior vena cavography offers a double interest:

on one hand, in case of very small tumors, it shows early signs since it is very easily deformed, and, on the other hand, in case of voluminous tumors, it allows to rule out eventual thrombosis and hence to avoid the risk of postoperative pulmonary embolism.

References

Abdelsayed MA (1978) Renal tumors involving the inferior vena cava: plan for management. J Urol 120:153–155

Anselmi G (1970) Wilm's tumour propagated through the inferior vena cava into the right heart cavities. Br Heart J 32:575–578

Aytac A (1976) Metastatic Wilm's tumor in the right atrium propagated through the inferior vena cava. Vasc Surg 10:268–274

Beck AD (1977) Renal cell carcinoma involving the inferior vena cava: radiologic evaluation and surgical management. J Urol 118:533–537

Ben Menachem Y (1969) Inferior venacavography as an aid in the diagnosis of space-occupying lesions of the pancreas. Isr J Med Sci 5:1198–2205

Berges W (1977) Pancreatic pseudocyst of head: compressing of vena cava inferior with lethal embolism of pulmonary artery. Gastroenterology 15:747–750

Bugge-Asperheim B (1977) Aortic-caval fistula from ruptured abdominal aortic aneurysm. Ann Chir Gynaecol 66:108–112

Cahill PJ (1977) Inferior vena caval involvement by adrenal cortical carcinoma. Urology 10:604–607

Da Costa H (1977) Frequency of inferior vena caval abnormality due to a juxtaposed pathology. Nuklearmedizin 16:71–75

Dardik H (1976) Intravenous rupture of arteriosclerotic aneurysms of the abdominal aorta. Surgery 80:647–651

Datta DV (1978) Diagnostic value of combined transhepatic venography and inferior vena cavography in chronic Budd-Chiari syndrome. Am J Dig Dis 23:1031–1041

Dreze (1974) Pathology of the inferior vena cava. Compression of the inferior vena cava by the renal artery. Rev Med Liege 29:433–437

Gosink BB (1978) The inferior vena cava: mass effects. AJR 130:533–536

Gregoir W (1973) Cavography in cancer of the kidney. Acta Urol Belg 41:325–336

Harris RD (1976) The etiology of inferior vena caval obstruction and compression. CRC Crit Rev Diagn Imaging 8:57–86

Hietala SO (1977) Cavography in the management of malignant abdominal tumors. Acta Radiol 18:217–224

Jaffe RB (1969) Localization of metastatic pheochromocytoma in pregnancy by caval catheterization. Including urinary catecholamine values in uncomplicated pregnancies. J Obstet Gynecol 104:939–944

Kaswin R (1977) Rupture of a subrenal abdominal aortic aneurysm into the inferior vena cava. Ann Chir 31:533–536

Lippey ER (1978) Concurrent extraperitoneal and intracaval rupture of an abdominal aneurysm. Med J Aust 1:517–518

Lymperopoulos S (1973) Diagnostic value of the cavography in urology. Z Urol Nephrol 66:401–412

McCoy RM (1969) Use of inferior venacavography in the evaluation of renal neoplasms. J Urol 102:556–559

McCullough DL (1974) Inferior vena caval extension of renal carcinoma: a lost cause? Roentgenographic and pathologic findings in surgical patients. AJR 121:819–826

Musiani U (1977) Hypernephroma of the right kidney with inferior vena caval and right atrial thrombosis: case study and successful removal. J Urol 118:472–473

O'Halloran JF (1969) Concomitant aortography and inferior venacavography in patients with abdominal masses. Arch Surg 98:341–343

Okuda K (1977) Angiographic demonstration of growth of hepatocellular carcinoma in the hepatic vein and inferior vena cava. Radiology 124:33–36

Palmer J (1975) Diagnosis of venous extension in renal cell carcinoma. The value of routine inferior venacavography. Australas Radiol 19:265–271

Reckless JP (1972) Aorto-caval fistulae: an uncommon complication of abdominal aortic aneurysms. Br J Surg 59:461–462

Resnick MI (1973) Testicular tumor presenting as inferior vena caval thrombosis. J Urol 109:656–658

Rignault D (1976) Budd-Chiari syndrome caused by a membranous stenosis of the inferior vena cava. Chirurgie 102:913–920

Samuels S (1970) Alveolar hydatid disease involvement of the inferior vena cava. Am Surg 36:698–701

Schechter LS (1974) Venous obstruction in pelvis lipomatosis. J Urol 111:757–759

Seal PV (1970) Rupture of an abdominal aortic aneurysm into the inferior vena cava. A report of 3 cases. Br J Surg 57:904–906

Spayregen S (1973) Anterior displacement of the inferior vena cava by hepatic masses. Angiology 24:619–626

Svane S (1969) Tumor thrombus of the inferior vena cava resulting from renal carcinoma. A report of 12 autopsied cases. J Urol Nephrol (Paris) 3:245–256

Vix VA (1972) Elevated inferior vena cava pressure in ascites. Therapeutic implications in portocaval shunt. Am J Surg 123:721–723

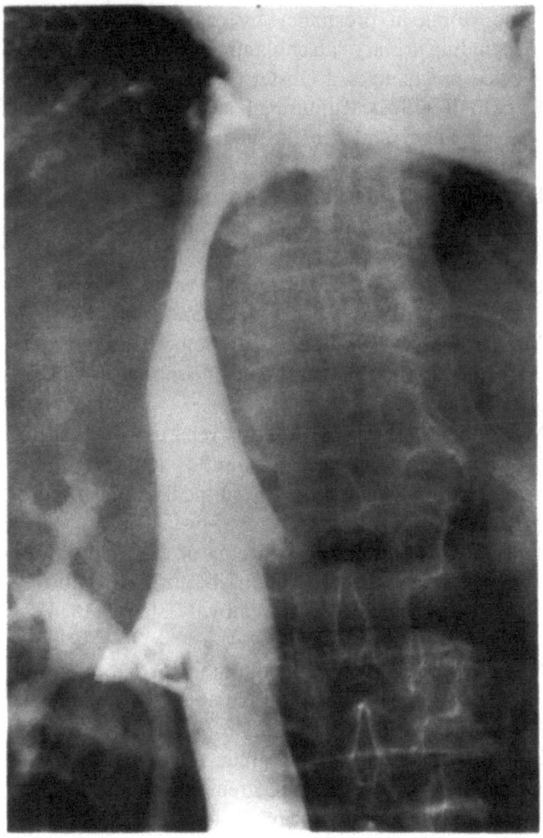

Fig. 8.1. Cirrhosis. Stenosis of the retrohepatic segment of the inferior vena cava: this stenosis is regular but slightly asymmetrical; it begins on the intrahepatic segment and finishes with a mild dilatation of the suprahepatic juxta-auricular part of the inferior vena cava

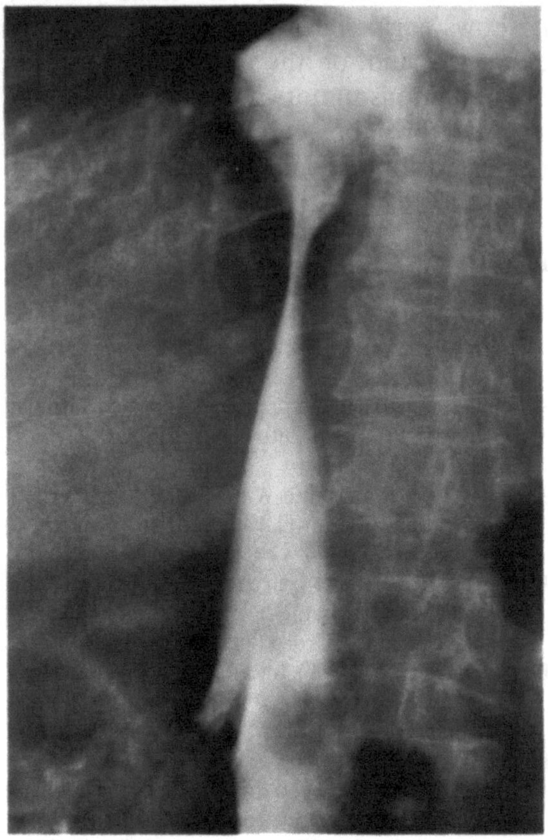

Fig. 8.2. Atrophic cirrhosis. Note the tight stenosis of the retrohepatic segment of the inferior vena cava. The stenosis is regular with clear-cut borders and there is an important dilatation of the infrahepatic segment of the inferior vena cava. The lateral view often shows anteroposterior dilatation of the cava

Fig. 8.3. Cirrhosis. There is sometimes dilatation of the retrohepatic segment of the vena cava as in this case of atrophic cirrhosis. The cava is quite normal up to the level of the renal veins and then undergoes clear right-left distension ▷

Fig. 8.4. Ascites. Note the narrowness of the infrarenal segment of the inferior vena cava which has nevertheless perfectly parallel walls. From the renal veins on, the caliber of the inferior vena cava decreases progressively and becomes extremely tiny. This stenosis is quite regular. The suprahepatic segment of the inferior cava is normal. After the ascites has been punctured, the inferior vena cava regains normal appearance

Fig. 8.5a, b. Ascites. a Frontal view in the supine position. There is a very progressive, regular and perfectly symmetrical narrowing of the inferior vena cava above the renal veins. b Right lateral decubitus. The inferior vena cava regains its normal diameter since the hydrostatic pressure exerted by the ascites upon the inferior vena cava is lesser in this position. On a lateral view in the supine position the same narrowing would be visible as on the frontal view

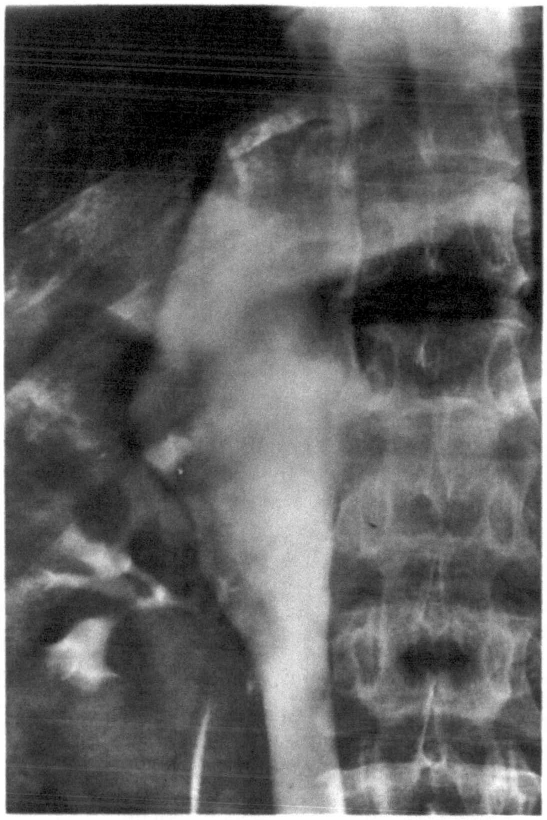
8.3

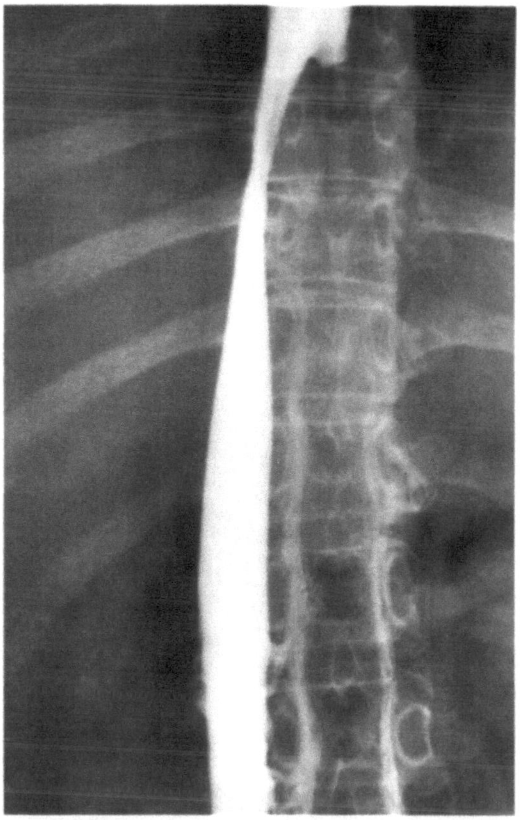
8.4

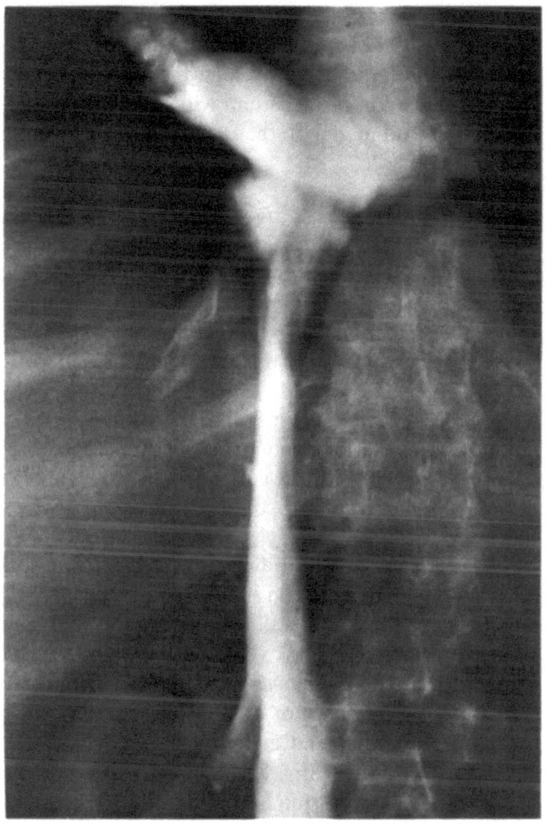
8.5a

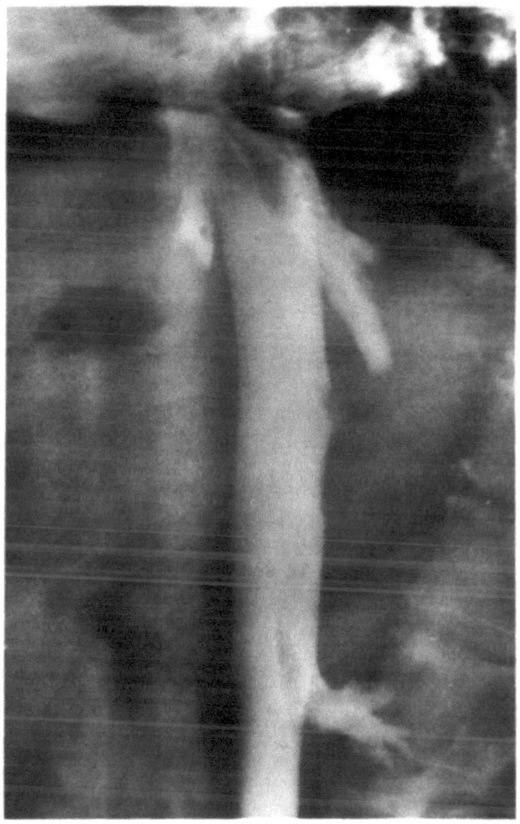
8.5b

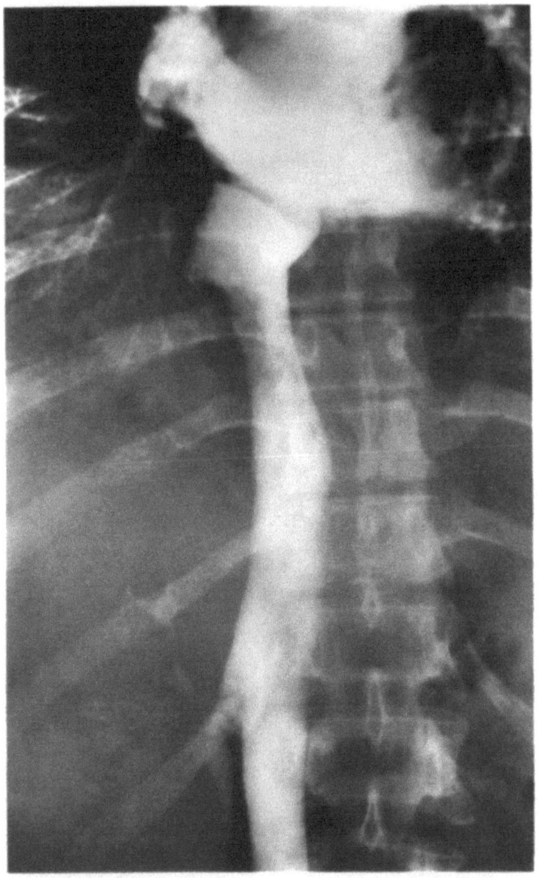

8.6a

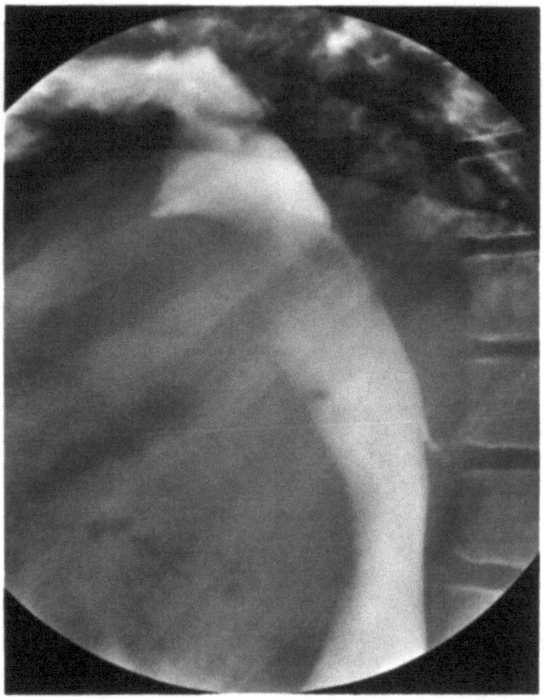

8.6b

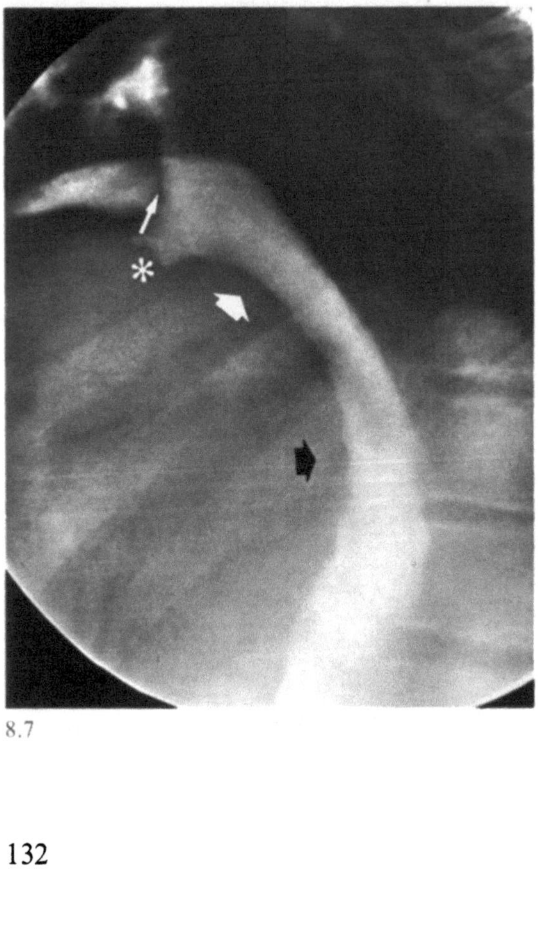

8.7

Fig. 8.6a, b. Inferior vena cavography in a Budd-Chiari syndrome. a Frontal view. b Lateral view. There is a compression of the right anterolateral aspect of the inferior vena cava due to hypertrophy of the caudate lobe in a Budd-Chiari's syndrome. Moreover, note the "beaklike" appearance of the terminal segment of the large hepatic vein which corresponds to the opacification of its ostium without dilution of the contrast medium, due to the beyond located thrombosis

Fig. 8.7. Inferior vena cavography in a Budd-Chiari syndrome. A lateral view shows the extrinsic compression of the retrohepatic segment of the cava by the hypertrophic caudate lobe (↗); "funnellike" appearance due to the opacification of the obstructed large hepatic vein (*). Note the Eustachian valvule (↗)

Fig. 8.8a, b. Hydatid cyst of the left liver lobe. Desaxation of the inferior vena cava, with compression of its anterior wall in the lower segment of its retrohepatic course by the hydatid cyst ▷

Fig. 8.9a, b. Huge hydatid cyst of the right liver lobe: a High centered cavogram shows extrinsic compression onto the right lateral wall of the inferior vena cava. Due to a huge cyst, this vessel is markedly displaced toward the left. b A lower centered cavogram demonstrates the presence of an absolutely misknown intracaval thrombus (*). Cavography is an indispensable investigation in cases with voluminous hydatid cysts. Indeed, any compression onto the cava produces stasis and possibly thrombosis (risk of postoperative embolism) ▷

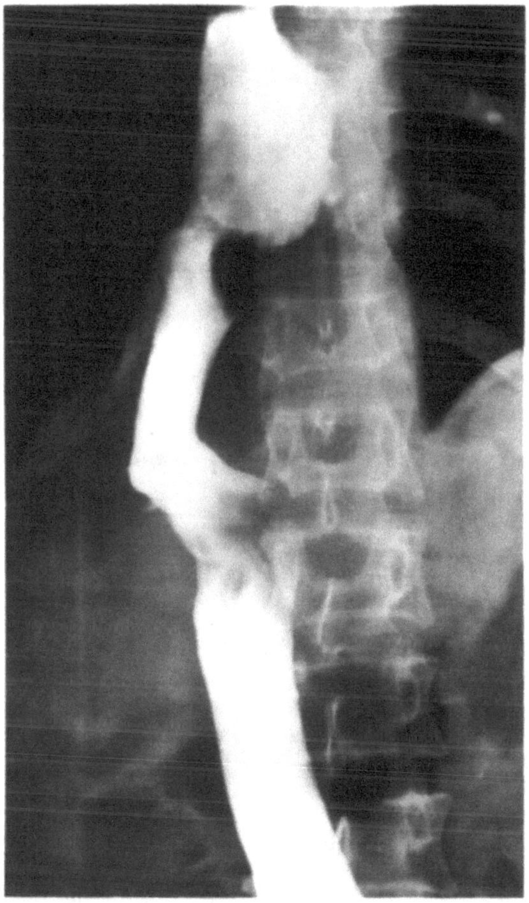

8.8a

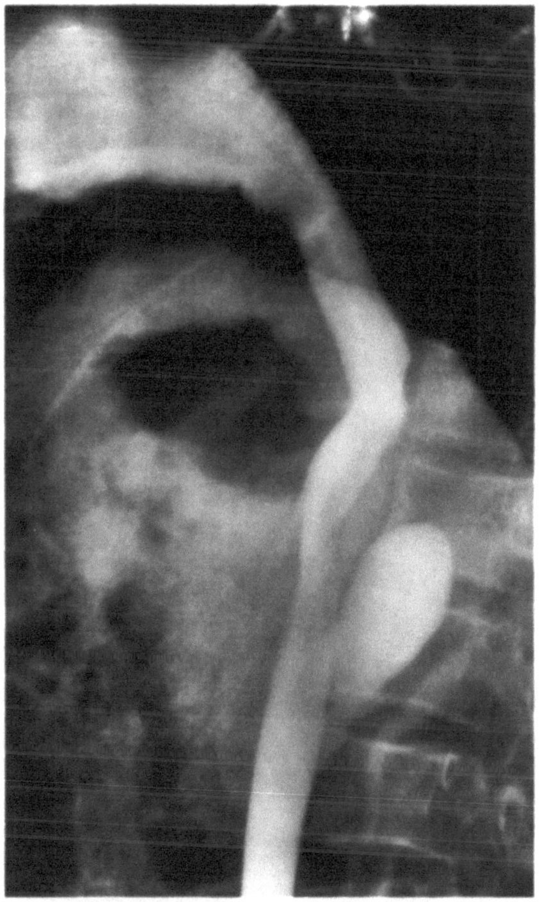

8.8b

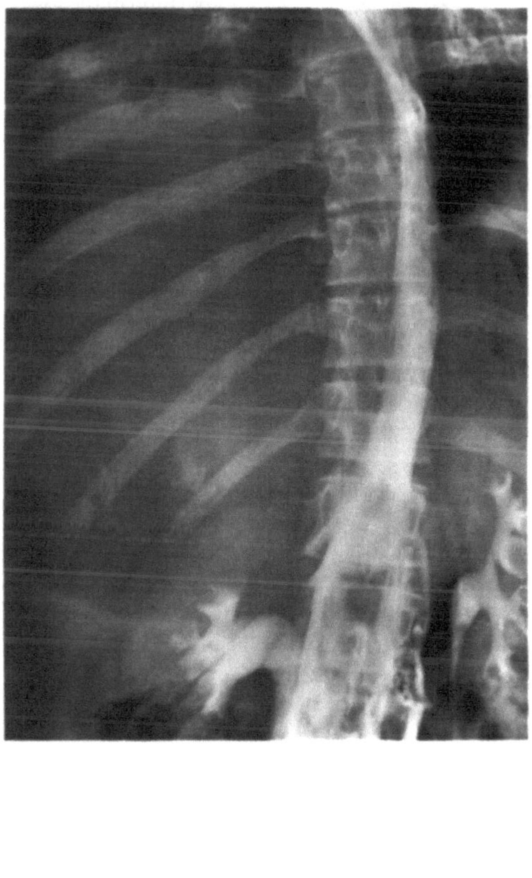

8.9a

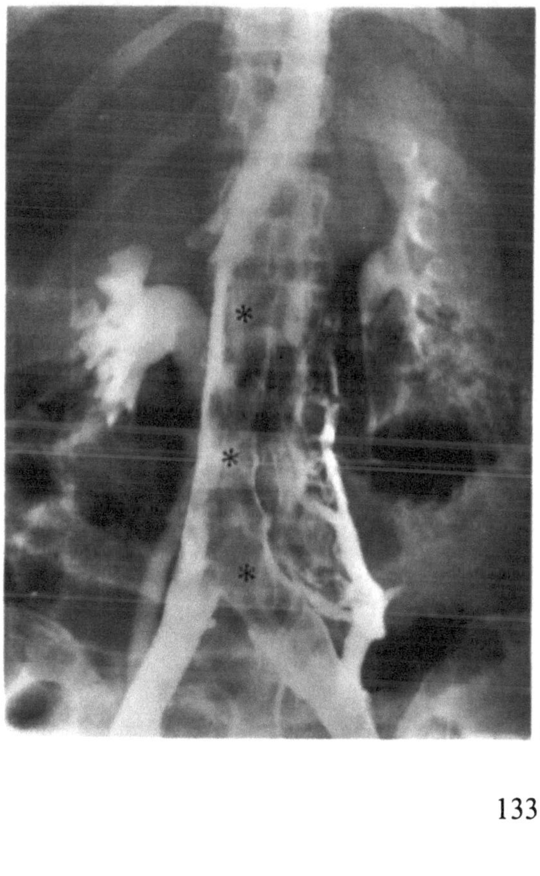

8.9b

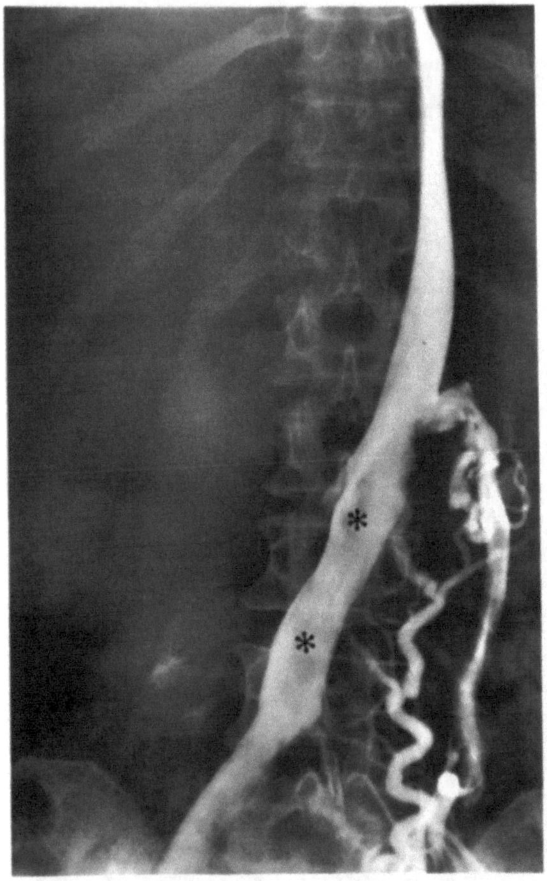

8.10a

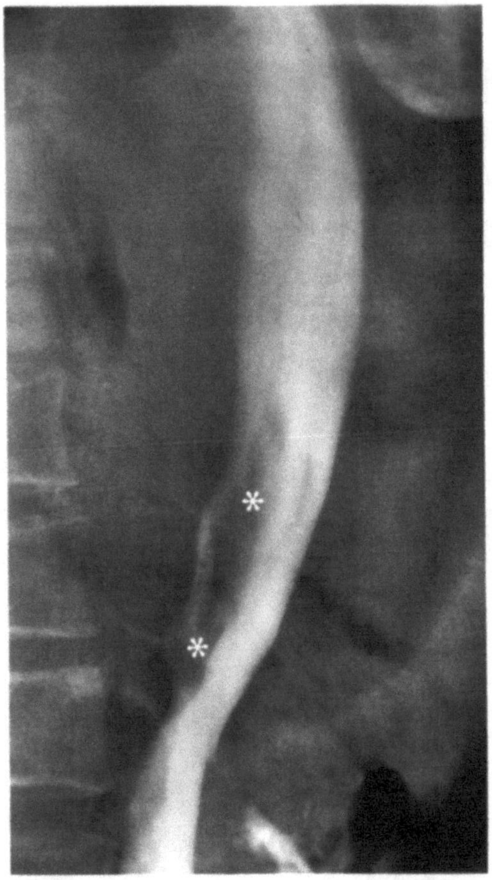

8.10b

Fig. 8.10a, b. Huge simple biliary cyst of the right liver lobe. Extended extrinsic compression of the inferior vena cava, which is displaced to the left of the spine. Note that due to the importance of the compression and of the stasis, the presence of an intracaval thrombus has been completely missed (*). Besides, there is a thrombosis of the left common iliac system (a: frontal view). The lateral view (b) shows particularly well the thrombus (*). Note the anteroposterior dilatation of the inferior vena cava which drapes over the biliary cyst. Orthogonal projections are indispensable to appreciate venous compressions and invasions

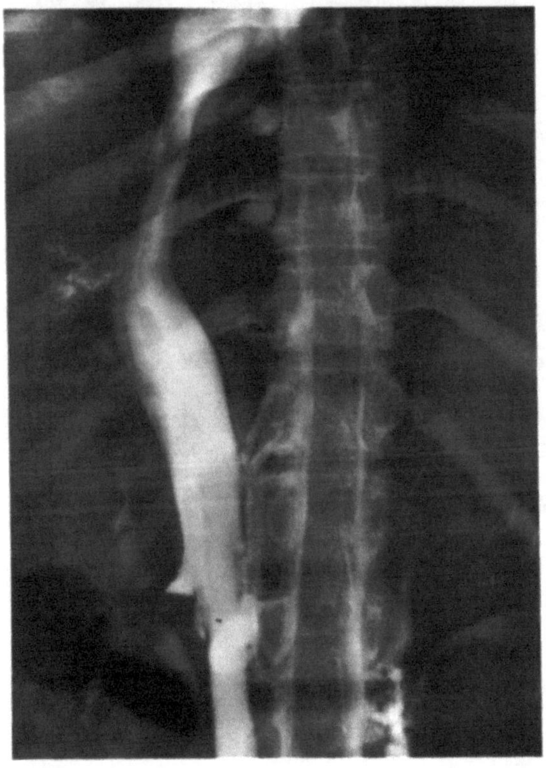

Fig. 8.11. Hepatoma of the left liver lobe. Note the compression and displacement of the vena cava. But since there is only extrinsic compression, the caval walls remain perfectly regular. There is already some mainly intraspinal collateral circulation

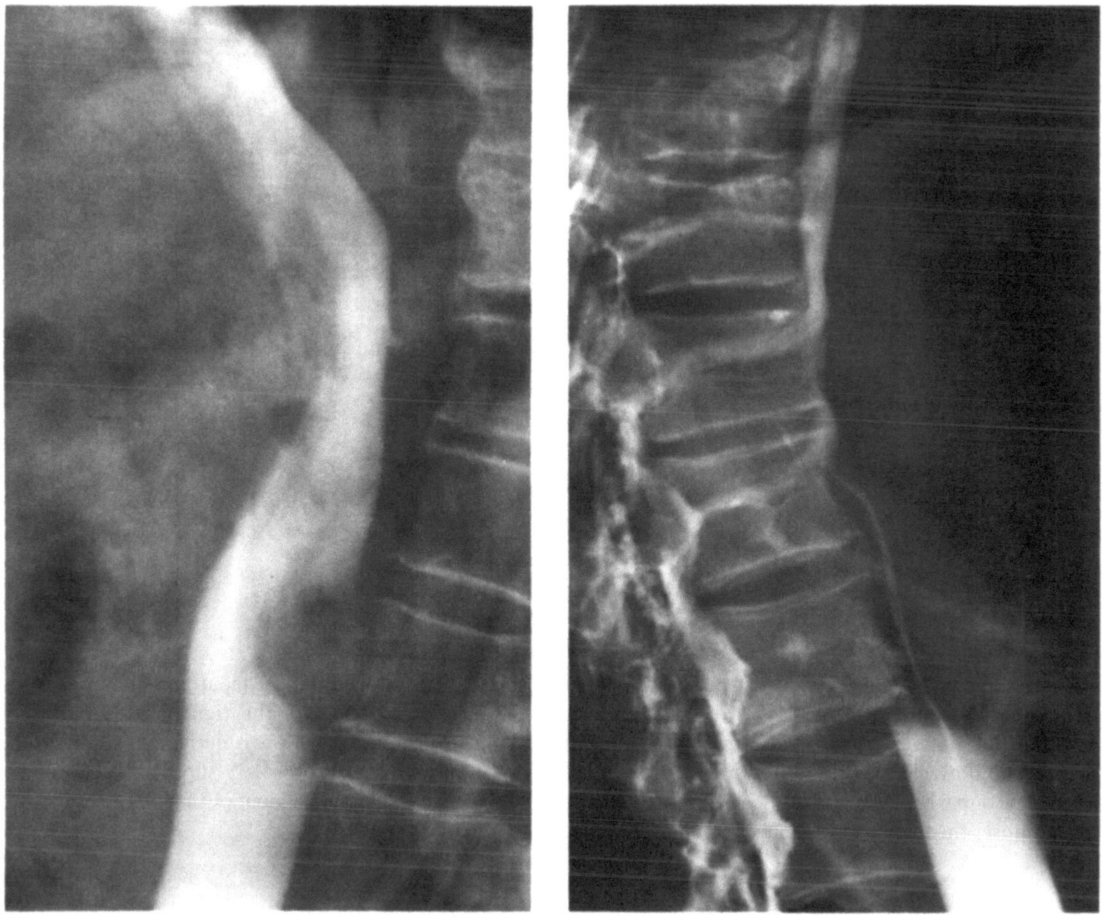

8.12a 8.12b

Fig. 8.12a, b. Extrinsic compression due to a hepatoma of the right liver lobe. a X-ray in right lateral decubitus: very clear impression of the hepatic neoplastic nodules on the inferior vena cava. b X-ray in left lateral decubitus: Clearly increased compression of the inferior vena cava. Complete obstruction of the retrohepatic segment of this vessel; drainage occurs via the peri- and intraspinal plexuses

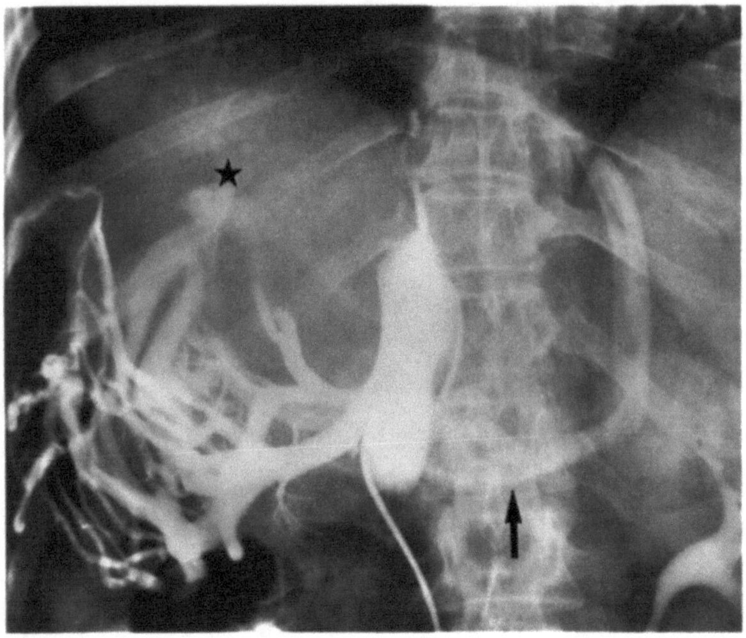

Fig. 8.13. Extrinsic compression of the inferior vena cava by a hepatoma in segment VIII of the right liver lobe. The inferior vena cava is flattened: to circumvent the hepatic obstacle, the blood flows first through the accessory suprahepatic veins, then via intrahepatic anastomoses through distal branches of the right large suprahepatic vein. But the hepatoma compresses also the terminal segment of the right large suprahepatic vein (∗). Therefore the flow is derivated, via interlobar anastomoses, toward the left suprahepatic vein (↗) and the suprahepatic segment of the inferior vena cava

Fig. 8.14. Invading of the inferior vena cava by a hepatoma of the right liver lobe. The hepatoma invades directly the wall of the inferior vena cava and causes irregularity on the right lateral wall of its retrohepatic segment (→) ▷

Fig. 8.15. Tumoral invasion of the hepatic segment of the inferior vena cava by a hepatoma. The intracaval bud is much larger and causes partial obstruction of the inferior vena cava. Some contrast material around this irregular bud provides it a somewhat "vermicular" appearance (→)

Fig. 8.16. Extrinsic compression of the inferior vena cava by a large hepatic hemangioma. This hemangioma involves the whole liver and more particularly the left lobe, causing extrinsic pressure on the anterior and left lateral wall of the postrenal segment of the inferior vena cava. Any intra-abdominal mass, whether of hepatic origin or not, reaching a certain volume, may affect the inferior vena cava

Fig. 8.17. Compression of the infrahepatic segment of the inferior vena cava by a tumor of the quadrate lobe. This mainly intraperitoneal tumor compresses and displaces the inferior vena cava

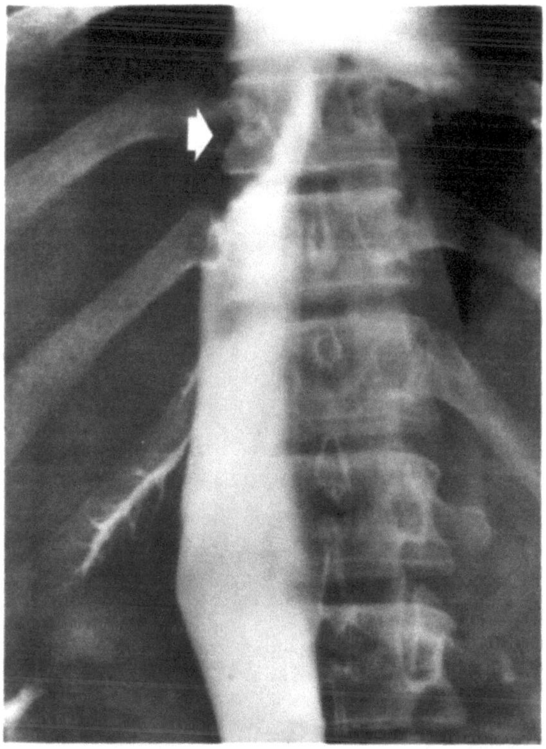
8.14

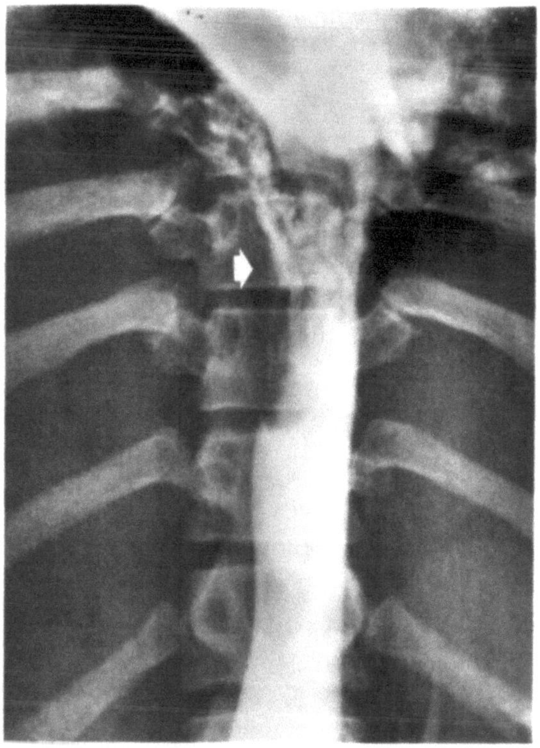
8.15

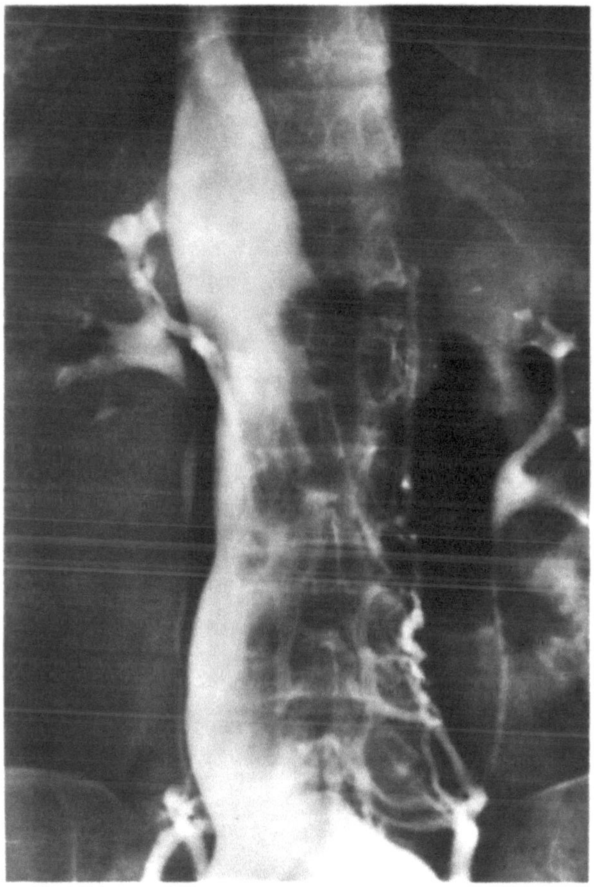
8.16

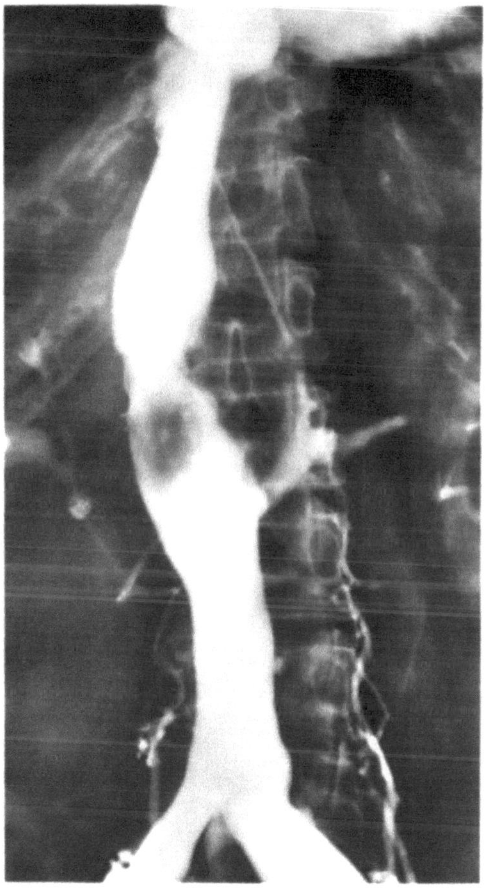
8.17

Chapter 9. Renal Venography

Catheterization of the renal veins has been used for years to obtain blood samples, but it was only in 1956 that Harrisson performed the first renal phlebographies for diagnosing renal vein occlusion. Since then numerous indications have been proposed: renovascular hypertension (Abrams), extensions of renal and retroperitoneal masses (Kahn), vascular impressions (Nebesar). However, due to the inconstant opacification of the intrarenal veins, some authors consider this investigation to have very few indications. It is currently regaining interest thanks to technical improvements allowing more constant opacification. Among these, use of occlusive catheters with balloons has been almost completely given up, whereas the pharmacoangiographic method, proposed by Olin, is now frequently employed. Thanks to this improvement, renal venography can be considered as an easy and safe method affording valuable data for the diagnosis of renal diseases and of renal vein involvements.

9.1 Anatomy (Fig. 9.1)

The anatomy of the renal veins is characterized by absence of symmetry of the trunks and identical intrarenal disposition.

9.1.1 Right Renal Vein

The right renal vein is short, about 3 cm from the hilus to the inferior vena cava, and courses anteriorly, medially and cranially. It is located ventrally to the renal artery. It receives the veins of the perirenal venous ring, the pyelic and ureteral veins, the right gonadal vein in 10% of cases, and, exceptionally, an accessory adrenal vein. Duplication of the renal vein is seen in about 25% of cases and does not always correspond to multiple renal arteries. These double renal veins usually have the same caliber and are superposed. They communicate extensively inside the kidney.

9.1.2 Left Renal Vein

The left renal vein is rather long (mean value: 8 cm), horizontal, orientated medially, and located anteriorly to the renal artery. It courses ventral to the aorta and dorsal to the superior mesenteric artery. It usually receives the gonadal vein on its inferior surface and the left adrenal vein on its superior surface. There are also communications with the ascending lumbar vein (renoazygolumbar arcade). The left renal vein enters the inferior vena cava perpendicularly.

Variations on this side are different from the right side. Duplication of the left renal vein is rare (1%). There exist abnormal courses, e.g., the retroaortic course (3%), uncommonly opening onto the iliac vein.

The most common anomaly is the periaortic ring, which is seen in 17% to 20% of cases. At the level of the hilus a single vein splits into two branches at the lateral aspect of the aorta: the main, horizontal branch passes in front of the aorta and the smaller branch courses obliquely downward and laterally and passes behind the aorta.

9.1.3 Intrarenal Venous System

This system is similar on both sides and quite analogous to the arterial system. It arises at the level of the peritubular capillary networks to form on the one hand the cortical interlobular veins, and on the other the medullar venae rectae. These veins form Verheyen's star, situated at the base of the pyramids and constituted by the arcuate veins. The latter bend at the level of the renal columns to form the interlobular veins, the lobular veins, and finally, the trunk of the renal vein.

9.2 Technique

In order to overcome inadequacies of opacification of the intrarenal veins, a number of different methods have been proposed; some of them have been abandoned or are only used by some phlebographers. In fact the most-used technique is retrograde selective renal venography by femoral approach. The following techniques are used:

1) Renal venography by percutaneous puncture (Leger and Gilranz) (Fig. 9.2).
2) Renal venography by cutdown of the left spermatic vein (Peluffa).
3) Renal venography by catheter with balloons: a) *Occlusive renal venography,* with a catheter placed in the inferior vena cava (Gillot, Thalheimer). This technique necessitates the placement of a catheter with one balloon above and the other below the renal veins. Injection is made between the inflated balloons during temporary blockage of the caval return (Fig. 9.3). b) *Selective renal venography* by catheter with balloons (Galmarini, Takaro).
4) Selective renal venography, performed by retrograde femoral catheterization or by puncture either of a vein of the arm or of the jugular vein in cases of iliac or caval obstruction. a) *Technique described by Kahn.* This is the most commonly used. Retrograde opacification of a vein with a high forward flow rate necessitates the injection of large amounts of contrast material in a short time (Fig. 9.4). The technical principles are:

Utilization of a relatively large catheter (outer diameter 8–9 French) with side holes and a 180° bend at the end, the distance across the bend being about 50% greater than the diameter of the inferior vena cava. The catheter must be placed at the level of the renal hilus, without entering a branch of the renal vein (Fig. 9.5).

Injection of a large amount of contrast material at a high rate: 40 to 60 ml delivered at 20 to 30 ml/s.

Rapid but short serial filming: two to three films per second for 5 s.

This technique provides opacification of the entire renal venous system up to the arcuate veins in 70% of cases.

As concerns renal transplantation, the technical principles are the same, but the catheter used has a different bend (Fig. 9.6). b) *Technical improvements.* Pharmacoangiography has brought improvements. The method has was proposed by Olin and Reuter and has been used by numerous authors. It consists in diminution of the arterial blood flow with ensuing better retrograde opacification as far as the cortical veins. It necessitates arterial catheterization, but numerous indications for renal venography are also indications for arteriography. Renal venography under arterial blockage is thus often possible. It consists of the injection of a small dose of epinephrine into the renal artery (from 5 to 15 µg, depending on the weight of the patient, injected in 30 s), immediately prior to a renal venography performed according to the technique described above (Fig. 9.7).

5) Sampling in the renal veins has been performed for a long time especially for estimation of the renin plasmatic activity and for determination of extraction of *p*-aminohippuric acid. The catheterization technique is the same. For the interpretation of the results one must take into account the phlebographic data and particularly the anatomic anomalies. Sampling in the trunks of the renal veins is easy. The catheter must be placed at the level of the hilus, beyond the gonadal and suprarenal veins on the left. Strong aspirations lead to impure samples and should thus be avoided, and spontaneous outflow preferred. Segmental sampling requires catheters with a long intermediate portion and a distal tip curved upward or downward. Catheter guidance systems are useful for the placement. In this case, spontaneous outflow is a compulsory condition.

The renal venographic technique is usually quite simple, the investigation is practically harmless. Venous complications at the puncture site are rare. Perforation of a vein with the guide wire or subintimal injections of contrast material may occur; elementary precautions should however help to avoid them.

9.3 Normal Findings

9.3.1 Right Renal Vein (Figs. 9.8 and 9.9)

The right renal vein's short course and almost anteroposterior axis account for its incomplete visualization on a frontal view. Its diameter is about 15 mm, and it is seen to make an angle of 45° with the inferior vena cava, which it enters at the level of the first lumbar vertebra. The extrarenal branches are only rarely opacified.

9.3.2 Left Renal Vein (Figs. 9.10 and 9.11)

The left renal vein has a frontal course. Its diameter is about 2 cm, but it becomes wider in its terminal portion, ventral to the aorta. It forms an angle of 80° to 90° with the inferior vena cava, which it enters at the L1–L2 interspace. The adrenal vein is frequently opacified (70% of cases) as well as the gonadal vein (80%) and the renoazygolumbar arcade (47%).

The injection also demonstrates in most cases a periaortic ring with its inferior branch oblique downward and medially, of smaller caliber and entering the inferior vena cava at the L3–L4 interspace.

9.3.3 Intrarenal Veins

The best phlebographic techniques demonstrate the interlobular veins which join to form a closely anastomosed corticomedullar plexus corresponding to the arcuate veins. These form the interlobular veins which drain into three trunks on the left (superior, median, and inferior) and into two trunks on the right. On the left side the trunks join at the level of the hilus. On the right, joining may occur very close to the inferior vena cava.

The interpretation of a renal venogram depends on the quality of the opacification, so that nonvisualization of the peripheral veins must be interpreted critically.

9.4 Pathologic Findings

Renal venography is carried out in most of cases to demonstrate either a pathologic condition of the renal vein itself, most often obstruction; or renal or extrarenal conditions affecting the renal vein, in order to orientate the diagnosis or to appreciate the extent of the lesion.

9.4.1 Pathology of the Vein Proper

Thrombosis of the Main Renal Veins

Thrombosis of the renal veins is most often considered in adults presenting with a painful acute abdominal syndrome or with a nephrotic syndrome. It may also be a chance finding. The radiologic diagnosis may sometimes be suspected from the intravenous urography, but it requires arterial and venous investigations carried out at the same time for the following reasons:

The arteriogram provides indirect but nonnegligible signs. It also makes it possible to demonstrate certain etiologies and to rule out a tumoral process.

It allows one to perform a phlebogram with pharmacologic arterial blockage, which makes it possible to suppress false images.

Renal phlebography cannot always be performed, especially when there is obtruction of the inferior vena cava. Arteriography is then the only available investigation.

The radiologic investigation has two aims: diagnosis, and demonstration of the extent of the disease in view of a possible surgical procedure.

The radiological results depend on the anatomic type:

a) *Thrombosis of the Renal Veins of Peripheral Origin.* This type of thrombosis is most often secondary to a renal parenchymal disease. It extends more or less to the renal venous trunk. Phlebography is the only radiologic investigation that gives evidence of peripheral renal vein occlusion. It may show a *direct sign.*: the intraluminal defect characterized by a radiolucent lacuna delineated by contrast material (Fig. 9.12). This is the fundamental sign, the site of which depends on the extension of the disease. The presence of a dome-shaped cutoff of the vein is difficult to interpret since a filling defect may present similar images (Figs. 9.13 and 9.14). Alternatively, *indirect signs* may be seen: stagnation of the contrast material, and evidence of perirenal collateral circulation (Fig. 9.15).

b) *Occlusion of the Trunk of the Renal Vein* (Fig. 9.16). This is most often due to invasion or to extrinsic compression (adenopathy, retroperitoneal tumors, cancer of the pancreas, retroperitoneal fibrosis). More rarely it is an intrinsic obstruction, secondary to a trauma or to a tumor. When the inferior vena cava is patent, renal venography should be carried out with great caution, so as to avoid dislodging a thrombus. It will then allow differentiation of extrinsic from intrinsic obstruction. Intrinsic obstruction presents as described above. Extrinsic obstruction causes a more or less marked narrowing of the vein, which has irregular walls due to the tumoral infiltration. Sometimes, there is total cutoff of the vein. The vein is often abnormally located, for instance displaced anteroposteriorly. These anomalies are especially informative for the appreciation of the tumoral extension.

c) *Occlusion of the Inferior Vena Cava Involving the Renal Veins.* This may occur in thromboembolic disease or be due to a tumor (adrenal, retroperitoneal, hepatic, or of the opposite kidney). Inferior vena cavography suffices. The only technique for the opacification of the renal veins would be a percutaneous puncture, but it does not seem necessary for these cases.

Other Venous Diseases

Traumatisms of the renal vein most often pass undetected; they are only rarely seen at the time of the injury.

Venous malformations should be suspected when there are vascular impressions on the renal pelvis, especially associated with hematuria; in such cases, renal venography should be performed, to search for pyelic or ureteral varices (Fig. 9.17).

9.4.2 Tumoral Pathology

Renal venography is performed either for diagnosis or to determine the tumoral extension.

Diagnostic Renal Phlebography

This investigation is seldom used for the differential diagnosis of renal cysts and hypernephromas. A noncharacteristic tumoral syndrome may be seen in both cases. The presence of a venous cutoff would suggest a malignancy (Fig. 9.18). There are two conditions for which the phlebogram orientates the diagnosis:

Tumors of the excretory system for which the diagnosis is difficult (infiltrative tumor without renal symptoms or obstruction). In this case, renal venography is often more informative than arteriography, since it demonstrates infiltration of the walls and cutoff of veins.

Infiltrative renal lymphomas. The outspread and stretched appearance of the veins would be evocative. According to Kahn, renal venography would be a simple method for following up treatment of such lymphomas.

Renal Phlebography for Determining the Extension of Hypernephromas

When it is cautiously carried out after verification of the patency of the inferior vena cava, renal phlebography makes it possible to ascertain the patency of the renal vein (Figs. 9.19 and 9.20). There will be either total cutoff, or cutoff of a branch at the level of the tumor, or a defect corresponding to an intraluminal thrombus (Fig. 9.21).

However, renal phlebography may at times be less appropriate than selective arteriography, which besides establishing the diagnosis of hypernephroma, allows one to appreciate venous involvement.

9.4.3 Other Renal Parenchymal Diseases

Renal Atrophies and Hypoplasiae

The renal venogram gives clues for the differential diagnosis between renal agenesia and a small nonfunctional kidney, acquired or hypoplastic. The differentiation varies according to the diseased side. *On the left side,* in case of agenesia of the kidney, there is a venous trunk, from which the gonadal and adrenal veins arise, but no renal vein beyond. Contrariwise, when there is a parenchymatous primordium, the renal phlebography demonstrates a network of intrarenal veins (Fig. 9.22). *On the right side,* there is no renal vein in cases of agenesia. But failure of catheterization may also be responsible for its nonvisualization, so that a conclusive diagnosis cannot be made. On both sides, the caliber of the vein, in its terminal segment on the right and before the suprarenal and gonadal veins on the left, will suggest whether a small kidney is acquired or congenital (Figs. 9.23 and 9.24).

Hypertension of Renal Origin

Abrams proposes combining renal venography with the withdrawal of samples in patients with obstructive lesions of the renal artery. Renal phlebography permits study of the venous washout of the contrast material. Normally the injected contrast material disappears within 2–3 s. Diminution in the arterial flow, whatever its origin – stenosis of the trunk or peripheral nephroangiosclerosis – causes prolonged washout, lasting 6 s on average. This test is useful mainly for assessing the condition of the kidney contralateral to the one with arterial stenosis.

Chronic Nephropathies

For these cases renal phlebography is of less value. According to Kahn and Rosch it would give clues as to the etiology and permit differentiation between chronic pyelonephritis, chronic glomerulonephritis, and nephroangiosclerosis.

Traumatic Lesions of the Renal Parenchyma

According to Braedel, renal phlebography is indicated for the study of the parenchyma in the vicinity of an arterial stenosis. It shows either nonopacification with or without extravasation, when the parenchyma is destroyed, or almost normal opacification with prolonged washout, when there is isolated arterial occlusion.

9.5 Indications

According to certain authors the indications for renal phlebography are very restricted. For others, however, they are very large. For the discussion one must take into account that the method is easy and safe, and that some diseases have early venous lesions.

9.5.1 Thromboses of the Renal Veins

Suspicion of thrombosis of the renal veins is the main and unanimously recognized indication for renal phlebography.

Renal venography associated with arteriography is the only method that will demonstrate thrombosis of the intrarenal veins. It must always be coupled with inferior vena cavography and is contraindicated as soon as the thrombosis of the renal veins extends to the inferior vena cava.

9.5.2 Appreciation of the Extension of Renal and Retroperitoneal Tumors

With renal tumors, the invasion of the renal vein is appreciated in most cases by the study of the venous return in the arteriogram. Renal venography will be performed in doubtful cases. However, the important sign is the opacification of the inferior vena cava; opacification of the renal vein is interesting for the prognosis. As concerns retroperitoneal tumors, tumors of the body of the pancreas and adrenal tumors, renal phlebography is rarely performed (Fig. 9.25).

9.5.3 Silent Kidneys

A renal venogram may help to determine the etiology in cases of silent kidney. It permits diagnosis of renal agenesia, especially of the left kidney, and, in some cases, differentiation of major hypoplasia and nonfunctional atrophy. If there is an obstructive silent kidney, renal phlebography may provide clues suggesting a malignant tumor of the excretory system stenosing the renal pelvis.

9.5.4 Intraparenchymal Infiltration Processes

Renal phlebography may give arguments in favor of an invasive renal tumor or of lymphomatous involvement of the kidney.

9.5.5 Hematuria with Irregularities in the Renal Pelvis

The existence of pyelic irregularities may be consistent with extrinsic vascular impressions or with an invasive tumor of the renal pelvis. Renal phlebography may show varices around the renal pelvis, and collateral venous circulation associated with thrombosis of the renal veins. It provides an argument in favor of tumors of the excretory system.

9.5.6 Miscellaneous

Other uses of renal venography may be mentioned. It can provide detailed knowledge of the renal vascular anatomy in a donor for renal transplants. It can also be used in studying the patency of some splenorenal anastomoses (Fig. 9.26). Indications for renal vein sampling fall outside the scope of radiology.

9.6 Conclusion

Renal venography is an easy and safe investigation. Inconstant results and difficult interpretation are its main drawbacks. These may be eliminated by use of perfectly adapted techniques. Renal phlebography after blockage of the arterial flow gives the best results; although it requires arterial catheterization, this should not be considered a drawback, since the main indications for renal venography also necessitate an arteriogram. Carrying out both investigations simultaneously does not increase the risks, permits more reliable diagnosis, and improves the quality of the venogram.

References

Abrams HL, Baum S, Stamey T (1964) Renal venous washout time in renovascular hypertension. Radiology 83:597–609

Ahlberg NE, Bartley O, Chidekel N, Wahlqvist L (1967) An anatomic and roentgenographic study of the communications of the renal vein in patients with and without renal carcinoma. Scand J Urol Nephrol 1:43–51

Anson BJ, Kurth LE (1955) Common variations in the renal blood supply. Surg Gynecol Obstet 100:157

Anson BJ, Caudwell EW, Pick JW, Beaton LE (1947) The blood supply of the kidney, suprarenal gland and associated structures. Surg Gynecol Obstet 84:313

Beres JA, Zboralske FF, Wilson SD, Amberg JR (1964) Percutaneous transrenal venography in experimental renal vein obstruction and human renal vein thrombosis. Radiology 83:587

Braedel HU, Moeller JF (1974) La phlébographie rénale rétrograde dans les traumatismes fermés du rein. J Radiol Electrol Med Nucl 55:867–873

Braedel HU, Haage H, Moeller JF, Schindler E (1976a) Differential diagnostic importance of retrograde phlebography in cases of unusual ectasia and renal pelvic deformity. Radiology 119:65–69

Braedel HU, Schindler E, Moeller JF, Polsky MS (1976b) Renal phlebography: An aid in the diagnosis of the absent or non functioning kidney. J Urol 116:703–707

Caron J, Bonte G, Ribet M (1963) Technique de phlébographie rénale. J Radiol Electrol Med Nucl 44:329–332

Chait A, Stoane L, Moskowitz H, Mellins HZ (1968) Renal vein thrombosis. Radiology 90:886–896

Chuang VP, Mena CE, Hoskins PA (1974) Congenital anomalies of the left renal vein. Angiographic consideration. Br J Radiol 47:214–219

Cope C, Isard HJ (1969) Left renal vein entrapment. A new diagnostic finding in retroperitoneal disease. Radiology 92:867–872

Dalla Palma L, Servello M (1956) La phlébographie rénale. Presse Med 64:150

Ferris EJ, Hipona FA, Kahn PC, Phillips E, Shapiro J (1969) Venography of the inferior vena cava and its branches. Williams and Wilkins, Baltimore

Fitz A (1967) Renal venous renin determinations in the diagnosis of surgically correctable hypertension. Circulation 36:942–950

Galmarini D, Forti D, Fassati LR, Pisani F, Rossi R (1966) La phlébographie rénale sous blocage rénal; nouvelle technique d'exploration. Presse Med 74:503–506

Gillot C, Stuhl L (1966) La phlébographie rénale occlusive; documents pathologiques obtenus en sériographie. Presse Med 74:1041–1046

Gillot C, Stuhl L, Ecoiffier J (1965) La phlébographie rénale occlusive; technique et résultats normaux. Presse Med 73:2215–2220

Gilsanz V, Estrada R, Anaya A (1965) Transparietal renal phlebography. A new method. Lancet 1:179–183

Gray RK, Katz RM (1969) Epinephrine-assisted renal venography in renal vein thrombosis: Report of two adolescents with nephrotic syndrome. Radiology 93:793

Harrison CV, Milne MD, Steiner RE (1956) Clinical aspects of renal vein thrombosis. J Med 25:285

Haverling M (1966) Renal phlebography – an experimental study in the pig. Acta Radiol [Suppl] (Stockh) 251, 1–74

Hipona FA, Crummy AB (1966) The roentgen diagnosis of renal vein thrombosis. Clinical aspects. AJR 98:122–131

Itzchak Y, Adar R, Mozes M, Deutsch V (1974) Renal venography in the diagnosis of agenesis and small contracted kidney. Clin Radiol 25:379–383

Kahn PC (1969) Selective venography in renal parenchymal disease. Radiology 92:345–350

Korobkin M, Glickman MG, Schambelan M (1976) Segmental renal vein sampling for renin. Radiology 118:307–315

Leger L, Proux C, Duranteau M (1957) Phlébographie rénale et cave inférieure par injections intraparenchymateuses. Presse Med 65:141

March TL, Halpern M (1963) Renal vein thrombosis demonstrated by selective renal phlebography. Radiology 81:958

Michel JR, Moreau JF, Chevrot A (1974) Choix d'une méthode angiographique dans l'exploration du cancer rénal. J Urol Nephrol 80:605–620

Michelakis AM, Foster JH, Liddle GW, Rhamy RK,

Kuchel O, Gordon RD (1967) Measurement of renin in both renal veins. Arch Intern Med 120:444–448

Mitty HA (1975) Circumaortic renal collar. A potentially hazardous anomaly of the left renal vein. AJR 125:307–310

Nebesar RA, Pollard JJ, Earley EE (1967) Renal vascular impressions. AJR 101:719–727

Padovani J (1971) Confrontation des différentes méthodes d'opacification des veines rénales. J Radiol Electrol Med Nucl 52:279

Peluffo JC, Paez BL (1963) Phlébographie rénale gauche par la veine spermatique. J Urol Nephrol 69:16

Pick JW, Anson BJ (1940) Renal vascular pedicle; anatomical study of 430 body-halves. J Urol 44:411

Rosch J, Antonovic R, Goldman ML, Dotter CT (1975) Epinephrine renal venography. ROEFO 123:501–515

Ross JA, Samuel E, Millar DR (1961) Variations in the renal vascular pedicle (an anatomical and radiological study with particular reference to renal transplantation). Br J Urol 33:478

Seldinger SI (1953) Catheter replacement of the needle in percutaneous arteriography. A new technique. Acta Radiol 39:368

Takaro T, Dow JA, Kishev S (1970) Selective occlusive renal phlebography in man. Radiology 94:589–596

Thalheimer M, Gillot JC (1962) La cavographie segmentaire. J Int Coll Surg 38:561

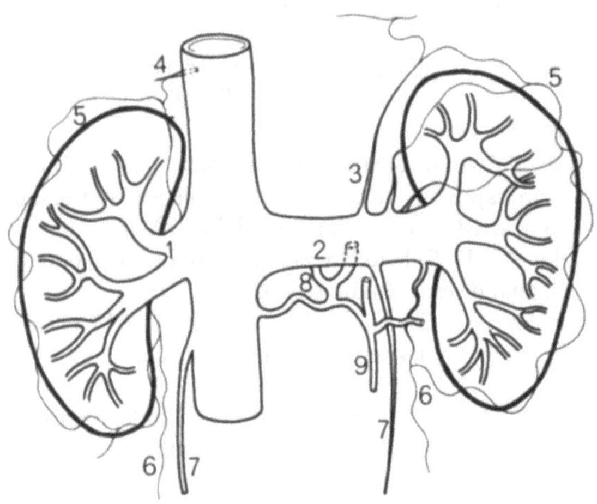

Fig. 9.1. Schema of the renal veins.

1 Right renal vein
2 Left renal vein
3 Left suprarenal vein
4 Right suprarenal vein
5 Perirenal veins
6 Ureteral vein
7 Gonadal vein
8 Renoazygolumbar arch
9 Ascending lumbar vein

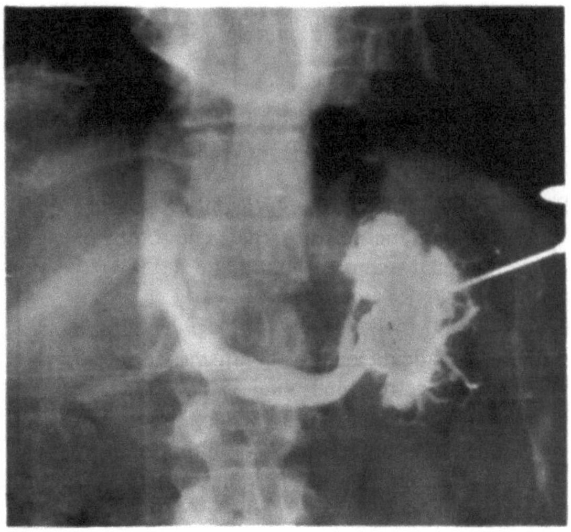

Fig. 9.2. Percutaneous renal venography. Good opacification of the left renal vein

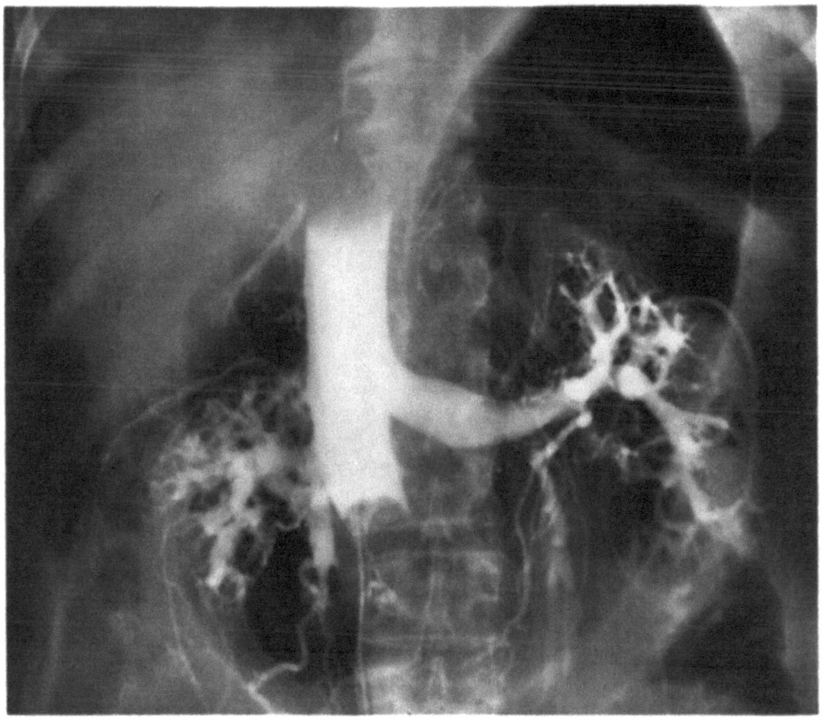

Fig. 9.3. Occlusive renal venography (Gillot's technique). Opacification of the entire retroperitoneal venous system

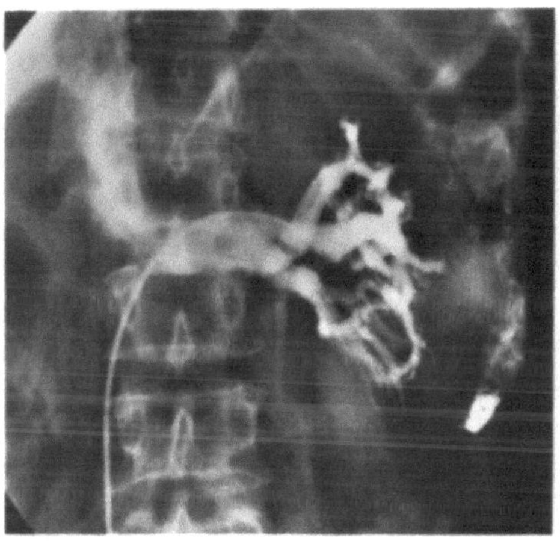

Fig. 9.4. Selective left renal venography. Opacification of the renal venous system up to the interlobular veins

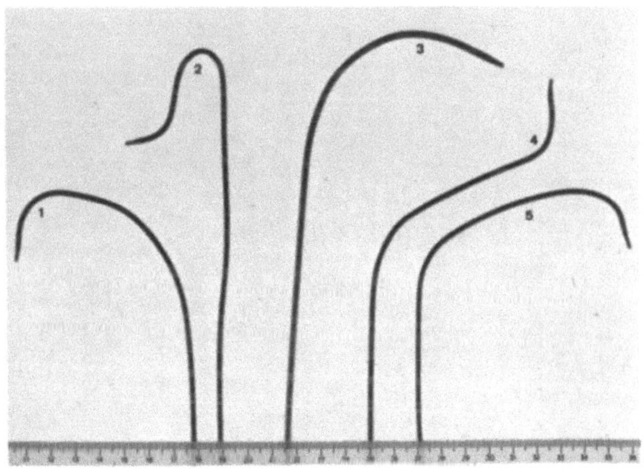

Fig. 9.5. Diagrammatic representation of catheters for renal phlebography and sampling.
1 Segmental sampling in the right inferior pole
2 Segmental sampling in the right superior pole
3 Right and left renal venography (side holes)
4 Segmental sampling in the left superior pole
5 Segmental sampling in the left inferior pole

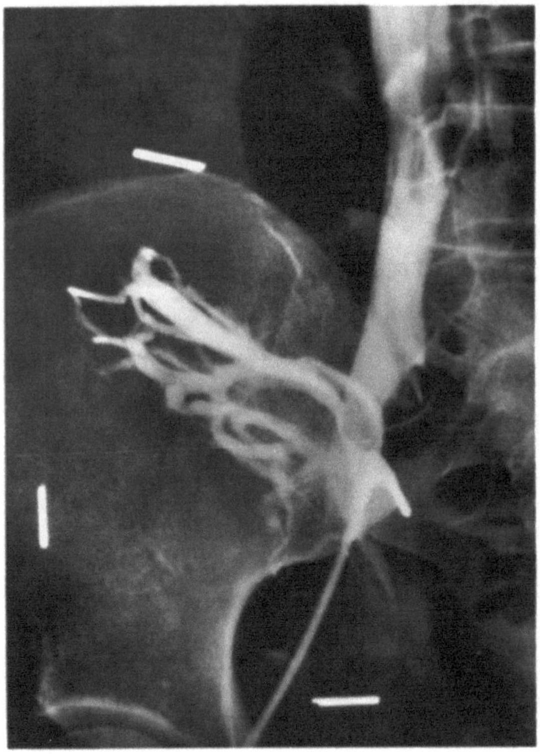

Fig. 9.6. Selective renal venography in a transplanted kidney. Correct opacification up to the interlobular veins

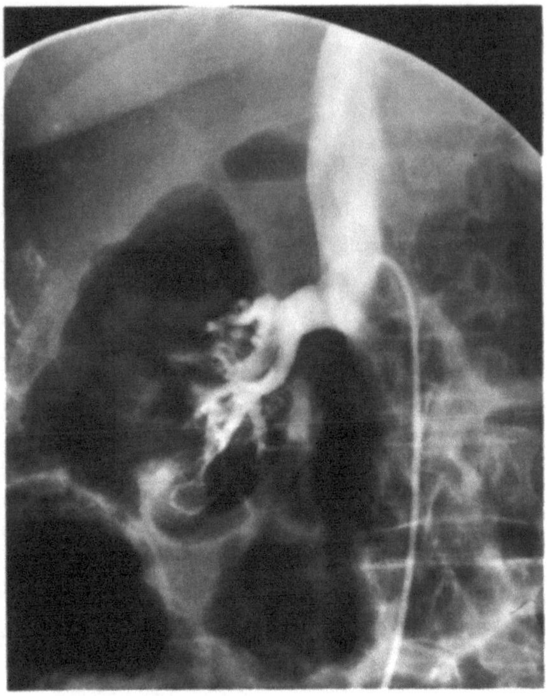

Fig. 9.8. Right renal venography. Insufficient opacification

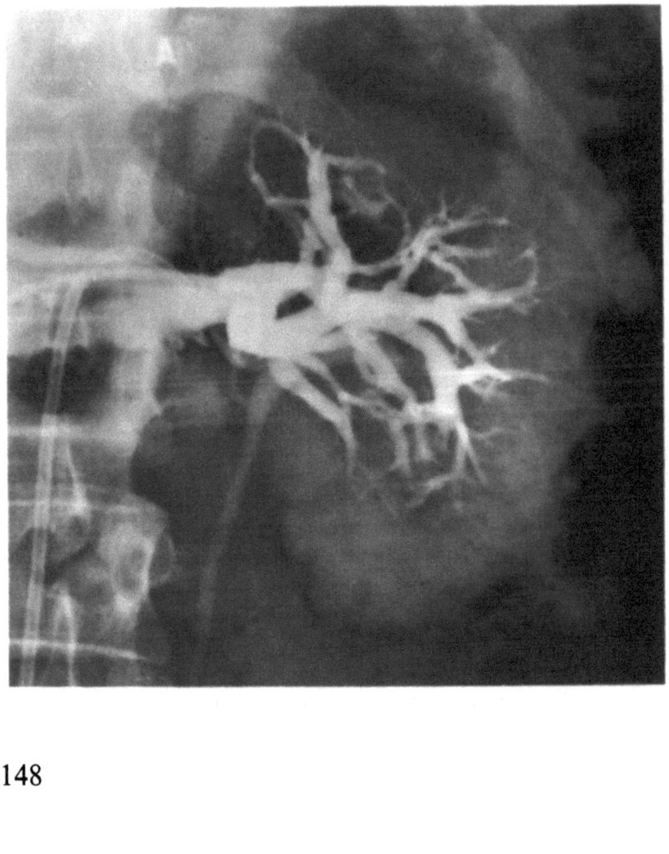

Fig. 9.7. Selective left renal venography (intra-arterial injection of adrenalin). Opacification of the whole renal venous system up to the inter-lobular veins

Fig. 9.9. Right renal venography. Presence of a double renal vein with lumbar anastomosis of the inferior renal vein

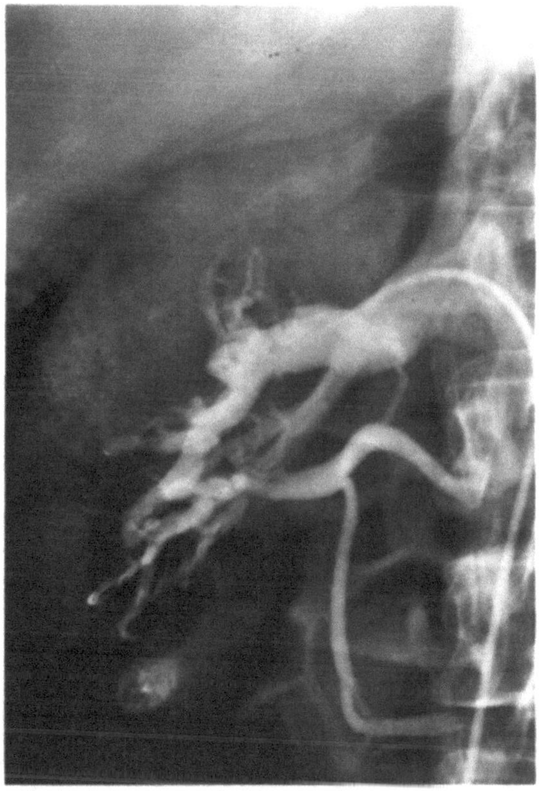

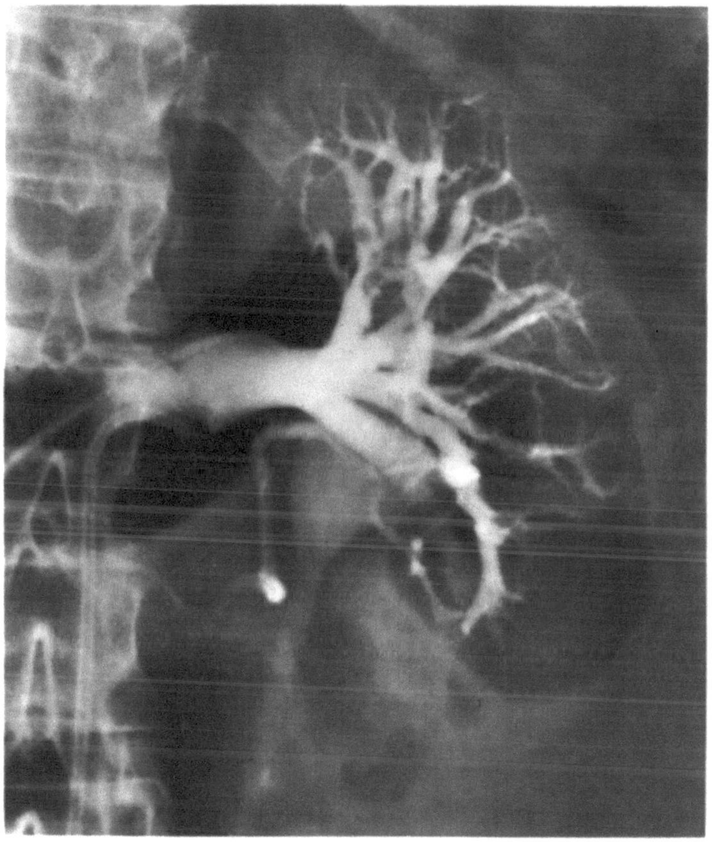

Fig. 9.10. Intra-arterial adrenalin-assisted left renal venography. Opacification of the peripheral renal veins (interlobular veins). Incomplete opacification of the lower pole due to wrong position of the catheter

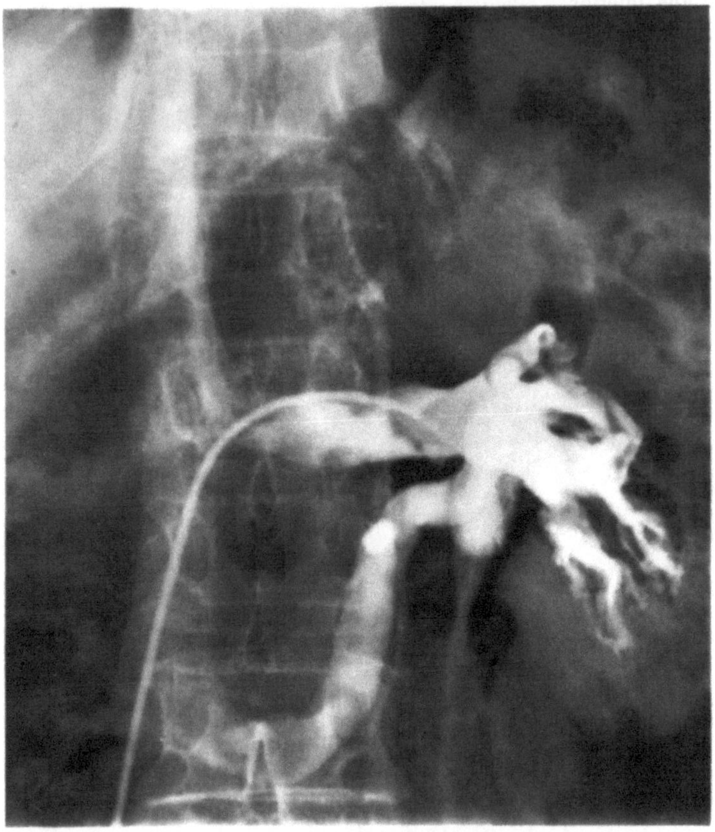

Fig. 9.11. Left renal venography. Periaortic venous collar

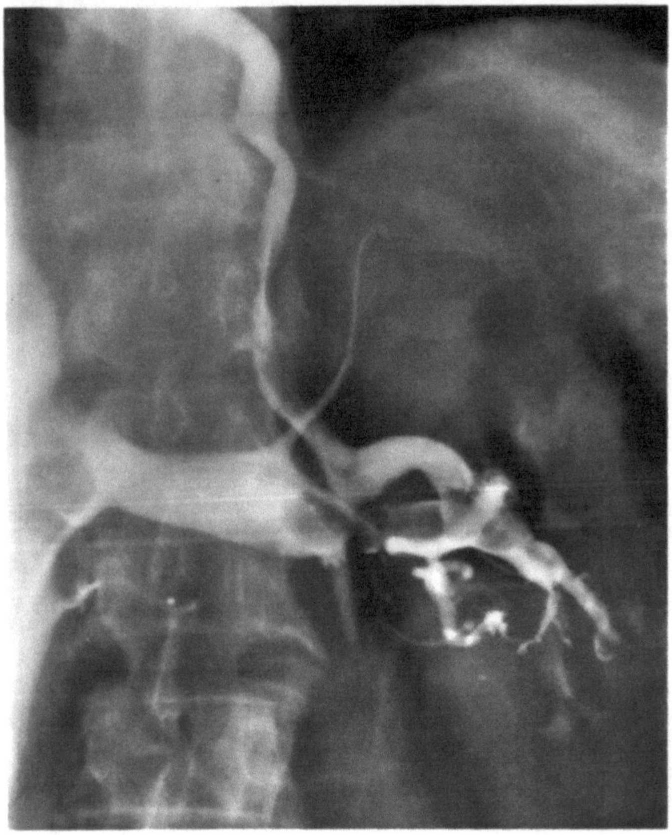

Fig. 9.12. Thrombosis of the renal vein. Nephrotic syndrome. Normal cavogram. Selective renal venography shows a distal thrombosis: intraluminal filling defect. Note drainage toward the azygos system

Fig. 9.13. Adrenalin-assisted left renal venography. Thrombosis of the intrarenal veins: no opacification, irregular, heterogeneous and "laminated" appearance of the renal vein trunk

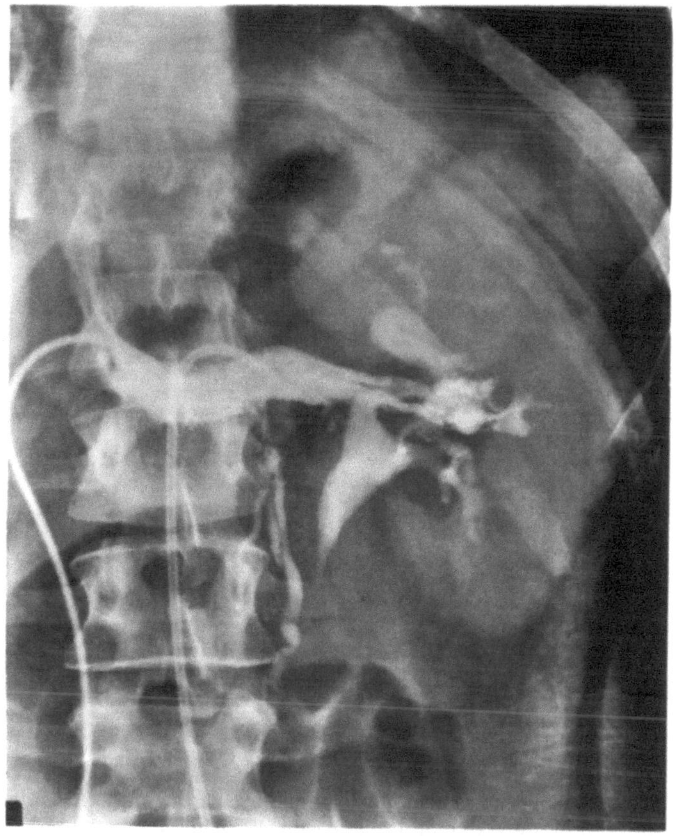

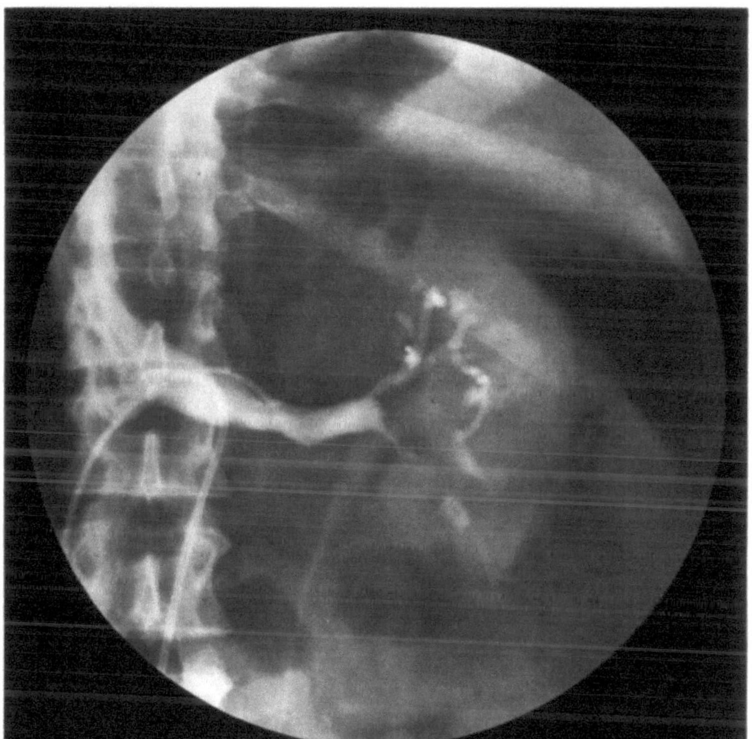

Fig. 9.14. Left renal venography. Thrombosis of the intrarenal veins. The renal vein is obstructed at the level of the hilus; the intrarenal veins fail to opacify

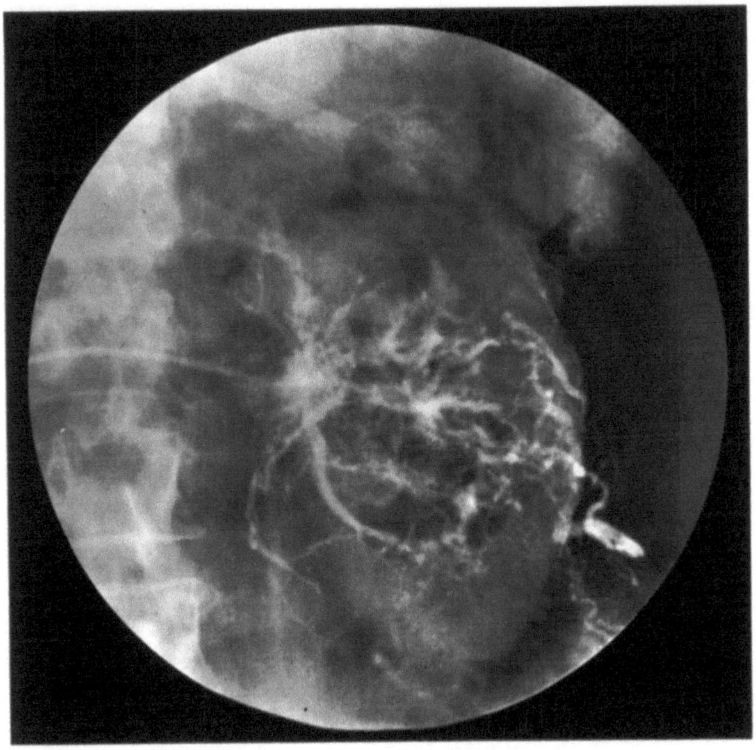

Fig. 9.15. Left renal venography. Thrombosis of the intrarenal veins. Opacification of a marked intra- and perirenal collateral circulation

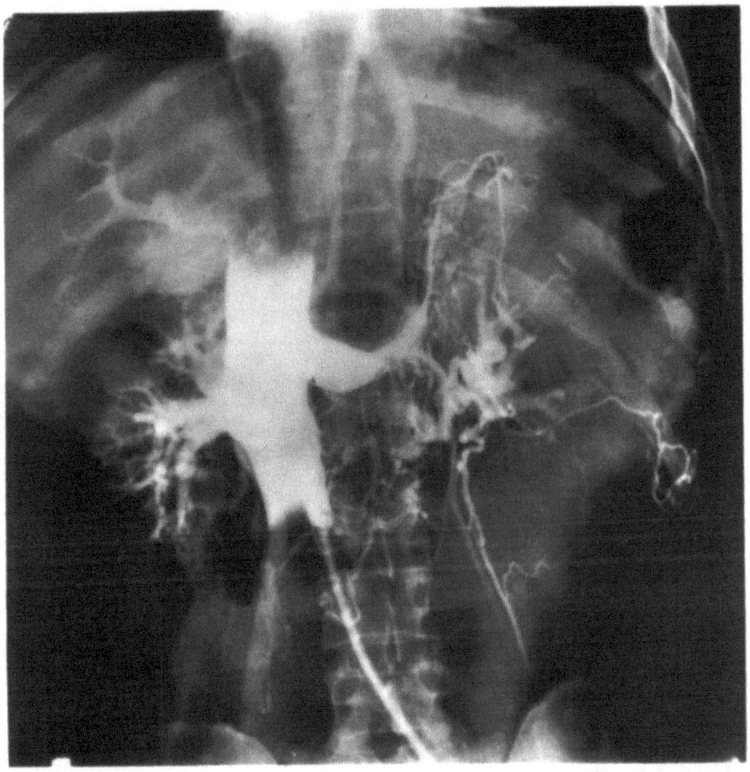

Fig. 9.16. Occlusive renal venography. Thrombosis of the trunk of the left renal vein (postoperative). Opacification of the intrarenal veins via collateral channels

Fig. 9.17. Adrenalin-assisted selective renal venography. Peripyelic varices in a patient with extrinsic pressure deformities at the level of the pelvis

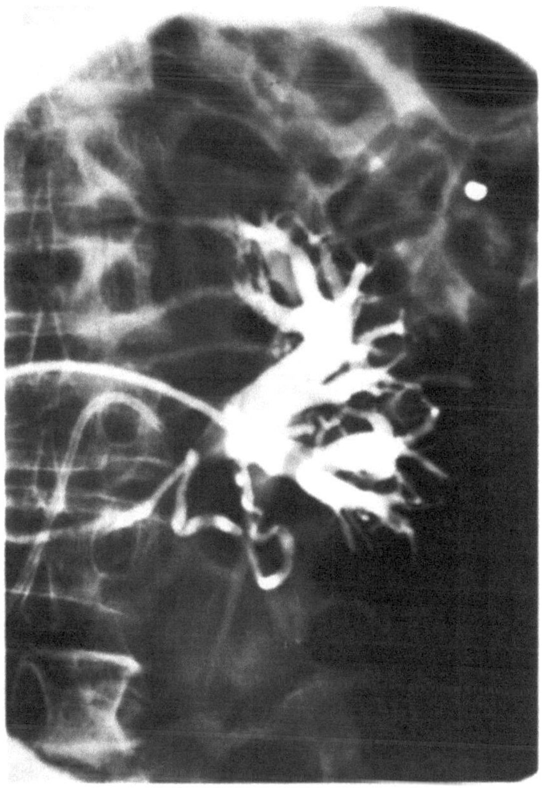

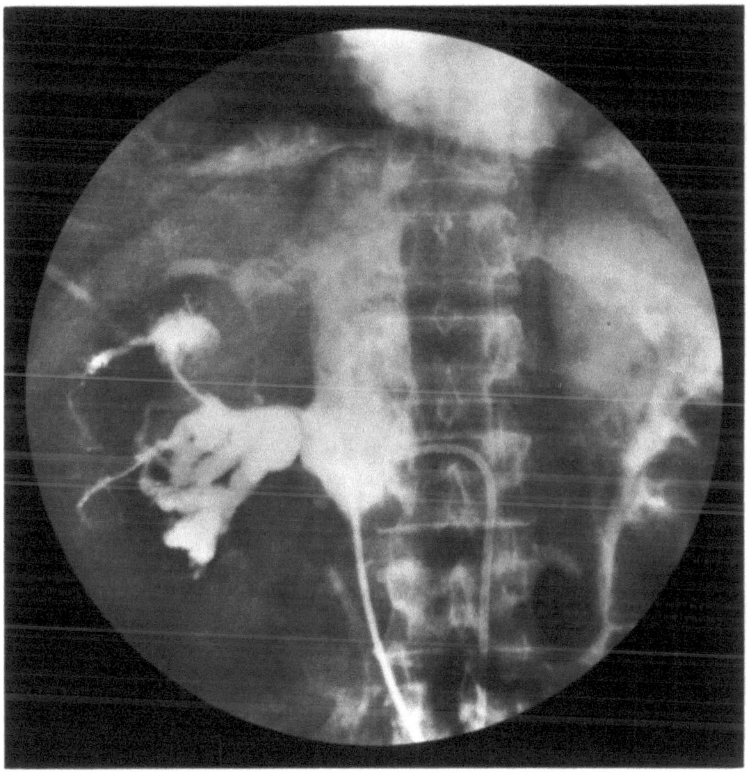

Fig. 9.18. Selective right renal venography. Partial obstruction and invasion of the veins of the upper renal pole suggesting a malignant tumoral syndrome

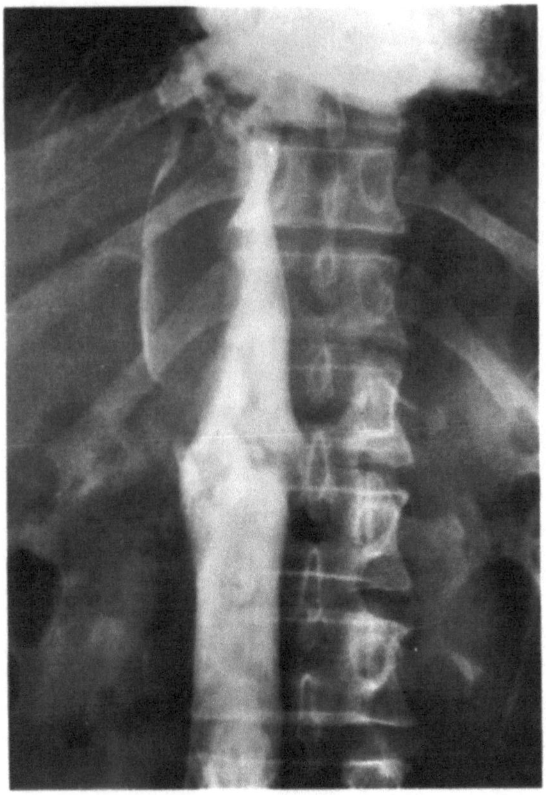

9.19

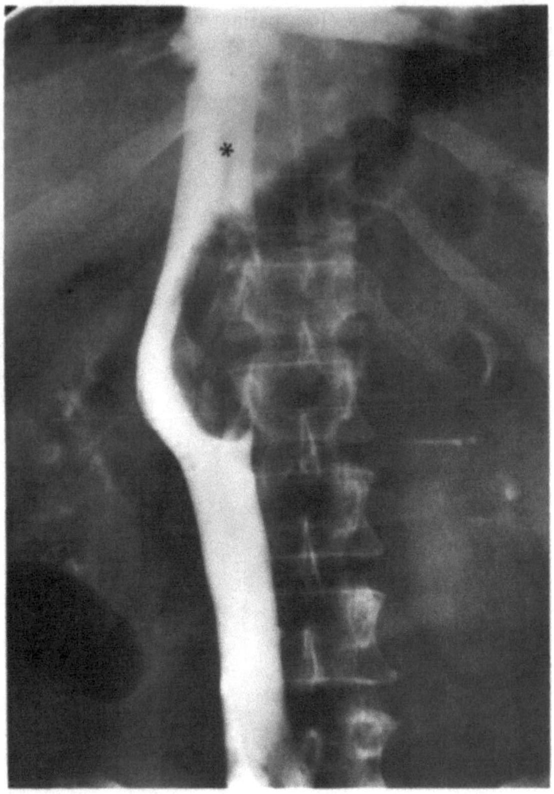

9.20

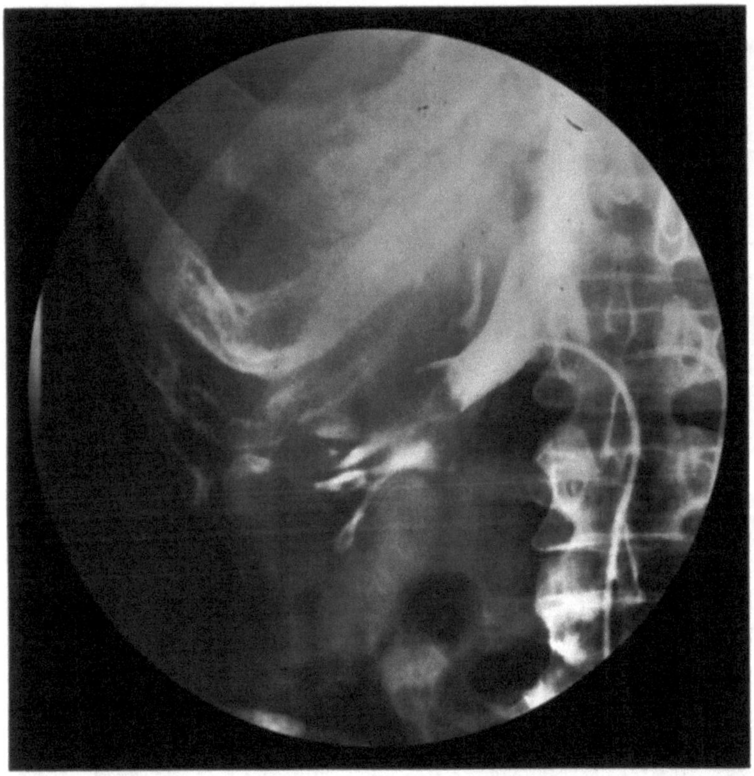

9.21

Fig. 9.19. Inferior vena cavography. Presence of a tumoral thrombus originating from the right renal vein and extending up to the right atrium. About this case, we would like to point out the necessity of a centering including the atrium in order to visualize the upper part of the thrombus. This thrombus is not adhesive, whence the necessity, as concerns tumoral pathology, to perform an inferior vena cavography prior to any selective renal venography

Fig. 9.20. Inferior vena cavography. Intracaval tumorous thrombus originating from the left renal vein. Note the large size of the intracaval thrombus topped by a small fibrinocruoric free thrombus (*)

Fig. 9.21. Epinephrine-assisted selective right renal venography. Irregular cupuliform stop consistent with the extension of a hypernephroma to the renal vein

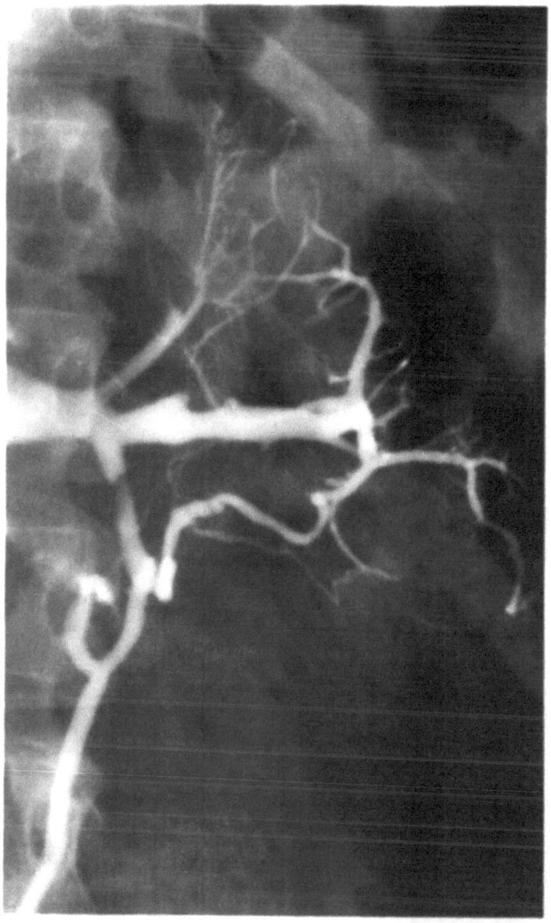

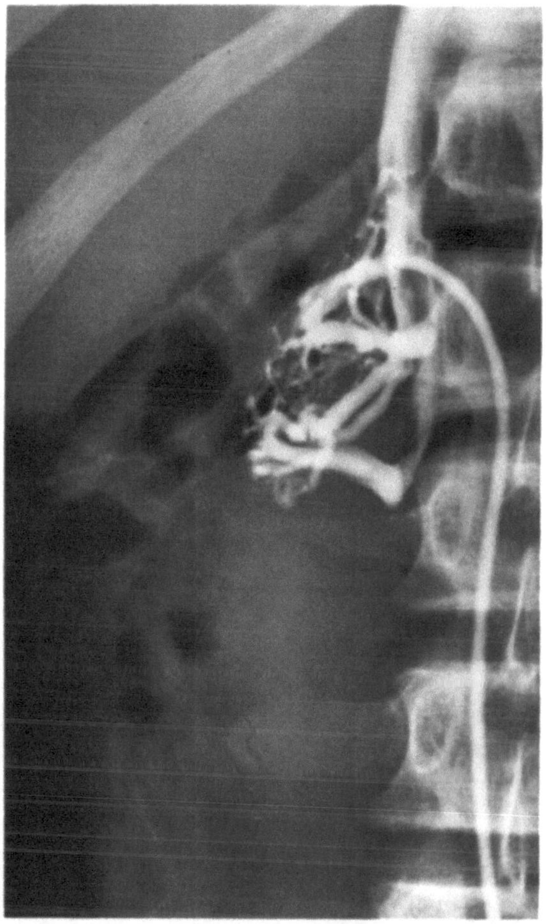

9.23

9.22

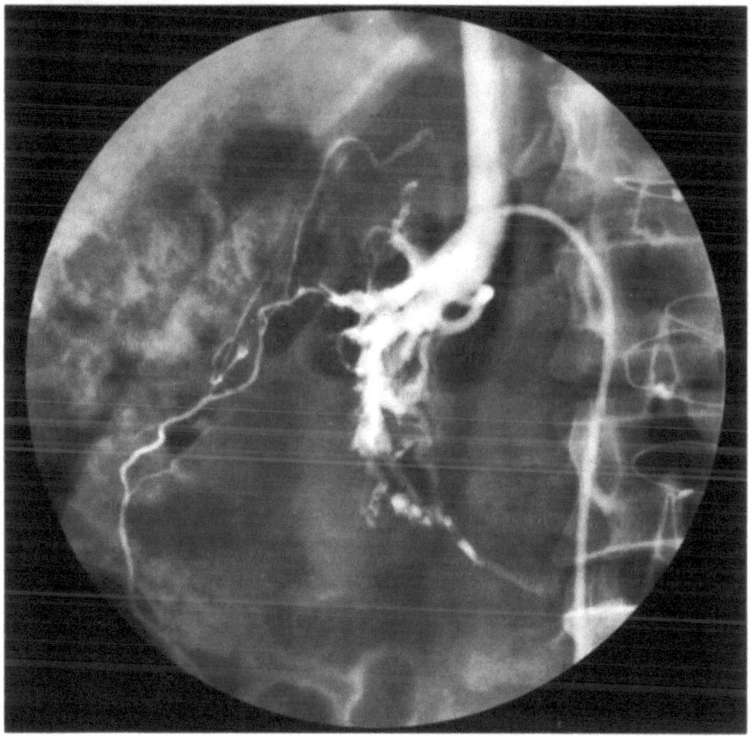

Fig. 9.22. Selective left renal venography. Opacification of veins beyond the suprarenal veins allows to affirm the presence of a renal primordium and to rule out agenesis

Fig. 9.23. Selective right renal venography. Congenital-type, small right kidney, with hypoplastic venous system (note the presence of three renal veins)

Fig. 9.24. Right renal venography. Venographic features consistent with atrophy: the trunk of the renal vein has a normal size, the perirenal venous ring is visualized at some distance from the external border of the kidney

9.24

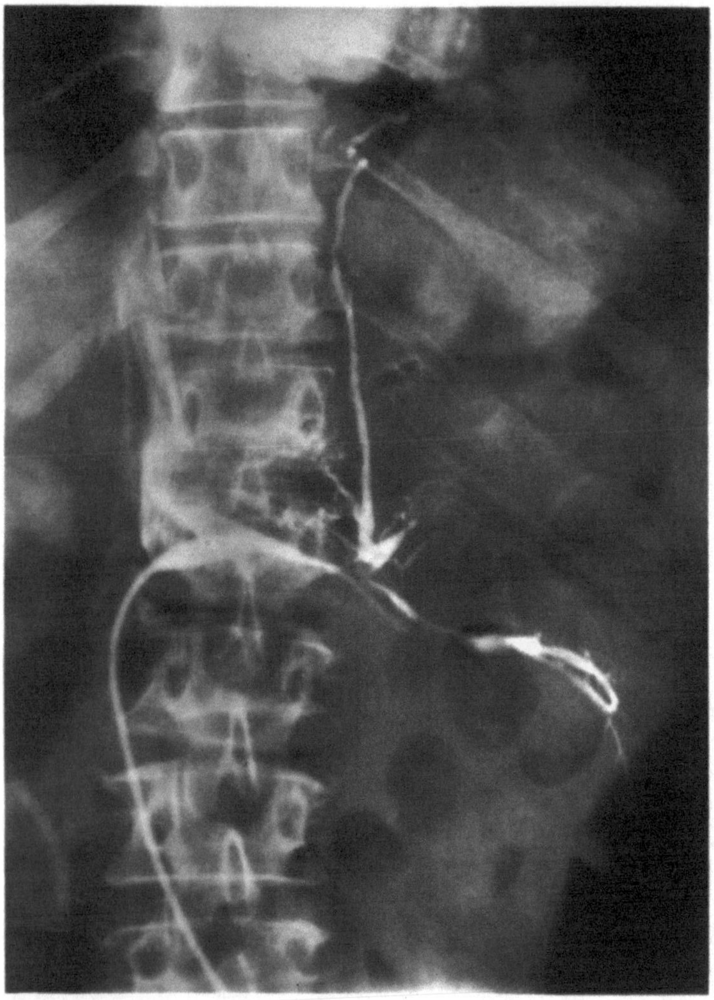

Fig. 9.25. Left renal venography. Invasion of the left renal vein by a retroperitoneal malignant tumor

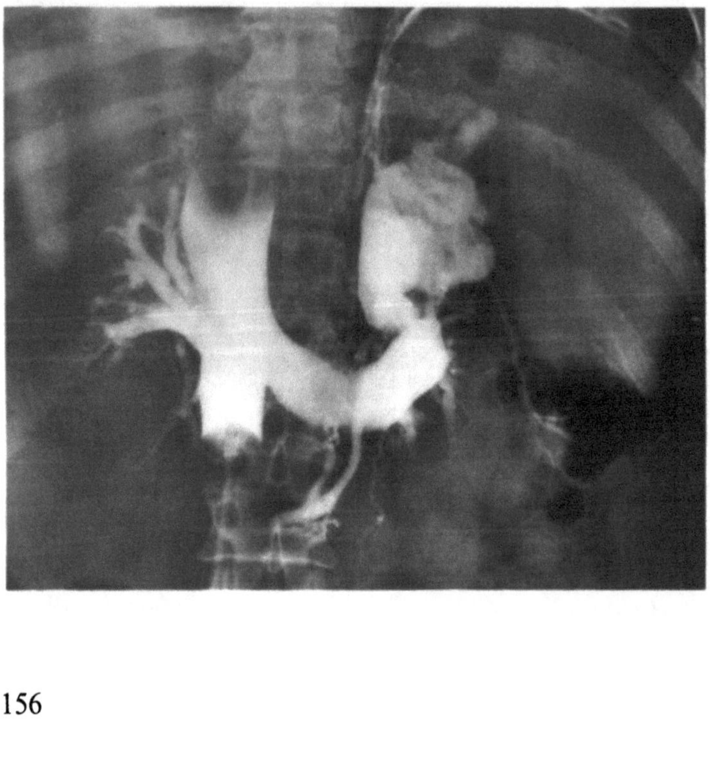

Fig. 9.26. Occlusive renal venography. Back-flow opacification of a spontaneous splenorenal anastomosis

Chapter 10. Adrenal Venography

Among the branches of the inferior vena cava, the adrenal veins are the most recently investigated radiologically. Masoni in 1957 performed the first catheterization of the right adrenal vein for biologic purposes. Subsequently, the first attempts at adrenal venography reported by Bucht and by Starer were often unsuccessful or entailed complications. In 1967, finally, the works of Mikaelson and of Reuter placed this technique among the various radiologic methods for the exploration of the adrenal glands. The anatomy of the adrenal veins is suitable for an investigation with twofold purpose: venous opacification allows the size and contours of the veins and the internal morphology of the adrenal glands to be appreciated, while withdrawal of blood samples permits separate measurements of hormone concentration.

10.1 Review of the Anatomy

(Fig. 10.1)

The greater part of the venous blood of the adrenal gland is drained by a main deep system. This system arises at the level of a corticospinal plexus. The deep veins converge toward the hilus and form the adrenal vein.

The right adrenal vein is anteriorly and medially oblique and slightly ascending. It joins the right posterior surface of the vena cava, 2 to 6 cm above the renal vein. Its caliber is about 2 to 3 mm. The left adrenal vein forms at the top of the gland and traverses it obliquely downward and medially, entering the superior surface of the left renal vein about 4 cm from the inferior vena cava. Its caliber is 2.5 to 3.5 mm. The accessory venous system in theory drains the blood from the glomerular zone toward the periadrenal veins. In fact, in normal subjects, the principal venous drainage seems to be toward the deep system.

10.2 Technique

Because of the fragility of the adrenal veins, adrenal venography must be performed with the greatest precautions. The technical problems mainly concern the right side, because of the smaller caliber of that vein and because of the difficulty of locating it.

The catheters (Fig. 10.2) must have a small caliber and be carefully tapered and preshaped. Adrenal vein catheterization is most often performed by retrograde femoral vein approach with Seldinger technique.

10.2.1 Right Adrenal Vein Catheterization

Preshaped catheters with a sharp bend at the distal centimeter or with a 'cobra-type' curve are used. Catheters with more complex loops permitting successive left and right adrenal vein catheterizations, are also used (Fig. 10.2). The right adrenal vein is searched for at the level of the costotransverse articulation, on the right posterior surface of the inferior vena cava. The catheterization is difficult; the test injection will be painful and should opacify a small triangular venous territory. These factors confirm that one has not opacified a small accessory hepatic vein, since in this latter case the injection is not painful and it produces prolonged opacification of a larger area draining into other hepatic veins.

However, the right adrenal vein and a small hepatic vein may have a common point of entry into the cava.

With some practice, catheterization of the right adrenal vein is successful in 70% to 80% of cases.

10.2.2 Left Adrenal Vein Catheterization

Coaxial catheters or preshaped catheters are used. The technique proposed by Bucht is easy to carry out: it uses a catheter with a principal bend and then a terminal reverse bend; the catheter is mounted on a guide wire, which is placed beforehand in the left renal vein (Fig. 10.2).

The left adrenal vein must be searched for at the level of the superior border of the left renal vein, along the left aspect of the spine. Failures are rare and due mainly to a malformation of the left renal vein.

The test injection is slightly painful. Identification of the left adrenal vein, including its differentiation from the inferior phrenic vein, is easy.

10.2.3 Withdrawal of Blood Samples

Blood samples should be taken prior to injection. For correct sampling the catheter must be strictly parallel to the venous axis. As far as possible, aspiration with the syringe should be avoided.

10.2.4 Filming

The contrast medium is injected by hand. Amount and delivery rate depend upon the size of the vein and of the gland, and on the reflux of contrast. Usually 2 to 3 ml for the right side and 4 to 5 ml for the left are injected at an average rate of 2 ml/s. It is a good idea to perform a first series with moderate delivery rate, which is often sufficient, at the risk of having to perform a second series with a higher rate when opacification proves insufficient. If severe pain should occur, the injection must be stopped. It may also be useful to perform additional series in other projections (frontal, oblique).

10.2.5 Incidents and Accidents

It is wrong to consider adrenal venography as a harmful investigation. Thrombosis of the adrenal vein is an uncommon complication. It is sometimes responsible for acute adrenal insufficiency, but this is usually regressive. Adrenal hematomas occur more frequently, but are less dangerous; they most often cause regressive lumbar pain syndromes. Intra- or extra-adrenal extravasation of contrast material may be seen; its main drawback is that it impedes interpretation of the films, and hence may adversely influence a surgical procedure. The frequency and severity of these complications are diminished by use of fine catheters and low delivery rates.

10.3 Results

10.3.1 Normal Findings

Right Adrenal Venography

The right adrenal gland is usually rather triangular, mainly situated above the kidney, and has a tapering superior pole. The adrenal vein is usually horizontal; it results from the convergence of several intra-adrenal veins which are difficult to distinguish individually (Fig. 10.3).

Almost as commonly, the right adrenal gland is found to have a drop-shaped appearance, with tapered superior extremity, globulous lower extremity, and prerenal development. In this case the adrenal vein is vertical and receives branches distributed like the veins of an elm leaf (Fig. 10.4). The accessory adrenal veins drain toward the perirenal venous ring.

Left Adrenal Venography

The left adrenal gland is situated between the kidney and the spine; it is roughly egg-shaped, with a tapering superior extremity and a globulous inferior extremity. The adrenal vein originates from the top of the gland and has a rectilinear, downward and medially oblique course. The intra-adrenal veins have a regular distribution comparable to the veins of an elm leaf. Numerous peripheral anastomoses are seen, and the inferior vein of the left crus of the diaphragm is often opacified, either completely or partly, at the level of its valve (Figs. 10.5 and 10.6).

The size of the adrenals is difficult to appreciate because of the morphologic variations depending on the projection in the frontal plane. Only the long axis seems constant and ranges from 2.5 cm to 3.5 cm on the right, and from 4.5 to 5.5 cm on the left.

10.3.2 Pathologic Findings

Aldosteronism

Primary aldosteronism results usually from the development in the adrenal cortex of a small tumor, 8 to 12 mm in diameter. Only adrenal venography permits diagnosis of such tumors. In a considerable number of cases it will also allow diagnosis when the aldosteronism is secondary to bilateral, nodular or diffuse, hyperplasia of the adrenal glands.

Adenomas. The venogram shows a rounded avascular area producing an arciform displacement of the intra-adrenal veins. In some more voluminous tumors the veins are flattened, mimicking tumoral opacification. In the event of very small tumors or of tumors with exoadrenal development, diagnosis is difficult. In such cases the levels of aldosterone are high on the involved side and there is a significant gradient relative to the uninvolved gland (Figs. 10.7–10.9).

Adrenal hyperplasia. Whether it is a matter of simple diffuse hyperplasia or of microadenomatosis, such lesions are not always radiologically detectable. The gland may be increased in volume, globulous and richly vascularized. Intraparenchymal lacunae may be seen. The aldosterone level is always very high in both adrenal veins (Figs. 10.10 and 10.11).

Adrenal venography makes a radiological diagnosis possible in 85% of cases. Diagnostic accuracy is increased with the help of adrenal function studies of the adrenal blood (95% of cases). Adrenal venography permits determination of the type of lesion concerned and hence provides the therapeutic indication. In case of adenoma, phlebography guides the surgeon and contraindicates operation in case of hyperplasia.

Cushing's Syndrome

The role of the radiologist is to differentiate cortical tumors from hyperplasias. Hyperplasias are the more frequently occurring; they have quite characteristic features: the gland has a long axis of more than 6 cm on the left, and of more than 4 cm on the right. Usually adrenalography permits a good appreciation of the volume of the gland. The vascularization is rich but of normal pattern (Figs. 10.12 and 10.13). Venography is rarely used to investigate tumors, apart from adenomas. These have similar features to those of Conn's adenoma, but they are often more voluminous (Figs. 10.14–10.16). On account of the etiologic orientation provided by the various adrenal function tests, indications for adrenal venography are restricted in patients with Cushing's syndrome. Only cases in which a tumor is suspected justify use of this method.

Adrenogenital Syndromes

These are usually secondary to a huge malignant corticoadrenoma. The venogram shows markedly hypertrophied adrenal veins and a mass syndrome which displaces the veins, which are multiplied, flattened, and sometimes cut off. Apart from such cases, when the investigation is not very useful for diagnosis, adrenal venography has revealed the peculiar effect of minor forms of congenital adrenal hyperplasia in patients presenting isolated hirsutism. The venographic appearance is quite similar to that of adrenal hyperplasia.

Pheochromocytoma

Adrenal venography is generally used as a possible second investigation in pheochromocytoma patients; i.e., it is only carried out in case of failure of arteriography when one is looking for a nonexpansive intra-adrenal pheochromocytoma. The radiologic appearance is that of a lacunar expansive syndrome with displacement and flattening of the intra-adrenal veins (Fig. 10.17). Bookstein, however, suggests a different attitude. He considers that 90% of pheochromocytomas involve the adrenals and that segmental blood sampling in the inferior and superior caval systems is the best method for demonstrating multiple ectopic and metastatic localizations. He therefore proposes bilateral adrenal venography associated with samplings from the caval system, prior to arteriography, in each case with a positive diagnosis.

Nonfunctional Adrenal Tumors

The radiologic appearance is the same as in the tumoral syndrome without peculiarity. As in the previous cases, it is difficult to ascertain whether the mass is benign or malignant (Fig. 10.18).

10.4 Indications

Adrenal venography is a second investigation in the radiologic investigation of the adrenals. Whether it is indicated depends on the clinicobiologic data and the findings of nephrourotomography. Schematically, one can say that adrenal venography is indicated in all patients presenting a syndrome of cortical or medullar hyperfunction secondary to an adrenal tumor without nephrourographic signs. It should thus be performed mainly to demonstrate small adrenal lesions, particularly adenomas. The only technique that could compete with it is selective adrenal arteriography, but the latter is more difficult and longer, and does not allow blood sampling. A comparative study made by Kahn of 20 cases of Conn's adenoma is significant: the diagnosis was made by selective adrenal arteriography in 60% of the cases, by adrenal phlebography in 85%, and in 95% when the phlebography was associated with adrenal function tests.

10.5 Conclusion

Adrenal phlebography represents a step forward in the diagnostic accuracy of the radiologic investigations of the adrenals. It is now possible to determine the indications for this method, and its place is now well assessed in the cortical hyperfunction syndrome. Only its usefulness in the topographic diagnosis of a pheochromocytoma is still under discussion. It is certainly a delicate examination, requiring skill and a strict and painstaking technique in order to diminish as far as possible the risk of complications. The accuracy of the data provided justifies its role among the radiologic investigations of the adrenal glands.

References

Bayliss RI, Edwards OM, Starer F (1970) Complications of adrenal venography. Br J Radiol 43:531–533

Bookstein JJ, Walter FJ (1975) The role of abdominal radiography in hypertension secondary to renal and adrenal disease. Med Clin North Am 59:169–200

Bucht H (1962) Percutaneous catheterization of the left adrenal vein in man. Scand J Clin Lab Invest [Suppl 64] 14:27–38

Joffre F (1973) La phlébographie surrénalienne. Ann Radiol (Paris) 16:581–596

Kahn PC, Kelleher MD, Egdahl RH, Melby JC (1971) Adrenal arteriography and venography in primary aldosteronism. Radiology 101:71–78

Kyaw MM (1972) Simplified technique of bilateral adrenal vein catheterization using a simple preshaped catheter. Radiology 105:203–205

Masoni A (1957) Catheterization of the right adrenal vein in man. Acta Med Scand 159:225

Mikaelsson CG (1967) Retrograde phlebography of both adrenal veins: A preliminary report. Acta Radiol [Diagn] (Stockh) 6:348–354

Mitty HA, Nicolis GL, Gabrilove JL (1973) Adrenal venography: Clinical roentgenographic correlation in 80 patients. AJR 119:564–575

Reuter SR, Blair AJ, Schteigart DE, Bookstein JJ (1967) Adrenal venography. Radiology 89:805–814

Starer F (1965) Percutaneous suprarenal venography. Br J Radiol 38:675–681

Suc JM, Joffre F, Conte J, Carcy JB, Bec P, Boulard C (1970) Le cathétérisme et l'opacification radiologique des veines surrénaliennes. Presse Med 78:589–593

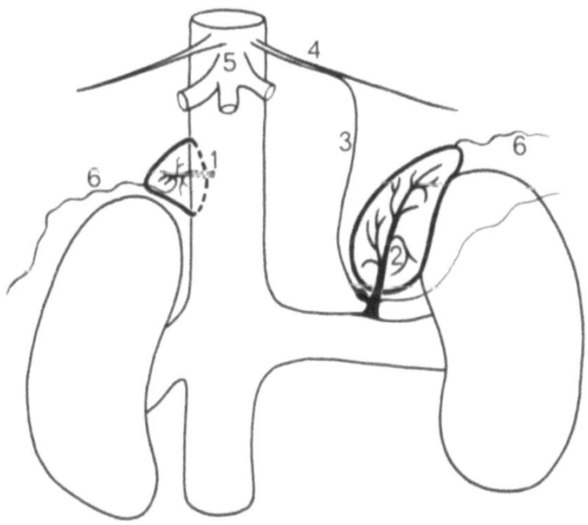

Fig. 10.1. Anatomy of the adrenal veins.
1 Right adrenal vein
2 Left adrenal vein
3 Inferior vein of the left crus of the diaphragm
4 Inferior phrenic vein
5 Hepatic veins
6 Perirenal veins

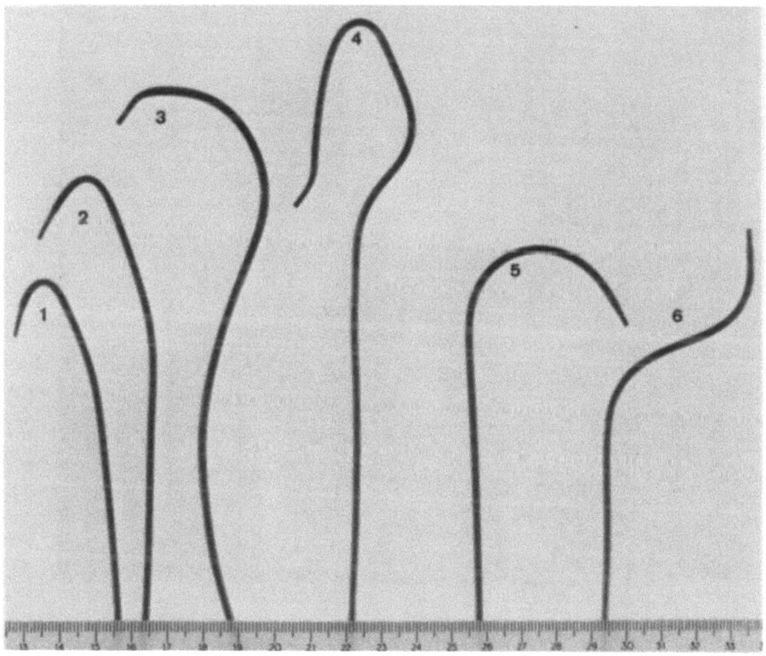

Fig. 10.2. Catheters used for adrenal venography.
1 Right adrenal vein (small vena cava)
2 Right adrenal vein (large vena cava)
3 Right adrenal vein (Cobra catheter)
4 Right and left adrenal veins (KYAW)
5 Left renal vein (1)
6 Left adrenal vein (2)

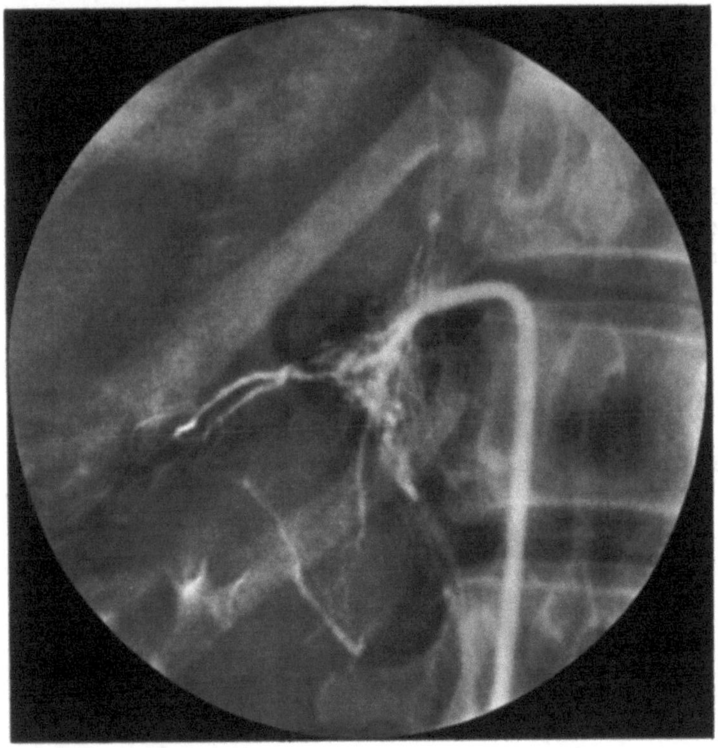

Fig. 10.3. Normal right adrenal venogram. Horizontal adrenal vein. Triangular adrenal gland

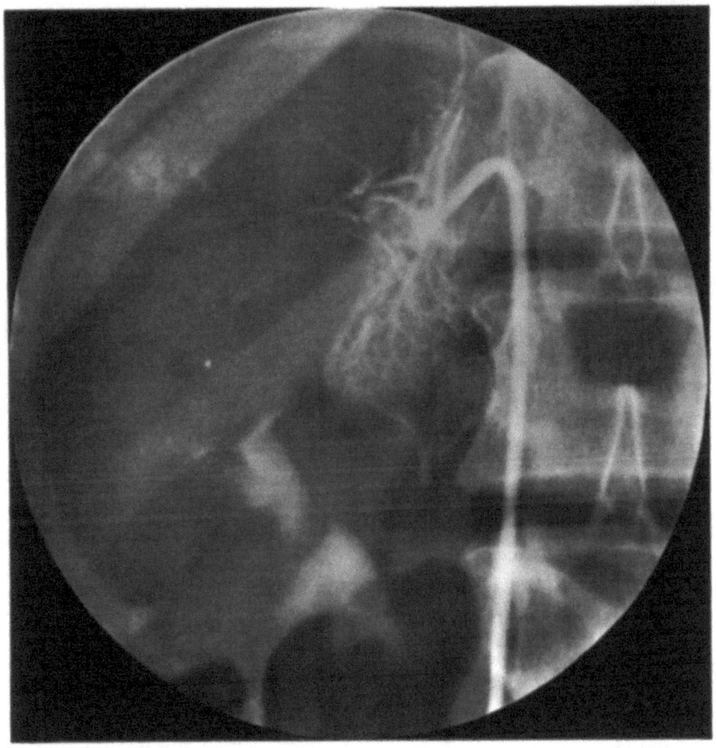

Fig. 10.4. Normal right adrenal venogram. Drop-shaped adrenal gland

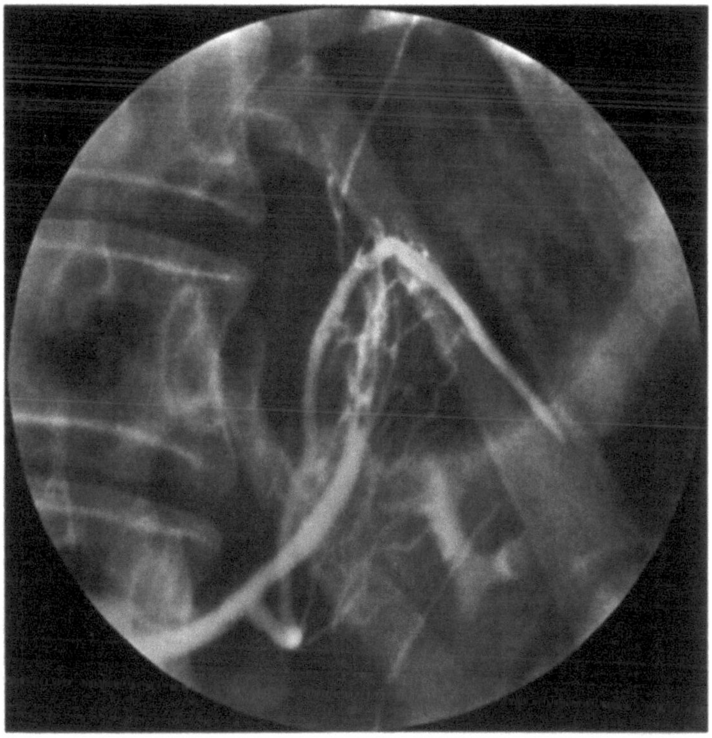

Fig. 10.5. Normal left adrenal venogram

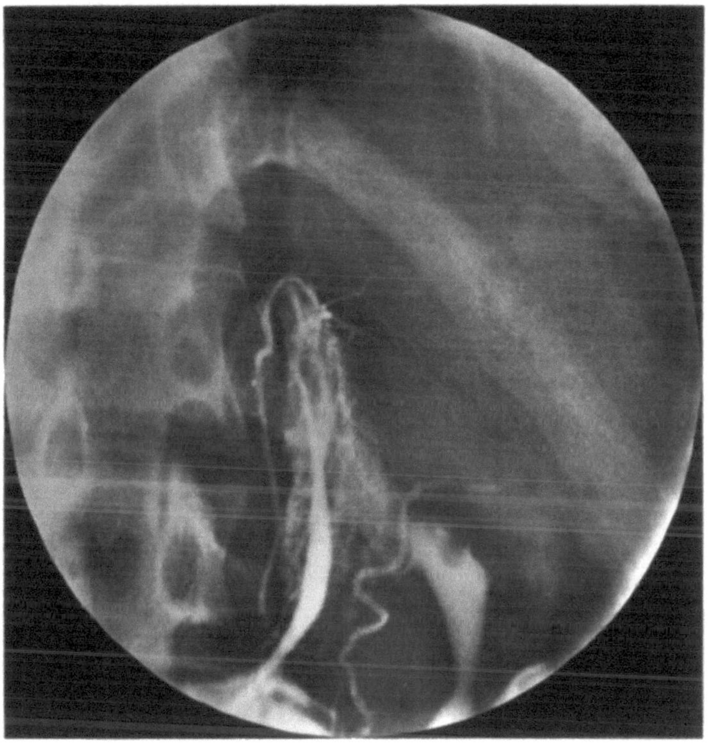

Fig. 10.6. Normal left adrenal venogram

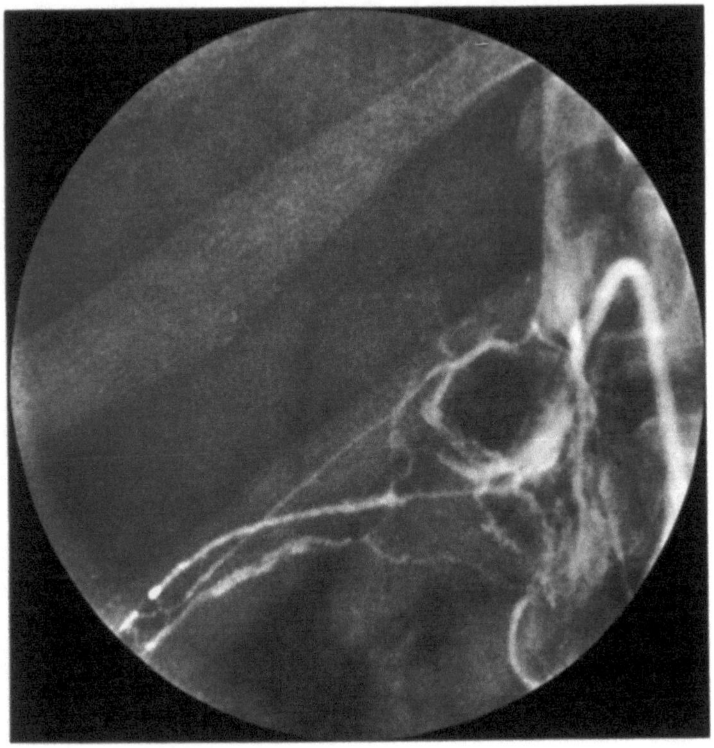

Fig. 10.7. Right adrenal venogram: Conn's adenoma

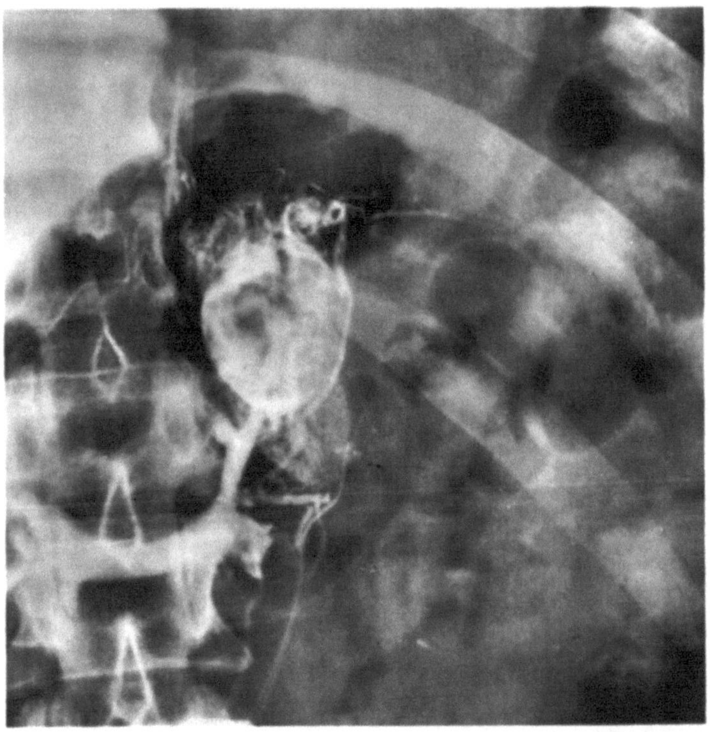

Fig. 10.8. Left adrenal venogram. Large adenoma in the median part of the gland

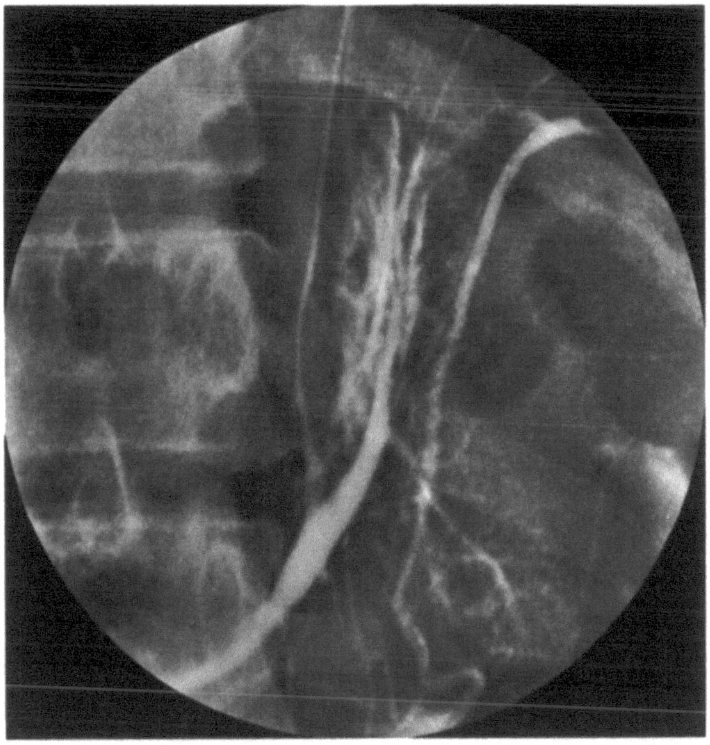

Fig. 10.9. Left adrenal venogram. Small adenoma of the inferior pole of the gland. Surgery proves the presence of an adenoma of 4 mm in diameter

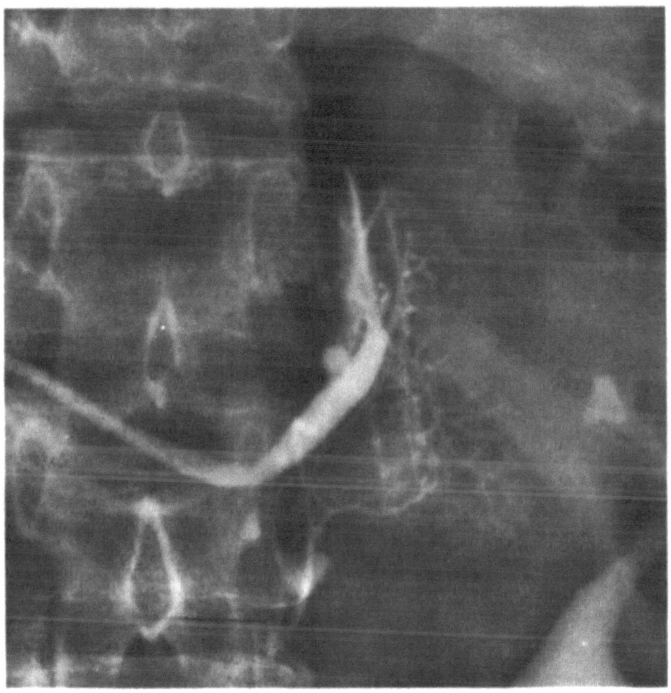

Fig. 10.10. Left adrenal venogram. Adrenal hyperplasia in primary hyperaldosteronism

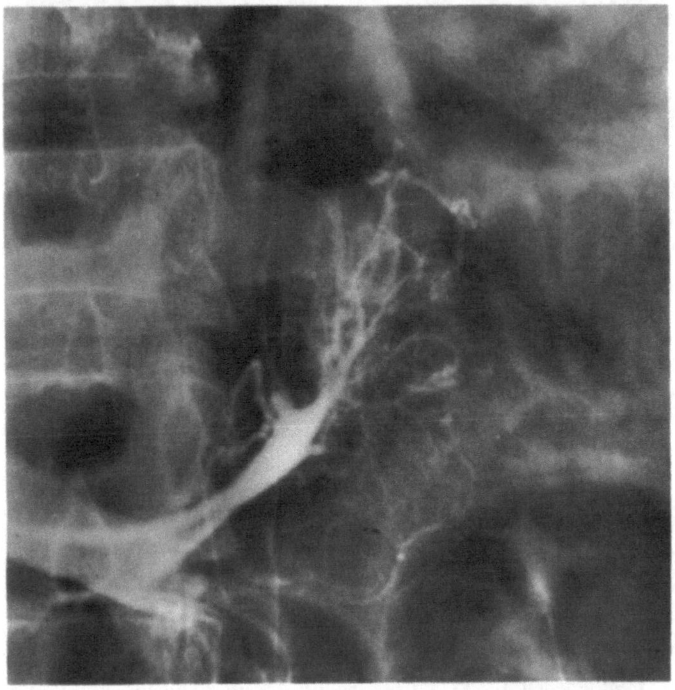

Fig. 10.11. Left adrenal venogram. Adrenal hyperplasia with glandular hypertrophy and hypervascularization. There are rounded, intraglandular nodules corresponding to microadenomatosis, which is responsible for primary hyperaldosteronism

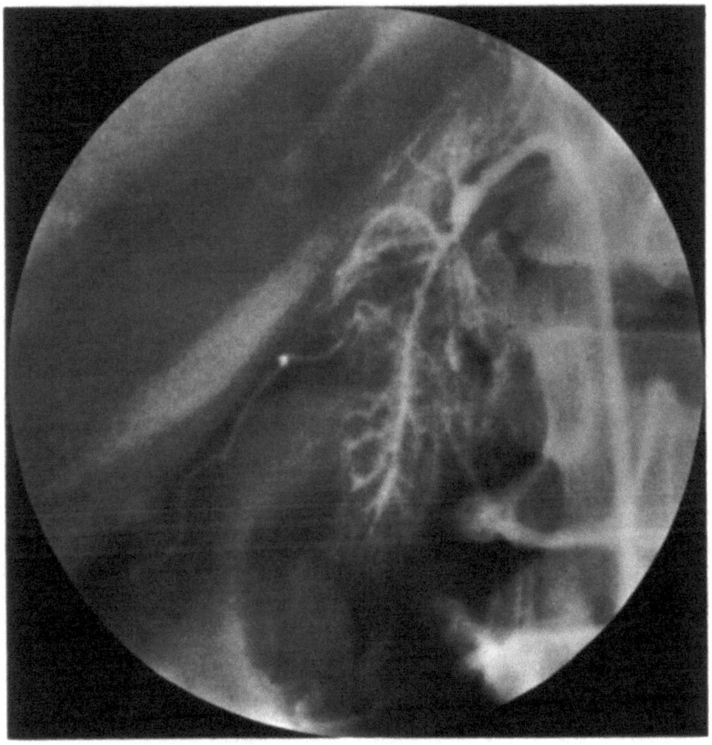

Fig. 10.12. Right adrenal venogram. Adrenal hyperplasia with glandular hypertrophy and hypervascularization in a Cushing's syndrome

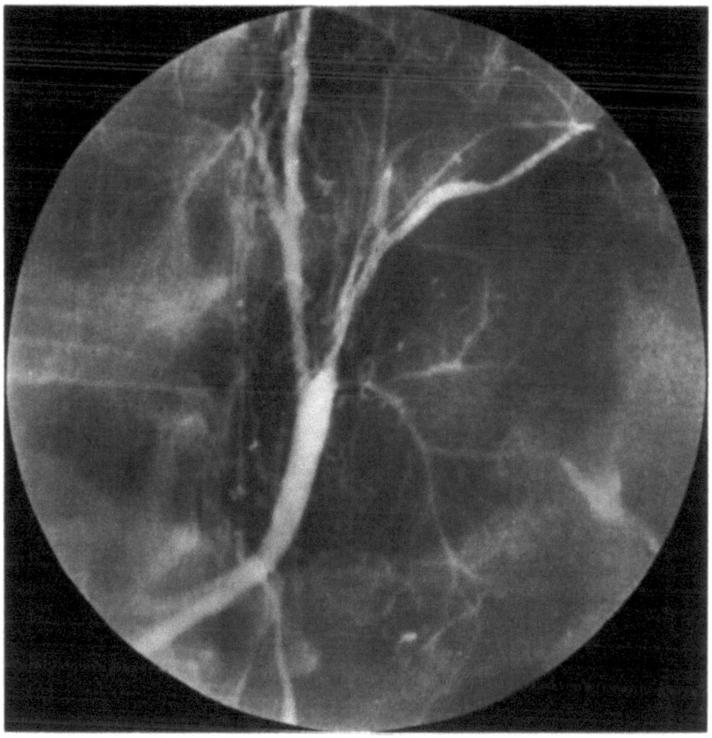

Fig. 10.13. Left adrenal venogram. Adrenal hyperplasia with major glandular hypertrophy (great axis = 8 cm) in a Cushing's syndrome

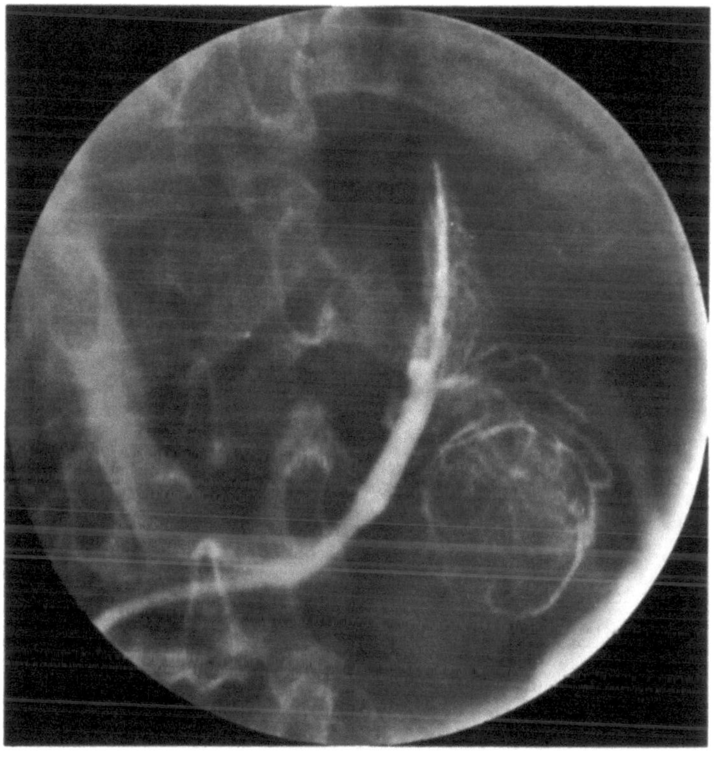

Fig. 10.14. Left adrenal venogram. Benign tumor features in a patient with Cushing syndrome. This was confirmed by surgery. Right adrenal venography could not be performed

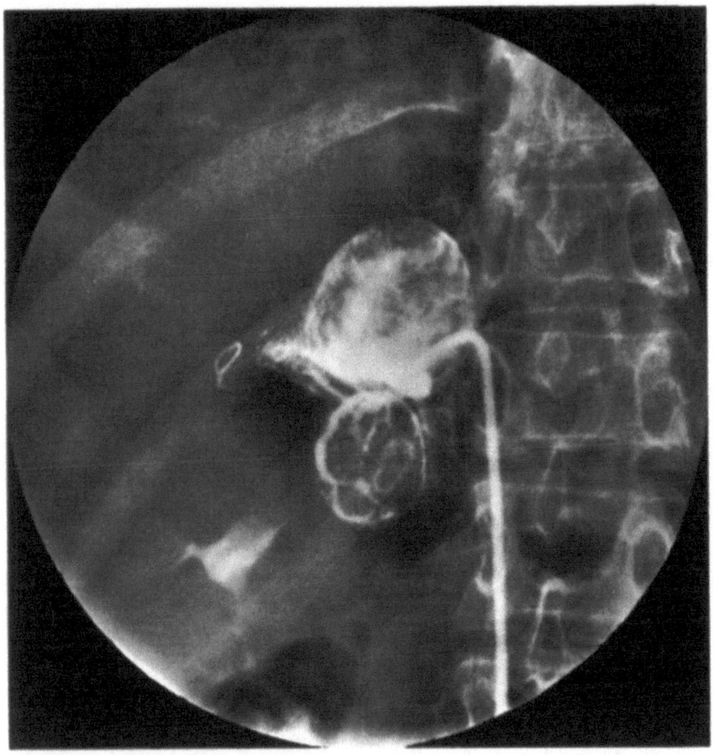

Fig. 10.15. Right adrenal venogram. This investigation was unnecessarily performed for recurrent endocrine syndrome

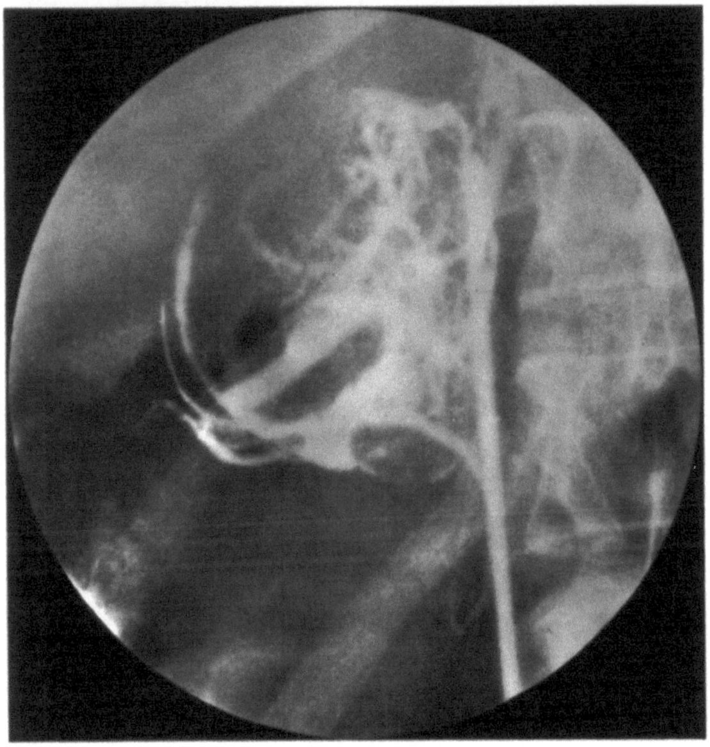

Fig. 10.16. Right adrenal venogram. Appearance of benign expansive process of the right adrenal gland in a Cushing's syndrome. It proved to represent a cortical adenoma at surgery

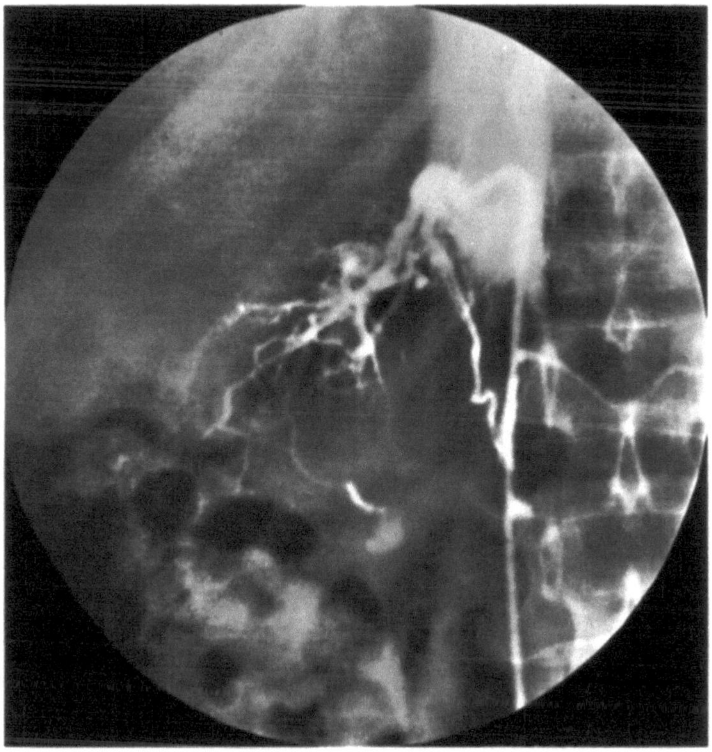

Fig. 10.17. Right adrenal venogram. Voluminous expansive process with hypervascularization corresponding to a pheochromocytoma

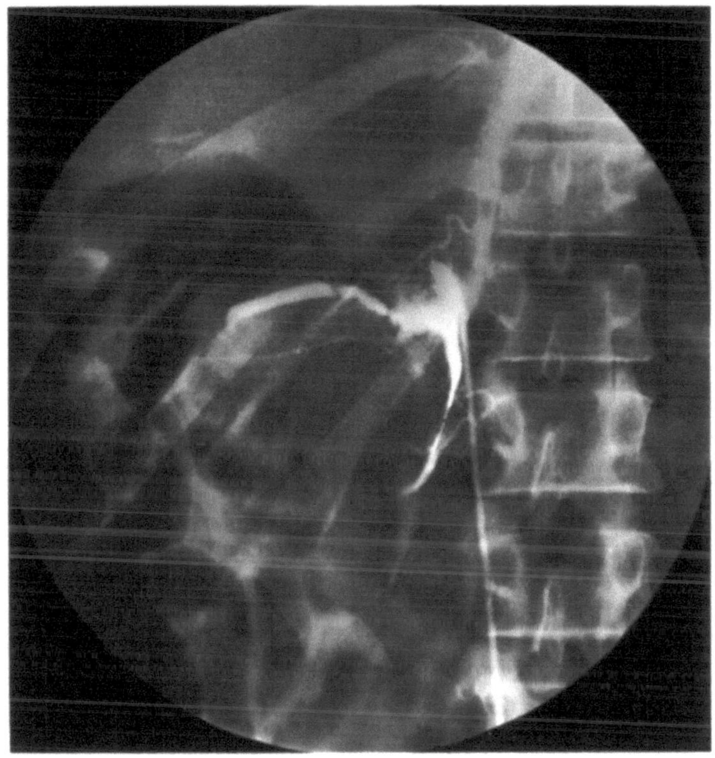

Fig. 10.18. Right adrenal venogram. Large expansive process with displacement and invasion of the peritumoral veins. Nonsecreting malignant adrenocortical tumor

Chapter 11. Spermatic Venography

It was only 20 years after Ivanissevitch, in 1918, applied surgical treatment to a testicular varicocele, that Souza Cortin, in 1937, performed peroperatively the first venography of the spermatic vessels, in the direction of the venous flow.

Since 1952, when Tulloch discovered the role played by varicoceles in male infertility, the range of operative indications has become wider. Retrograde spermatic venography by percutaneous approach, as performed by Ahlberg et al. in 1965, has become an exploratory and preoperative method. Left varicoceles being clinically by far the more frequent, surgical procedures have most often consisted in resection of the left spermatic vein alone, and venography, of which the first recognized role was to explain surgical failures and to prevent recurrences, was likewise mainly concerned with investigations of the left spermatic vein (Ahlberg, Amin, Brown, Comhaire, Diamond, Atriby, Frick, Glickman, Jacobs, Lien, Nataf, Ponthieu, Rolla, Vassilev).

Only recently (1978) has right retrograde spermatic venography been used in regular practice, in the same way as left spermatic venography (Bigot, Chatel).

11.1 Embryology

The embryogenesis of the spermatic veins must be considered in relation to the evolution of the inferior vena caval system as a whole in the embryo (Huntington, McClure, Paturet). Both spermatic veins derive from the subcardinal venous system. In the embryo the venous system is dorsal, paired, and symmetrical. It is constituted by a right and a left anterior cardinal system, and by a right and a left posterior cardinal system. The posterior cardinal veins and the anterior cardinal veins join to form the duct of Cuvier which empties into a single medial venous sinus. The blood from the embryonic paramedian renal anlage drains via the ventral subcardinal venous network, which has anastomoses on the midline, as do also the caudal ends of the posterior cardinal system (11-mm embryo).

These systems subsequently undergo asymmetrical atrophy: the posterior cardinal system persists only in its caudal part (the iliac veins); from the initially paired and symmetrical supracardinal system only the right part persists (the right inferior vena cava). The communication between the cranial and left part of the subcardinal network also disappears. The left renal vein has a double origin: its distal part derives from left anastomoses between the supra- and subcardinal systems, and its medial part derives from the subcardinal network.

The gonadal veins develop from the paramedian and anterior supracardinal system, so that the paramedian right and left gonadal veins are originally situated ventrally and to the left of the postrenal division of the inferior vena cava, which derives from the right lateral and posterior supracardinal system. The gonadal veins empty into the left renal veins. Subsequently, the right spermatic vein migrates and opens into the anterior aspect of the inferior vena cava, or in some cases into the right renal vein. This explains the variable termination of the right spermatic vein, which may join the left or right renal vein instead of the inferior vena cava, this last being the normal pattern. The lower frequency of anastomoses of the right spermatic vein with the adjacent venous networks is also due to this migration, which causes interruption of cranial venous communications, whereas they persist on the left.

11.2 Anatomy

11.2.1 The Spermatic Veins

The spermatic veins follow the path of their arteries. They have a long course and terminate in the interrenal area, owing to the primarily lumbar site of the gonads and the secondary descent. Their termination is asymmetrical, on the right joining the inferior vena cava, on the left the left renal vein.

They collect the venous blood from the testicles and the anterior part of the epididymis. The testicular and the anterior epididymal veins form the anterior spermatic plexus or pampiniform plexus, comprising six to eight large veins coursing in the spermatic cord. This plexus ascends in the cord in front of the ductus deferens and together with the spermatic artery. At the level of the deep inguinal ring the plexus is composed of three venous trunks, which coalesce into two veins in the iliolumbar region, to become a single vessel in the lumbar area: the spermatic vein. This configuration is the most perfect type of concentration of a venous system through numeric reduction that is encountered in the human organism.

The veins follow their arteries ventrally and, later, laterally; the arteries arise from the aorta in the interrenal area. They run upward in front of the psoas muscle, cross in front of the ureters and are covered by the right and left mesocolic fascias and by the posterior parietal peritoneum. On the peritoneum, anteriorly, course the right and the left colic vessels. On the left, the spermatic vein is related to Treitz's vascular arch (constituted by the left superior colic artery and the inferior mesenteric vein; Fig. 11.4).

The right spermatic vein accompanies its artery in coursing progressively closer to the midline. It terminates at an acute angle on the right anterolateral aspect of the inferior vena cava at the level of the second lumbar vertebra, always somewhat lower than the level of origin of its artery. The termination of the right spermatic vein is

Table 11.1. Anastomoses of the spermatic veins

	Left spermatic vein	Right spermatic vein
Anastomoses with the renal veins. Small anastomotic rami with the trunk of the renal vein	15.2%	4.7%
Anastomoses with the exorenal ring	20%	15.6%
Anstomoses with the inferior vena cava	1.6%	7.8%
Anastomoses with the intercostal veins	15.2%	4.6%
Anastomoses with the ureteric veins	19.2%	7.8%
Anastomoses with the lumbar and perivertebral systems	40.8%	7.7%
Anstomoses with the epigastric veins	12%	3.1%
Anastomoses with the hypogastric veins	4%	5%
Anastomoses with the colic veins	45.4%	37.5%
Vertical anastomoses between different spermatic segments	45%	25%
Anastomoses with the external pudendal system	23.2%	14%
Anastomoses between the two spermatic veins at the lumbar level		2.4%
Anastomoses between the spermatic systems at the level fo the scrotum		3%

in fact quite variable. It opens most often into the inferior vena cava (95% of cases), but may also join the right renal vein (5%; Bigot, Chatel) and exceptionally the left renal vein (Ahlberg). In some cases the termination consists of two trunks, one emptying into the inferior vena cava, the other into the right renal vein (18% of cases).

The left spermatic vein abandons its artery slightly below the inferior pole of the kidney and opens at a right angle into the left renal vein. Termination into the left renal vein is almost constant, apart from cases of left-sided inferior vena cava.

Valves are usually present in the scrotal and inguinal portions of the spermatic veins. Ostial valves may exist (Ahlberg, Anson, Rivington), nine times out of ten on the right, six times out of ten on the left, in a normal population. The gonadal veins receive peritoneal, ureteric (Fig. 11.5), adipous, and muscular veins. They have multiple and various anastomoses with the parietoabdominal veins, the colic veins (Fig. 11.6), the veins of the lumbar plexus through the psoas muscle, the renoazygolumbar veins, the ureteric veins, and the exorenal venous arch of Tuffier and Lejard (Fig. 11.3). These anastomoses are quite frequent, especially on the left (Table 1).

11.2.2 Venous Drainage of the Scrotum

The spermatic veins are only one of the drainage pathways of the scrotum (Fig. 11.11) and its contents. There are two main groups:

1) A deep group comprising, besides the anterior spermatic plexus (which is continuous with the spermatic vein and collects the venous blood from the testicle and the anterior part of the epididymis), (a) the posterior spermatic plexus, or group of the funicular veins which drain into the epigastric vein near its termination in the external iliac vein; and (b) the veins of the ductus deferens, which join the vesicoprostatic and seminal plexus, drained by the vesical veins toward the hypogastric vein.
2) A superficial group (Fig. 11.8) comprising the scrotal veins which join the internal saphenous vein via the external pudendal veins, and the hypogastric vein via the superficial perineal veins and the internal pudendal vein.

The deep venous system communicates on the one hand with the superficial system in the cutaneous covering of the scrotum and in the inguinal segment, and on the other hand with the contralateral venous system at the level of the spermatic plexus and the cutaneous covering of the scrotum.

11.3 Technique

Whereas it was first performed peroperatively by denudation of the spermatic veins and opacification in the direction of the physiologic blood flow (Souza-Cortin), spermatic venography is now a preoperative investigation, performed transcutaneously by transfemoral puncture, selective catheterization, and retrograde opacification (Ahlberg).

The main technical problem lies in the selective catheterization of the right spermatic vein. The termination site of this vein is variable (it joins the inferior vena cava at a variable level, on one of the aspects, or the right renal vein). Above all, this termination forms an acute angle, considerably impeding selective catheterization. It seems essential to use catheters with a sharp bend (Fig. 11.12). Since it is necessary to change the catheter when passing from investigation of the right side to the left, it is preferable to begin with the catheterization of the right spermatic vein, since the catheter which is used for the left spermatic vein can also, when necessary, be used for the right renal vein. When the right spermatic vein is not found in the inferior vena cava, it must be searched for in the right renal vein.

Usually two series are performed, beginning with a series centered on the lumbar segment (Figs. 11.2, 11.4, and 11.5), to demonstrate the presence or absence of valves in this segment. When no competent valve is clearly visible, a second series centered on the inguinal area and the scrotum is carried out, with the patient upright or with a Valsalva maneuver (Figs. 11.2c, 11.7, and 11.8). When on the first series the spermatic vein is seen to have a valve near its ostium, without collaterals or anastomoses, additional opacification of the renal vein can be achieved with the patient upright, using the same centering, which will show any anastomoses between the renal vein and the spermatic vein, feeding the spermatic vein below the valve (Fig. 11.3). A lower-centered, third series with the patient upright may then show whether these anastomoses cause a varicocele. Thus the investigation should be carried out as follows:

1) Femoral puncture, usually on the right side.
2) Introduction of the right spermatic catheter.
3) Catheterization of the right spermatic vein and right serial filming (Fig. 11.4).
4) Introduction of the left spermatic catheter (first along the same route, when the right spermatic vein has not been found, so that a series of the right renal vein may be carried out).
5) Catheterization of the left spermatic vein and left serial filming (Fig. 11.2).

The amount of contrast medium must be adapted to the size of the vein, as determined by fluoroscopy: about 2 to 4 ml/s for 5 to 9 s. The number of films must be as low as possible: two films per series, at the end of injection, i.e., usually eight films for the entire examination. Irradiation of the gonads is thus minimized.

11.4 Results

The main application of retrograde spermatic venography is currently in the detection of infraclinical varicocele. This should in fact be seen in broader terms, those of "spermatic venous insufficiency," a concept combining incompetence of venous valves with more or less developed varicocele. In some cases there is obvious venous anomaly: e.g., reflux into the left spermatic vein during opacification of the left renal vein with the patient upright (Figs. 11.1 and 11.3), or a spermatic vein of large caliber and voluminous varicoid formation covering the entire testicular surface (Figs. 11.2c and 11.8).

Opacification of the testicular venous network is sometimes difficult and requires dynamic maneuvers (Valsalva and upright position; Figs. 11.3 and 11.7). It may happen that the pressure of the contrast, owing to insufficient catheterization, fails to displace the blood column coming from the testicles and collaterals when the patient is reclining. Only direct visualization of a valve, with its characteristic shape, is conclusive evidence of the competence of the spermatic venous system. The varicocele may be fed by anastomoses between the renal system and the lumbar segment of the spermatic vein (Fig. 11.3) while the spermatic trunk has a competent valve.

Retrograde opacification of the spermatic vein as far as the testicle, even if the testicular plexus is small (Fig. 11.7), must be taken as indicating spermatic venous insufficiency (Comhaire). It is known that there is no correlation between the size of the varicocele and its influence on semen quality (Brown, Charny), and that the result of surgery is better the smaller the varicocele (Dubin).

According to a recent study (Bigot, Chatel), right spermatic venous insufficiency is almost as frequent as left (60% on the right, 76% on the left). Left varicoceles are usually larger, and easy to diagnose from the clinical and thermographic data, unlike right ones, where spermatic venous insufficiency usually produces a lesser degree of dilatation – which is no clue as to its repercussion on semen quality (Dubin).

Compared to thermography, spermatic venography is clearly a more sensitive method, especially for the right side. It provides the surgeon with precise anatomic data, which are useful in case of recurrence after surgical ligation (Fig. 11.9).

11.5 Other Indications

The preoperative location of *ectopic testicles* can be seen on a retrograde phlebogram (Figs. 11.10; Amin, Diamond, Glickman, Jacobs, Lunderquist, Vassilev, Vitale, Weiss). Retrograde investigation of the gonadal veins has been used by some authors (Kolbenstevdt, Lee, Lien) for the diagnosis of *retroperitoneal lymph node involvements*, as an adjunct to lymphography and inferior vena cavography.

Finally, in females, the ovarian veins may be the site of *phlebitic phenomena* (Lotze), especially in post-partum. These ovarian thrombophlebites may be responsible for pulmonary embolisms, the origin of which may well go undetected without radiologic investigation of the gonadal veins (Delorme).

References

Ahlberg NE, Bartley O, Chidekel N (1965) Circumference of the left gonadal vein. An anatomical and statistical study. Acta Radiol 3:503–512

Ahlberg NE, Bartley O, Chidekel N, Frijesson A (1966) Phlebography in varicocele scroti. Acta Radiol 4:517–528

Ahlberg NE, Bartley O, Chidekel N (1967) An anatomic and roentgenographic study of the communications of the renal vein in patients without renal carcinoma. Scand J Urol Nephrol 1:43–51

Amin M, Wheeler CS (1976) Selective venography in abdominal cryptorchidism. J Urol 115:760–761

Bigot JM, Chatel A, Dectot H, Helenon C (1978) Phlébographie spermatique rétrograde: Anatomie radiologique (à propos de 152 explorations). Ann Radiol (Paris) 21:515–523

Brown JS, Dubin L, Becker M, Hotchkiss RS (1967a) Venography in the subfertile man with varicocele. J Urol 98:388–392

Brown JS, Dubin L, Hotchkiss RS (1967b) The varicocele as related to fertility. Fertil Steril 18:46–56

Charny CW (1962) Effect of varicocele in fertility. Fertil Steril 13:47–56

Chatel A, Bigot JM, Helenon C, Dectot H, Rotman J, Salat-Baroux J (1978a) Intérêt de la phlébographie spermatique dans le diagnostic des stérilités d'origine circulatoire (varicocèle). Comparaison avec des données cliniques thermographiques et anatomiques. Ann Radiol (Paris) 21:565–570

Chatel A, Bigot JM, Dectot H, Helenon C (1978b) Anatomie radiologique des veines spermatiques. A propos de 152 phlébographies spermatiques rétrogrades. J Chir (Paris) 115:443–450

Comhaire F, Kunnen M (1976) Selective retrograde venography of the internal spermatic vein: A conclusive approach to the diagnosis of varicocele. Andrologia 8:11–24

Comhaire F, Monteyne R, Kunnen M (1976) The value of scrotal thermography as compared with selective retrograde venography of the internal spermatic vein for the diagnosis of the sub-clinical varicocele. Fertil Steril 27:694–698

Delorme G (1968) La phlébographie de l'utérus par la technique d'injection rétrograde de l'utéro-ovarienne gauche. Ann Radiol (Paris) 11:11–20

Diamond A, Ravitz G (1975) Venographic demonstration of a varicocele in a boy. J Urol 114:640–645

Diamond AB, Meng CH, Kodroff M, Goldman SM (1977) Testicular venography in the non palpable testis. AJR 129:71–75

Dubin L, Amelar RD (1967) Varicocele size and results of varicocelectomy in selected subfertile men with varicocele. Fertil Steril 18:666–671

Dubin L, Amelar RD (1971) Etiologic factors in 1294 consecutive cases of male infertility. Fertil Steril 22:469–474

Etriby AF, Ibrahim AA, Mahmoud KZ, Elhaggar S (1975) Subfertility and varicocele. I – Venogram demonstration of anastomosis sites in subfertile men. Fertil Steril 26:1013–1017

Frick J, Bandtlow K (1969) Die Angiographie der linken vena spermatica. ROEFO 111:241–245

Glickman MG, Weiss RM, Itzachk Y (1977) Testicular venography for undescended testes. AJR 129:67–70

Huntington GS, Mc Clure CFW (1920) The development of the veins in the domestic cat (felix domestica) Anat Rec 20

Ivanissevitch C, Gregorini H (1918) Una nueva operacion para curar el varicocele. Semana Med 25:575–576

Jacobs JB (1969) Selective gonadal venography. Radiology 92:885–888

Kolbenstevdt A, Lien HH, Miller A, Haveland H (1975) Antegrade spermatic vein phlebography in testicular tumors. A preliminary report. Radiology 114:461–463
Lee KF, Greening R, Kramer S, Kahn CA, Kuroda K, Lin S, Koslow V (1971) The value of pelvic venography and lymphography in the clinical staging of carcinoma of the uterine cervix: Analysis of 105 proven cases by surgery. AJR 111:284–296
Lien HH, Kolbenstevdt A (1976) Venography of the left renal and left gonadal veins as a supplement to lymphography. Report of four cases. Lymphography 9:23–28
Lien HH, Kolbenstevdt A (1977) Phlebographic appearances of the left renal and left testicular veins. Acta Radiol 18:321–332
Lotze EC, Kaufman RH, Kaplan AC (1966) Postpartum ovarian vein thrombophlebitis. Obstet Gynecol Surv 21:853–870
Lunderquist A, Sfure R (1967) Roentgenologic diagnosis of cryptorchism. J Urol 98:219–223
McClure EF, Butler EG (1925) The development of the vena cava inferior in man. Am J Anat 35:331–352
Nataf R, Leclere J (1975) Intéret de la phlébographie spermatique per-opératoire dans la cure des varicocèles. J Urol Nephrol 81:226–232
Paturet G (1958) Traité d'anatomie. Les veines, vol 3, 2nd edn. Masson Paris
Ponthieu A, Huguet JF (1976) Varicocèle gauche et stase veineuse iliaque. J Urol Nephrol 3:187–200
Rivington W (1973) Valves in the renal veins. J Anat Physiol 7:163
Rolla G, Corte ES, Goldsmith A, Viera Vera A (1971) Hysterophlebography in patients with intrauterine devices. Rev Chil Obstet Ginecol 36:210–214
Tulloch WS (1952) A consideration of sterility factors in light of subsequent pregnancies. Subfertility in male. Trans Edin Obstet Soc 104:29
Vassilev Y (1962) Etude radiologique de la veine spermatique gauche dans les varicocèles idiopathiques. Presse Med 70:704–705
Vitale PJ, Khademi M, Seebode JJ (1974) Selective gonadal angiography for testicular localization in patients with cryptorchism. Surg Forum 25:538–540
Weiss RM, Glickman MG, Lytton B (1977) Venographic localization of the non palpable undescended testis in children. J Urol 117:513–515

Fig. 11.1. Opacification of the left renal vein in the upright position. In case of valvular incompetence of the spermatic vein, there occurs during upright position important reflux in this vein. Its location is thus facilitated: it terminates on the left aspect of the second lumbar vertebra, at most 1 cm lateral to the extreme edge of the vertebra

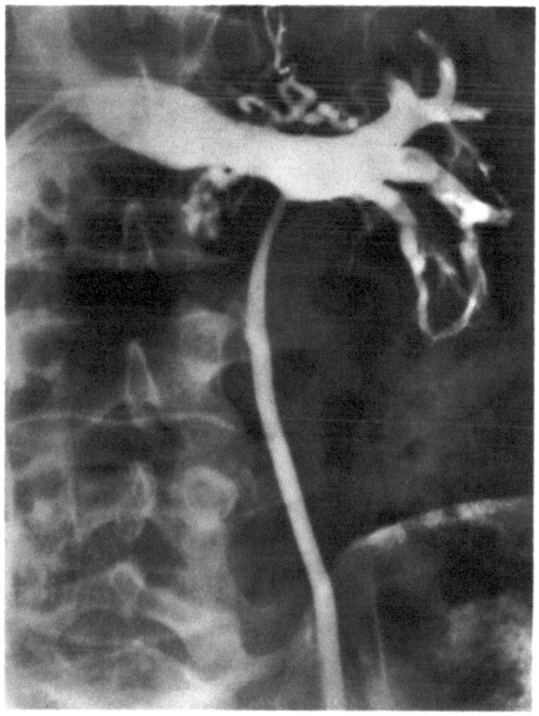

Fig. 11.2a–c. Incontinent left spermatic vein. a Frontal view. b Lateral view. From the inguinal canal on the spermatic vessels course along the concavity of the pelvis and become progressively posterior. At the median part of the ala ossis ilii the spermatic vein arises from two venous trunks. It has a very posterior course and projects along the anterior margin of the vertebrae on a lateral view. Note the small internal prevertebral anastomoses between the spermatic vein and the lumbar system. c Same patient with a large left varicocele which drains via the deferential system and the external pudendal veins

11.2a

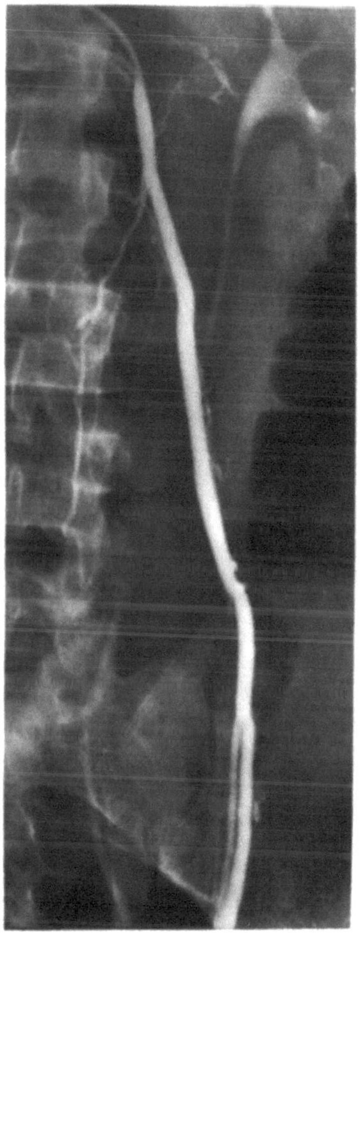

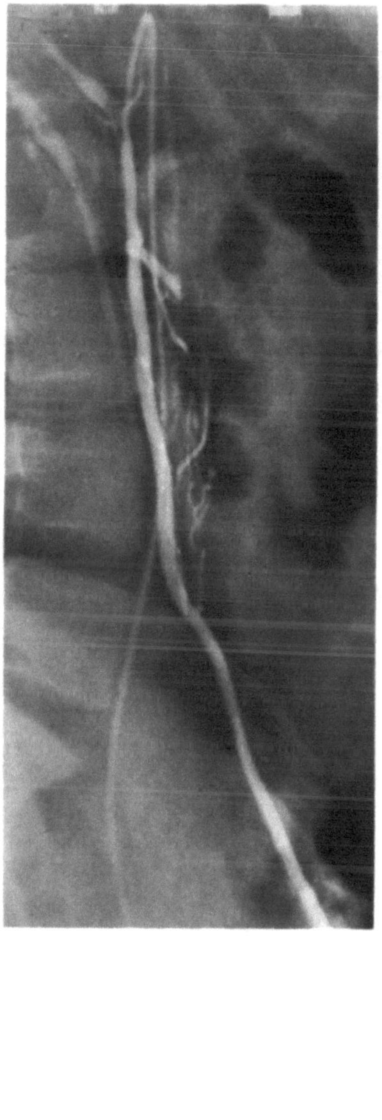

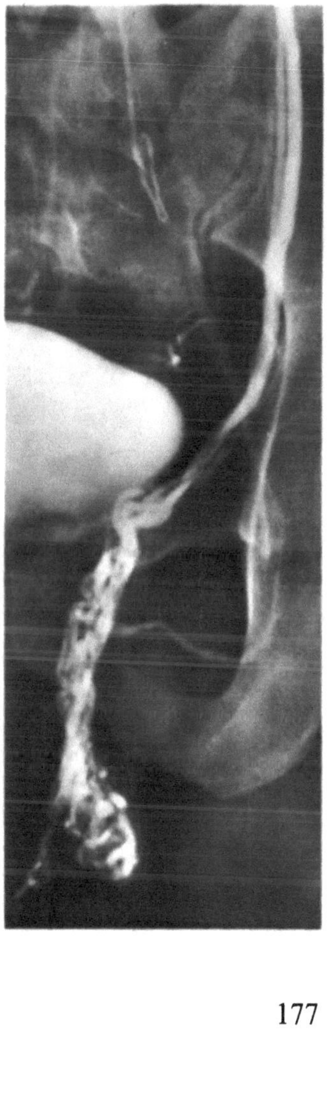

11.2b, c

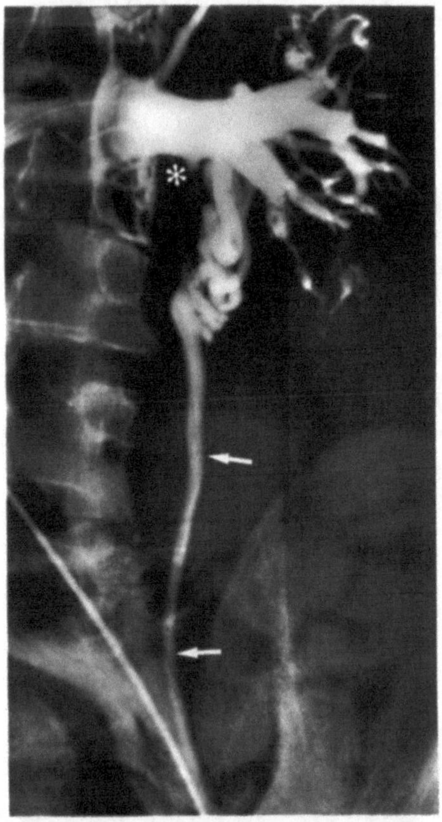

11.3a

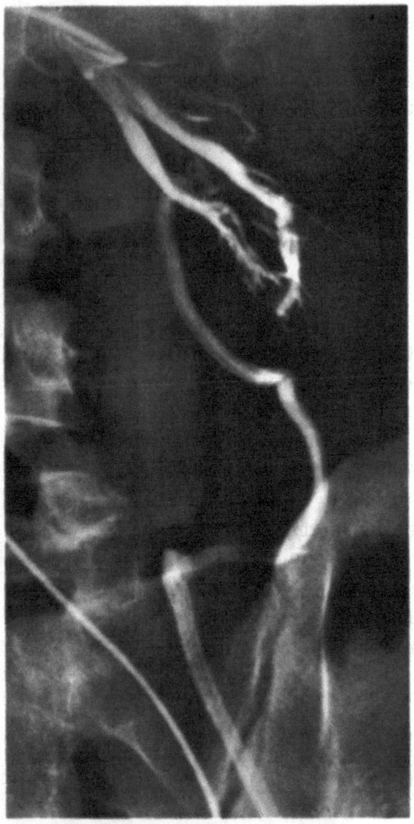

11.3b

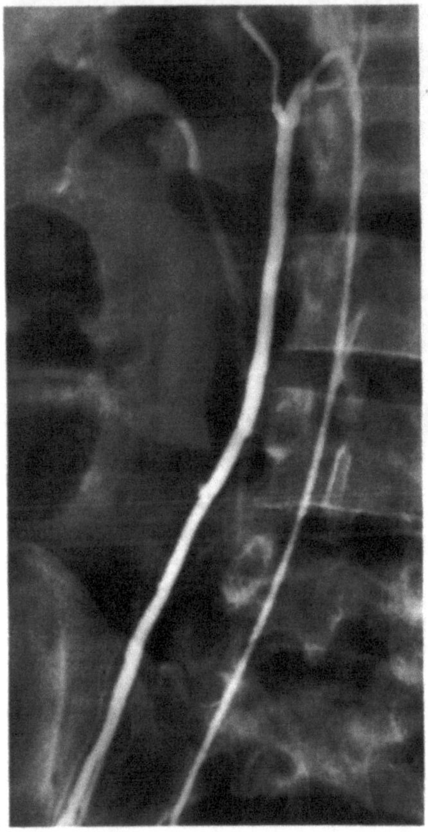

11.4

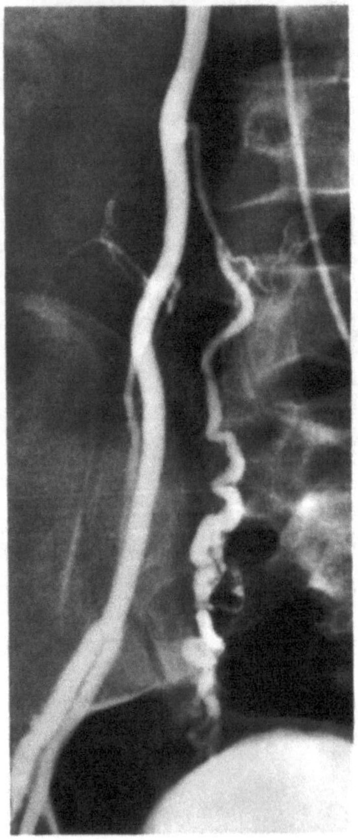

11.5

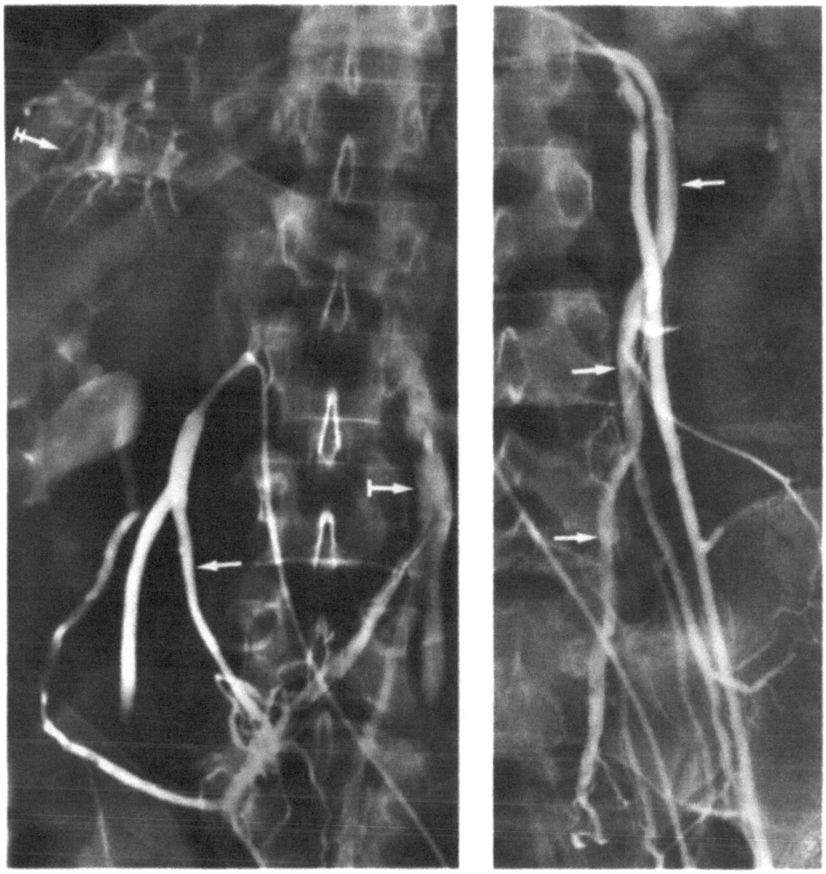

a b

Fig. 11.6. a Anastomoses between the spermatic veins and the portal system. Selective opacification of the right spermatic vein gives evidence of anastomosis (↗) with the mesenteric system. This anastomosis provides visualization of the superior mesenteric vein (↗) and then of the portal trunk and of the intrahepatic portal branches (↗). b Anastomoses between the left spermatic vein and the inferior mesenteric vein. Selective opacification of the left spermatic vein permits opacification of the entire inferior mesenteric vein (↗). The injection was performed in the upright position

---

◁ Fig. 11.3a, b. Opacification of the left spermatic vein via anastomoses of the renal system. a Injection into the left renal vein in the upright position. Faint visualization of the terminal portion of the spermatic vein due to the presence of a valve (*) which is competent. Important anastomoses arising from the hilus of the kidney allow retrograde opacification of the spermatic vein (↗) from the level of the L3 pedicle on. b Opacification of the left renal vein in the upright position. Very large anastomoses between the renal venous system and the spermatic system. The spermatic vein is competent near its origin, nonopacified in its lumbar segment, but opacified via the anastomosis at the level of the lateral masses of the sacrum. These two examples show that the existence of competent valves in the terminal segment of the spermatic vein does not exclude the presence of a varicocele. Only injection into the renal vein in the upright position allows to rule out lower located communications between the spermatic vein and anastomoses from the renal system

Fig. 11.4. Right spermatic venography. Vein with incompetent valves feeding a small varicocele. Note the anastomosis between the spermatic vein and the right renal vein

Fig. 11.5. Direct anastomosis between the right spermatic vein and the ureteral venous system. The right ureteral venous system is markedly developed and varicoid, and drains partly toward the hypogastric system. The right spermatic vein has an increased diameter. Presence of a large varicocele

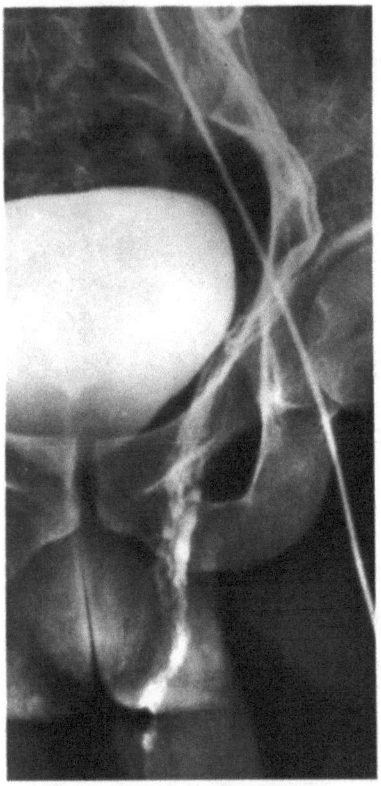

Fig. 11.7. Small right varicocele. In this patient who has a large varicocele on the left, thermography had not shown the smaller right varicocele. Only spermatic venography has given evidence of its presence

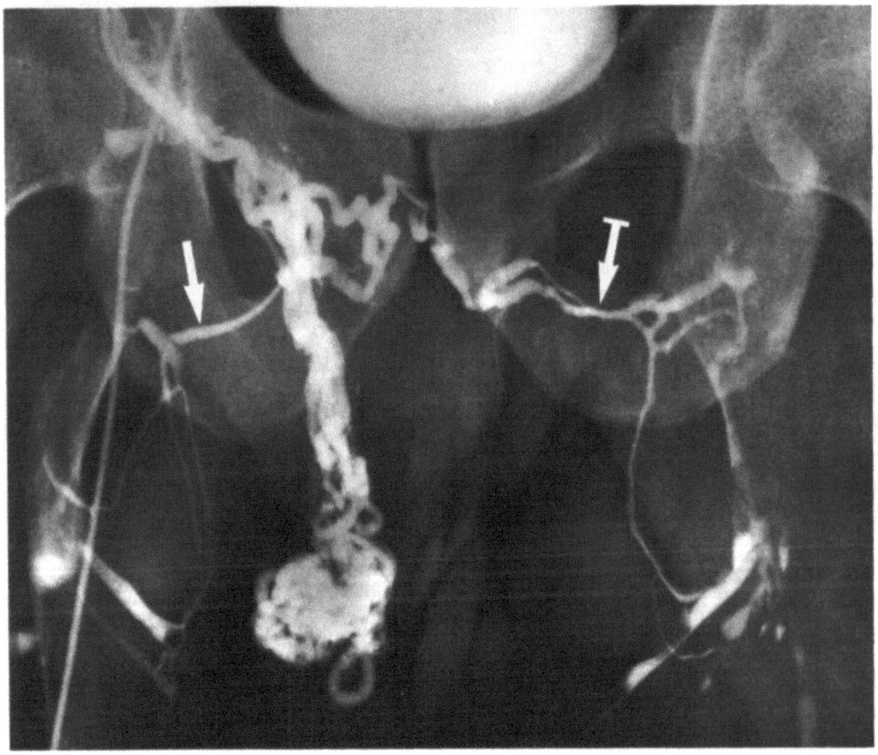

Fig. 11.8. Large right varicocele with bilateral drainage toward the external pudendal veins. The right spermatic vein feeds a huge right varicocele which empties partly into the right external pudendal system (↗) and into the left external pudendal system (↗)

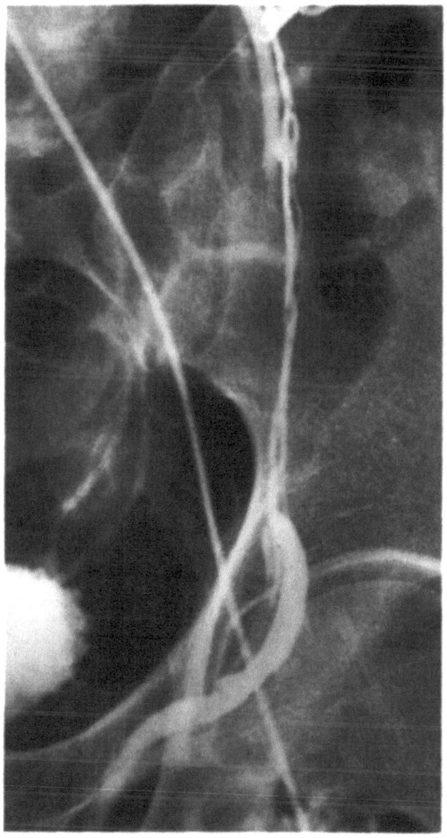

11.9

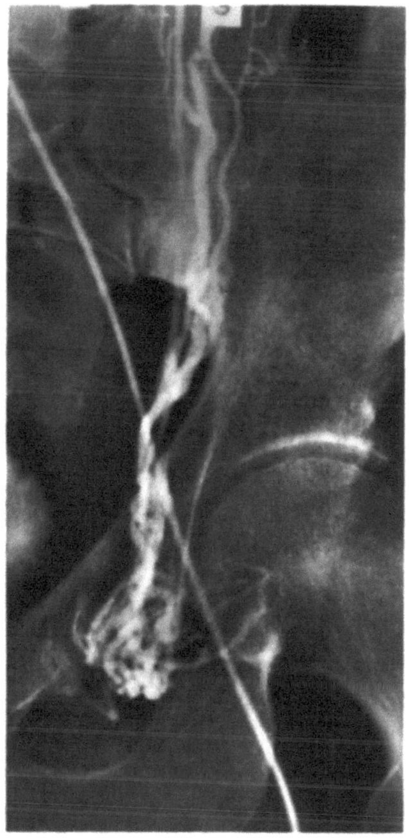

11.10

Fig. 11.9. Recurrent left varicocele after surgery. Selective retrograde opacification of the left spermatic vein demonstrates a filling defect in its main channel. But the spermatic venous trunk which has a large caliber below the ligature, is opacified through vertical anastomoses. Fine collateral channels that were overlooked at surgery become hypertrophic and cause recurrences

Fig. 11.10. Investigation of an ectopic testicle. Spermatic venography allows to locate ectopic testicles in case of incompetence of the valves (in this case at the level of the internal opening of the inguinal canal)

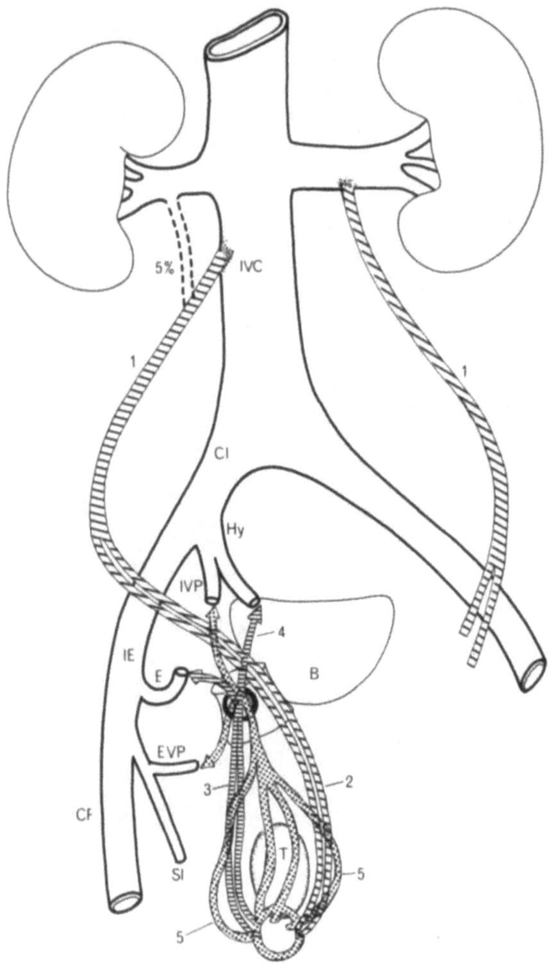

Fig. 11.11. Venous drainage of the scrotum.
1 Spermatic veins
2 Anterior spermatic plexus
3 Posterior spermatic plexus and vein of the deferent canal
4 Prostaticovesical and seminal plexus
5 Superficial group: scrotal veins
IVC Inferior vena cava
CI Common iliac vein
Hy Hypogastric vein (internal iliac vein)
IPV Internal pudendal vein
EI External iliac vein
E Epigastric vein
EPV External pudendal vein
CF Common femoral vein
B Bladder
T Testis

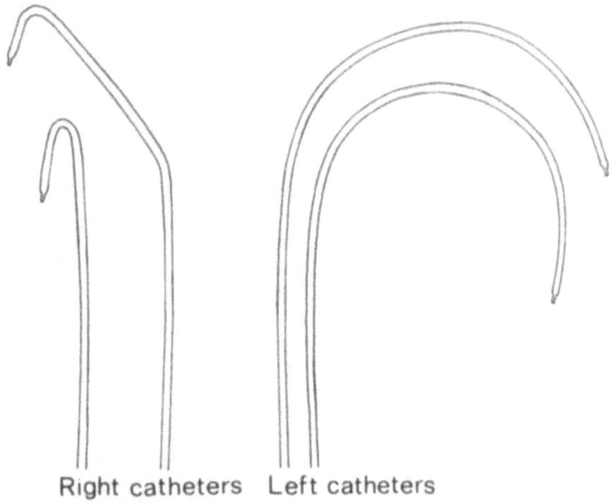

Fig. 11.12. Currently used types of catheters

Chapter 12. Hepatic Venography

12.1 History

The first hepatic vein catheterizations were performed in 1951 by Rappaport in dogs. In 1953 the technique was applied to humans by Tori for the diagnosis of neoplastic obstructions of the right hepatic vein. The same year, Norhagen obtained good opacification of the hepatic vein by inferior caval injection after occlusion of the inferior vena cava by a balloon placed in the atrium, and by increased intrathoracic pressure. Unfortunately this method brought severe complications, i.e., collapsus and arrhythmia. Also in the same year, Steinbach performed an inadvertent hepatic parenchymal injection by attempting splenoportography, and hence opacified the superior hepatic veins of the left liver lobe.

In 1954 Nunez obtained opacification of the hepatic veins through intraparenchymal injection of a contrast medium. He points out the possible value of this method for detecting obstructive lesions of the hepatic veins. In 1955 Brink and Botha diagnosed complete obstruction of the hepatic veins from the impossibility of catheterizing them and from their nonopacification on an inferior vena cavogram. The diagnosis was confirmed anatomically.

In 1963 Moreno carried out a hemodynamic and morphologic study by direct intrahepatic injection in 62 normal and cirrhotic patients. The intrahepatic injection rapidly filled the hepatic veins in normal subjects. It was the same in the cirrhotic patients, which allowed Moreno to conclude there was no postsinusoidal hemodynamic obstacle, the histologic lesions being compensated for by collateral circulation. Contrariwise, in the cardiac liver, the opacification showed a sinusoidal stasis and he noted delayed opacification of the hepatic veins (postsinusoidal obstacle). At the same time Britton reported the same conclusions with retrograde catheterization.

Since then numerous studies have been devoted to radiologic investigations of the hepatic veins.

12.2 Anatomy

The vascularization of the liver is constituted by two afferent pedicles, namely the hepatic artery and the portal system. There is a single efferent pedicle: the suprahepatic venous system.

The hepatic lobule is the circulatory unit of the liver. It is a hexagonal unit arranged around the smallest hepatic vessel, the centrolobular vein, and contains at each angle a portal vessel, a hepatic arteriole, a bile canaliculus, and a lymph vessel. The blood drained by the hepatic arteries and by the portal venules enters the sinusoidal circulation and flows centripetally, toward the centrolobular vein (Fig. 12.1). The total flow of the hepatic veins is considerable: it is about $1\,500 \pm 300$ ml/min.

The main anatomic characteristic of the hepatic veins is their morphologic variation. According to Couinaud, there are usually three main hepatic veins: the left hepatic vein, the sagittal or middle hepatic vein, and the right hepatic vein. The left and the sagittal veins are often united over a short distance before entering the inferior vena cava.

12.2.1 Left Hepatic Vein

The left hepatic vein drains the left liver lobe. It is formed by several veins which converge on the right posterior part of the left lobe; some of them are sagittal, the others almost sagittal. Sometimes a vein of the posterior surface of the liver is present. The trunk of the left hepatic vein is short and located in the left segmental fissure, crossing the Arantius canal. It courses transversely to the superior edge of the caudate lobe and enters the inferior vena cava.

According to certain authors (Nogueira) the left hepatic vein results from the confluence of an anteroposterior vein with a transverse left vein. Whatever the case, the left hepatic vein drains blood from the left lobe (segments II and III) and sometimes part of segment IV. Segment I is isolated and drains directly into the inferior vena cava.

12.2.2 Sagittal or Middle Hepatic Vein

This vein drains segment IV, and in part the right paramedian sector (segments V and VIII), which is a boundary area also drained by the right hepatic vein. The sagittal hepatic vein results from the confluence of veins proceeding from the anterior part of this segment. These venules are most often united into two main trunks, right and left. The sagittal hepatic vein occupies the main lobar fissure. This fissure is the base of the hepatic segmentation and of the division into right and left liver lobes (it separates the right and left territories of the portal distribution).

The sagittal hepatic vein joins the left hepatic vein above the caudate lobe (Spigelian lobe or segment I). Finally, it is a short and voluminous trunk which enters the left anterior wall of the inferior vena cava.

12.2.3 Right Hepatic Veins

The right hepatic veins are divided into inferior, middle, and superior veins. The inferior and the middle veins have a small caliber and are sometimes even absent. There are two or three inferior veins entering the anterior wall of the inferior vena cava where it courses dorsal to the liver. They drain a very small volume of parenchyma, located immediately to the right of the caudate lobe.

The middle veins course rather transversally on the posterior edge of the liver. They enter the right lateral wall of the inferior vena cava, cranial to the previous ones.

The right superior vein is often the largest of the hepatic veins. It occupies the right segmental fissure, which separates the lateral from the right paramedian sector. It drains the right lateral sector (segments VI and VII) and a part of the right paramedian sector (segments V and VIII). The veins of segment VII may form an isolated trunk. The vein enters the right anterior wall of the inferior vena cava above its intrahepatic course, close to the inferior phrenic veins. Its axis forms an angle of about 70° with the inferior vena cava.

12.2.4 Dorsal Veins

The dorsal veins drain segment I. There are one to four constant veins, which enter the lower third of the retrohepatic segment of the inferior vena cava. They are often termed "accessory hepatic veins."

12.2.5 Anatomic Variations

Sometimes all the veins are present according to the classical description, but their respective importance is different from the normal pattern. When the right superior vein is smaller, the inferior and middle veins are larger.

Sometimes the territory of the right superior vein as a whole is reduced. The following compensations are then seen:

Hypertrophy of the sagittal vein (it drains segment IV, segment V, and segment VI, totally or partly)

Hypertrophy of the right inferior vein, which then drains segment VI and a part of segment VII

Hypertrophy of the sagittal veins and right inferior veins, and reduction of the right superior vein

Hypertrophy of the inferior and middle veins

Other cases show marked morphologic variations:

Absence of a common trunk formed by the sagittal and the left hepatic veins

Duplication of the left lobar veins (there are then two venous trunks, an anterior and a posterior one)

Vein of the posterior edge of the left lobe

A vein of the umbilical fissure coursing in the left segmental fissure

A vein originating from segment VIII directly entering the inferior vena cava instead of joining the median vein.

Veins of segment IV emptying entirely into the sagittal vein

The left inferior phrenic vein emptying into the left hepatic vein

The superior right hepatic vein having a very short trunk

12.2.6 Anastomoses

According to Viamonte, the hepatic veins communicate both with one another (Fig. 12.9) – multiple anastomoses are seen between the main hepatic veins – and with the portal system. In the latter case, anastomoses are rare (Sabourin) and often pathologic. Sometimes the right hepatic vein communicates with the portal veins of segment VI. The right branch of the sagittal vein communicates with the portal vein of segment V. In cirrhoses, portohepatic communications are more frequent.

In conclusion, the superior hepatic venous system has three fundamental characteristics:

1) It is a venous plexus: each hepatic venous trunk receives multiple very fine rami coming directly from the parenchyma. This is the main difference from the portal system, which is of the dichotomous type; moreover, small vessels enter the inferior vena cava directly.
2) Anatomic variations are frequent, which makes it difficult to apply theoretical anatomic data in interpreting radiologic findings.
3) Finally, it is a very important venous system, since it drains the entire digestive territory (total flow 1500 ± 300 ml/min).

12.3 Technique

Opacification of the hepatic veins can be obtained by three methods:

1) By portal opacification, whereby the contrast material follows the normal blood flow and opacifies the hepatic veins after traversing the liver (afferent approach).
2) By hepatic puncture (direct approach), injection being performed at the level of the hepatic sinusoids and hepatic veins.
3) By retrograde opacification of the hepatic veins from the inferior vena cava, or by carboxyangiography (peripheral approach)

12.3.1 Afferent Approach

The hepatic veins are exceptionally seen on a late film of splenoportography by direct puncture.

After celiac or superior mesenteric arteriography, opacification of the hepatic veins is seen in about 1% of normal subjects (Glickman). This occurs in two circumstances:

1) Lack of drainage: compression of the distal part of a hepatic vein by a tumoral process renders drainage slower and thus allows a certain concentration of the contrast material into the hepatic veins.
2) Lack of nonopacified blood. Portal vein thrombosis or compression of the portal or splenic vein causes diminution or even suppression of the fraction of portal blood (which is not radiopaque). Thus, the arterial system takes over the entire hepatic vascularization and drains into the hepatic system without dilution. Two peculiar cases involve (a) hemangiomas in children, when the hepatic veins are massively and precociously opacified thanks to an arteriovenous shunt, and (b) arteriohepatic venous fistules, which are usually secondary to a puncture biopsy of the liver and are much more rare than hepaticoportal fistules.

Umbilicoportography, after repermeation of the round ligament of the liver, may opacify the hepatic veins that drain this segment. This method is mainly used in investigations of the portal vessels; it is somewhat difficult and is inconstant in achieving opacification of the hepatic veins. It involves the possibility of failure and requires the same aseptic conditions as surgery. The risks of pylephlebitis greatly restrict its indications.

12.3.2 Direct (Transhepatic) Approach (Figs. 12.18–12.21)

This rather simple method was described in 1958 by Paraf and Chalut. The trocar is the same as that used in percutaneous transhepatic cholangiographies. While the patient maintains apnea, the trocar is introduced on the median axillary line, at the level of the tenth right intercostal space, and level with the great axis of the liver. Due to its upward, medial, and posterior obliqueness, the puncture passes clearly above and dorsal to the hepatic hilus.

One may obtain dripping of venous blood right away – the test injection confirms that it comes from the hepatic veins – so that the pressure may be measured and the injection is performed. When there is no dripping, the catheter is slowly withdrawn until dripping occurs. A test injection may permit filling of the hepatic veins from the parenchyma. The hepatic veins are the most accessible to catheterization, so that opacification almost never fails. If it should fail, a second puncture can be performed. Sometimes thin portal rami are seen, but their smaller caliber and reverse direction toward the hilus allows one to recognize them readily. Nondilated bile ducts are usually not catheterized.

Direct puncture of the liver is used in investigation of the portal system. The catheter is given a different direction – more horizontal and more anterior. Apart from certain indications (embolization of varices, withdrawal of samples for assaying hormone levels), it is in fact preferable to explore the portal system by retrograde ileoportography, with injection of a large amount of contrast medium into the superior mesenteric artery. The direct transhepatic approach, though technically easy, has been abandoned in favor of retrograde phlebographic techniques because it has two limitations:

1) The puncture with a needle (the tip of which is either intraparenchymal or intravascular, or intrasclerotic in cases of sclerosis) makes the pressure measurements unreliable. When the injection is intraparenchymal, only a small area is analyzed, and interpretation of the image obtained at the puncture site is difficult.
2) It exposes the patient to the risks inherent in hepatic puncture: peritoneal hemorrhage (especially when several punctures

have been performed, with disturbances in the blood crasis or angiomatous malformations); intrahepatic arteriovenous fistula (mainly hepaticoportal or even hepaticohepatic); subcapsular rupture, usually uneventful; and choleperitoneum, which occurs only when there is dilatation of the bile passages.

Exploration of the hepatic venous system may be performed via a transjugular approach or by direct puncture of the parenchyma, in order to limit the risks of peritoneal and subcapsular rupture. At present, the only indication for direct puncture (transhepatic or transjugular) is the Budd-Chiari syndrome (Caroli). Opacification occurs above the thrombosis and allows the collateral circulation to be visualized.

12.3.3 Retrograde Approach

With this method the hepatic vascular system can be investigated in total or selectively.

Total

The hepatic veins are retrogradely opacified, thanks to inferior vena caval hyperpressure. With the contrainjection technique (Hernandez), concomitant injections of the inferior and superior venae cavae are performed (delayed by 2 s for the superior vena cava). This method requires bilateral femoral puncture and puncture of a vein at the bend of the elbow. When the liver is normal, it opacifies only the termination of the large trunks. Moreover, it does not permit manometric studies. Other methods have been proposed: auriculohepatic reflux; extended angiography (Viallet), which often produces opacification of the hepatic veins (especially in children or in cases of right ventricular insufficiency); and reflux by pulmonary hyperpressure obtained by a Valsalva maneuver. Occlusive methods with intra-atrial or intracaval balloons (Gillot) are no longer used.

Selective

This is the method most often used. Catheterization may be performed from above (vein of the bend of the elbow) or, more often, from below (femoral vein) (Figs. 12.2–12.6). The Seldinger technique is used. Usually the right superior hepatic vein is catheterized, since it is the easiest to approach. Sometimes, according to the clinical data, other areas are chosen (left veins, inferior right veins, middle veins, accessory veins).

A catheter 160 with a large bend, a single distal orifice, and no side holes is used. The patient is placed under electrocardiographic monitoring when the right atrium is to be traversed. Under fluoroscopic control the right main hepatic vein is searched for, very high near the inferior edge of the right atrium, at the level of the diaphragm, on the right aspect of the inferior vena cava. It is often necessary to bend the extremity of the catheter into the atrium. A test injection will verify the position of the catheter; this injection should be performed carefully, especially when the caudate veins are being sought (these latter veins are close to the suprarenal, lumbar, and inferior phrenic veins).

This method is always associated with a hemodynamic investigation. Pressures corresponding to the wedge position (sinusoidal pressure: hepatic sinusoidal pressure diminished by 1–2 mm Hg corresponds to the portal pressure), and free pressures (hepatic pressures) are recorded. Right atrial and inferior vena caval pressures are also recorded.

For each of the catheterized hepatic veins two successive injections are performed (Figs. 12.2–12.6), one with free flow (the hepatic vein is then opacified retrogradely as far as the fine rami of the fifth or sixth order), the other with the catheter in wedge position. Opacification of the hepatic parenchyma is then obtained.

Selective venography with a catheter with balloon allows opacification of an entire liver lobe (Fig. 12.7). It suffices to place it at the termination of one of the hepatic veins. Catheters with a balloon and a distal hole are employed. The balloon is inflated with diluted contrast medium in order to check whether its position is correct. The delivery rate and the amount of contrast material will depend on the volume of parenchyma drained by the hepatic vein (20 to 25 ml in the right major hepatic vein, 10 to 12 ml in a middle hepatic vein). Catheterization of the hepatic veins can be performed by lower or upper approach. This method does not permit hemodynamic studies, but it provides excellent opacification of the entire hepatic system of the area explored.

Incidents. The most frequent incident is intraparietal injection in the wall of the inferior vena cava. This happens most often during the test injections designed to show the position of the catheter tip when it has not entered a hepatic vein but is wedged into the inferior vena caval wall. This can easily be avoided by taking the precaution, prior to the injection, of verifying whether satisfactory reflux is obtained. Subcapsular injections cause persistence of an opaque stain corresponding to nonresorbed contrast material. When they are localized, they are harmless, but when they are more extended, they are responsible for detachment of Glisson's capsule.

Drawbacks. Failures are rare. Catheterization of a hepatic vein may be impossible to perform by lower approach when the inferior vena cava is not patent. Then, one must use the approach from above. A failed attempt at catheterization is not by itself conclusive proof of thrombosis. A high-pressure injection at the level of the hepatic ostium, assisted by a Valsalva maneuver and performed with a "pigtail" catheter, must then be performed.

Advantages. This method provides in one phase all the venous data for a hepatic disease and also allows hemodynamic study. The latter is unharmful and entails no major risks. It provides indispensable data in cirrhoses. After portocaval shunts it permits verification of the hemodynamic results and of the decrease of the portal hypertension. It is useful for the differential diagnosis, since it makes it possible to rule out cardiac diseases affecting the liver and malformations of the inferior vena cava.

Extensive Carboxyangiography

Bendib et al. use a gas contrast (carbon dioxide) without catheterization. The patient lies on his left side and carbon dioxide is injected into a vein of the upper limb. This gas fills the right hepatic veins, i.e., the highest-located area. This method is tolerated well and has the same indications as the total venographic techniques with positive contrast material. Nevertheless, the quality and morphologic precision are inferior to those obtained with the selective methods. Moreover, no hemodynamic measurements can be made.

Management

Inferior vena cavography. The techniques of retrograde catheterization of the hepatic veins are usually performed with an approach from below. The first step of the investigation, inferior vena cavography, is carried out by bifemoral percutaneous puncture.

Pressure measurements in the hepatic and in the portal venous systems. Different pressure measurements are made. One first performs catheterization of the right side of the heart with withdrawal curve of the right ventricle in the right atrium, then in the subauricular, retrohepatic, and, finally, infrahepatic inferior vena cava. The ventricular pressure is between 0 and 25 mm Hg; the right atrial pressure between 0 and 1 mm Hg; the pressure in the inferior vena cava is about 2 mm Hg.

Thereafter the tip of the catheter is placed in a hepatic vein (usually the right hepatic vein) in the wedged position. While the pressure is continuously being recorded, the catheter is returned to the free position; rapid decrease in pressure ensues. This procedure is repeated several times, in at least two different hepatic veins. The free hepatic pressure ranges between 1 and 5 mm Hg. The wedge hepatic pressure reflects the sinusoidal pressure and is about 5 to 10 mm Hg. In a normal subject, the difference between the free and the wedge pressure is about 5 mm Hg.

When hepatic veins of small caliber are catheterized, it may be worthwhile to substitute the pressure in the suprahepatic segment of the inferior vena cava for the free hepatic pressure, since it is often difficult to obtain the real free hepatic pressure, owing to artifacts. The difference between the sinusoidal pressures, appreciated by wedged catheterization, and the portal pressure is 1 to 2 mm Hg. The variation of these two parameters is corroborative: wedge injection thus provides a good estimate of the portal pressure.

Injection of the hepatic veins. The appearance varies according to the site of injection.

For *free injection* the rate is about 6 ml/s for 3 to 4 s. The hepatic vein is opacified retrogradely as far as fine rami of the fifth or sixth order (Figs. 12.2a, 12.3a, 12.4). The appearance is similar to the anatomic description. The hepatic venous system is dense, close, and grouped. The caliber of the hepatic veins is regular, without any dilatation. The branches course toward the inferior vena cava, a short segment of which is usually visible since it is opacified by reflux from the injected hepatic vein. Though it is transient, this opacification is of great interest since it makes it possible to check the ostia of the hepatic veins. The hepatic veins are rapidly washed through by nonopaque blood. The suprahepatic segment of the inferior vena cava is only partly opacified, owing to the dilution of the contrast material. The same phenomenon is seen at the level of the hepatic veins when the injection has been quantitatively insufficient.

Wedge injection (2 ml/s for 3 to 4 s) permits the opacification of a hepatic lobule (Figs. 12.3b, 12.5, and 12.6). The lobule appears as an opaque area several centimeters in diameter, with smooth, even contours. Filling of the adjacent hepatic veins from the injected lobule is frequently achieved. Communications between the hepatic veins are common, physiological and often poorly contrasted. While opacification of the hepatic veins is always very brief, parenchymal opacity persists longer. Portal filling is inconstant; when it occurs, it is only momentary, rapidly washed out in the hepatopetal direction and only seen with high-rate injections (5 to 8 ml/s).

When the injection is made using a *catheter with a balloon,* the balloon must be placed at the level of the termination of the hepatic vein, so as to permit retrograde opacification of the entire territory above. The balloon is inflated with contrast material diluted by half, in order to locate it accurately. The vein must be blocked, which necessitates often more than 5 ml of liquid. The amount of contrast material and its delivery rate will depend on the "volume" of the area to be explored. The usual amount for the main right hepatic vein is about 25 ml, with a delivery rate of 3 ml/s.

This method provides opacification not only of the trunk of the hepatic vein, but also of its origin branches and of the hepatic "parenchyma." Anastomoses with the adjacent lobar territories are easily opacified when there is no pathologic condition of the liver. No portal reflux is obtained with this method. No expansive process, even the smallest, located in the area explored can pass undetected with this method (Fig. 12.7).

12.4 Pathologic Findings

12.4.1 Cirrhosis

Hepatic venography is carried out for the hemodynamic investigation in portal hypertension. In cirrhoses, the increase of portal pressure is of either postsinusoidal or sinusoidal type. Hepatic venography is performed as a preoperative investigation or as a postoperative survey.

Preoperative Evaluation of Portal Hyperpressure

Wedge hepatic catheterization is the simplest method for detecting increased portal pressure and evaluating its degree. The wedge hepatic pressure reflects the intrasinusoidal pressure; it is increased, while the free hepatic pressure is normal. There is said to be portal hyperpressure when the gradient is greater than 7 mm Hg. Increase in this gradient is one of the elements from which the severity of the portal hypertension can be evaluated. The hypertension is mild when the gradient is between 7 and 14 mm Hg, moderate when it is between 15 and 30, and severe above 30 (Fig. 12.8).

The phlebographic patterns are variable. The hepatic lobule may be normal or appear heterogeneous, with irregular, jagged margins (Fig. 12.11). Schematically, there are two venographic patterns: one observes either a limited number of small veins, difficult to catheterize, producing a "dead tree" appearance, or veins of normal caliber but irregular and compressed. There may also be opacification of the efferent lymph vessels toward the liver hilus (Fig. 12.13), or retrograde portal opacification. But more significant than the mere fact of opacification are its intensity and the direction of the disappearance of the contrast, i.e., the direction of the washout.

According to Warren, four stages may be distinguished: Stage I: The venous sinusoidal network fills correctly in a homogeneous and regular fashion, without opacification of the portal veins. The dye drains into the hepatic veins. This is evidence of a still normal or very slightly reduced portal flow.

Stage II: There occurs retrograde opacification of the portal branches with hepatopetal blood flow in the opacified portal branches. Moderate peripheral portal vascular resistance is usually seen in this case (Fig. 12.10).

Stage III: The portal branches fill well, the contrast medium stagnates in the portal circulation. This pattern is found in late stages of hepatic cirrhosis and a fortiori in thromboses of the portal trunk (Fig. 12.11).

Stage IV: A portal trunk fills from the opacified portal branch thanks to reversed flow (hepatofugal). Hepatic venography thus permits differentiation between dynamic obstruction due to reversed flow and organic obstruction due to thrombosis in the course of cirrhoses at that stage. The reversed flow sometimes leads to filling of the collateral channels (Fig. 12.12).

Postoperative Survey

In this case the results depend upon the type of portocaval shunt that has been performed. In the case of terminolateral anastomoses, venography often demonstrates marked lymphatic circulation and the portal cul-de-sac. In laterolateral portocaval anastomoses, catheterization of the inferior vena cava demonstrates the patency of the portal trunk above the anastomosis. In both cases, the wedge pressures are markedly decreased (by about 50% to 60%). Laterolateral splenorenal anastomoses cause a lesser diminution in the pressure gradient, since the caliber of the renal vein accommodates sufficient portosplenic flow, only thanks to increased pressure. Diminution of the gradient is about 20%. In all cases, the presence of a portocaval anastomosis favors reversal of the portal flow and thus passage from stage II to stage III or IV of Warren's classification.

12.4.2 Budd-Chiari Syndrome

The Budd-Chiari syndrome consists of the clinical manifestations secondary to total or partial occlusion of the hepatic venous system or the suprahepatic segment of the inferior vena cava. Hepatic venography is useful to confirm the diagnosis, since the clinical and histological features are similar to those in cardiac liver or peliosis; it will also serve to demonstrate the presence of a surgically curable obstacle (diaphragm of the inferior vena cava, tumor in the neighborhood).

The choice of the technique depends upon existence or absence of associated inferior vena caval thrombosis. The order of the investigations is thus:

1) Inferior vena cavography.
2) Measurement of cardiac, inferior caval, and hepatic vein pressures.
3) Catheterization of the main or accessory hepatic veins or attempt at opacifying them.
4) In case of failure of the selective hepatic catheterization, transhepatic venography via transcutaneous approach.

12.4.3 Results

Inferior vena cava (see Chapt. 8). The inferior vena cavogram may be strictly normal, which occurs rarely. Most often, in case of a Budd-Chiari syndrome, there is a compensating hypertrophy of the caudate lobe causing *extrinsic compression* of the inferior vena cava on its retrohepatic segment. The compression is exerted to the detriment of the right anterolateral wall of the inferior vena cava. Moreover, when the hepatic veins are obstructed, a reflux of the contrast material most often occurs, toward the *ostia of the hepatic veins,* without secondary dilution flow (due to the inflow of nonopaque blood at this level). The obstructed ostium may have a beaklike appearance (Fig. 8.6). Sometimes the inferior vena cava is totally obstructed, so that approach from above must be attempted. Finally, there may be a *congenital membrane* occluding the inferior vena cava. This diagnosis should not be overlooked, since this disease process can be treated by surgery.

Hepatic vein catheterization. This is quite often impossible, at least as concerns the main trunks. Sometimes selective catheterization demonstrates the thrombus in the hepatic trunk and nonsystematized venules above (Fig. 12.22). In some cases, especially when there is compensating hypertrophy of the caudate lobe (Fig. 12.17), catheterization of accessory hepatic veins is possible, demonstrating their clearly increased caliber. There is of course no opacification of the adjacent lobes, since their hepatic veins are occluded.

In some cases it is possible to catheterize the venules from the inferior vena cava (Fig. 12.14–12.16). These veins are not systematized; they are proof of well-developed collateral venous channels. These cases have a quite good prognosis.

Transcutaneous venography (Figs. 12.18–12.21). When the inferior vena cava is occluded, this method provides radiologic proof of the Budd-Chiari syndrome and demonstrates the thrombosis of the hepatic veins and the presence of numerous collateral channels. This collateral venous network comprises the phrenic veins, the veins of the lesser omentum, the veins of the falciform ligament of the liver, and the intercostal veins. These collateral channels join the inferior caval system via the spinal plexuses and the azygos system. When the collateral circulation is not well developed, there occurs retrograde venous drainage into the portal system. When this drainage is massive, the prognosis is poor (Fig. 12.19). Sometimes a partial recanalization of a thrombosed vessel produces lacunar images at the level of the ostium (Fig. 12.21).

It must be kept in mind that suspicion of Budd-Chiari syndrome calls for a complete investigation of the hepatic system, since there may be an isolated lobar thrombosis (exploration of the right side only would risk failure to detect an involvement of the left side).

12.4.4 The Cardiac Liver

Usually, exploration of the hepatic veins is hardly necessary in patients with cardiac insufficiency, the clinical picture being evocative enough. Under certain circumstances (constrictive pericarditis), the hepatologic manifestations are prominent and the patient is suspected of having a Budd-Chiari syndrome or even cirrhosis (Fig. 12.23). The hemodynamic investigation will obviously be important. It will show increased pressures in the ventricle, right atrium, inferior vena cava, and hepatic veins (15 to 20 mm Hg). There is no gradient between the free and wedge hepatic pressures. This venous hyperpressure associated with anomalies in the right ventricular curve is sufficient to make the diagnosis. In this case inferior vena cavography shows stasis and dilatation of the hepatic vessels.

12.4.5 Intrahepatic Expansive Processes

Hepatic venography, especially the methods using the catheters with a balloon (Fig. 12.7), may be performed to demonstrate small intrahepatic expansive processes (Fig. 12.24), especially metastases.

Hepatic venography is not used for diagnosing larger expansive processes, whether benign or malignant. Such processes may produce compressions of the major hepatic veins, when they are located close to the veins' termination, and result in a localized pseudo-Budd-Chiari syndrome.

In hepatic polycystoses the hepatic veins are markedly deformed, since they wind around numerous cysts, and are therefore difficult to systematize (Fig. 12.25).

12.4.6 Perihepatitis Chronica Hyperplastica

Perihepatitis chronica hyperplastica, also called frosted liver, is an uncommon condition due to the development of a sclerous perihepatic covering below or above Glisson's capsule. The disease is encountered in portal hypertension; the obstacle is pre- or postsinusoidal (cirrhosis, idiopathic portal hypertension, cavernoma). Some very irregular, gnarled subcapsular vessels may be seen, with a network of the anastomotic type at the level of the fibrous covering (Fig. 12.26). Moreover, there may be additional specific changes due to other anomalies of the causal disease (cirrhosis).

References

Bendib M, Toumi M, Boudellab A (1974) La carboxy-angiographie élargie dans l'exploration de la sphère hépatique. Apport d'une nouvelle méthode de la phlébographie. Med Chir Dig 3:237–245

Brink AS, Botha D (1955) Budd-chiari. Diagnostic radiologique. Ann Radiol (Paris) 28:330–331

Britton RC, Brown CH, Shirey EK (1963) Intrahepatic veno-occlusive disease in cirrhosis with chronic ascites: Diagnosis by hepatic phlebography and results of surgical treatment. Ann Surg 158:370–382

Caroli J, Julien C (1966) Indication et résultats de la veinographie transcutanée transhépatique. Gaz Med Fr 6:2437–2460

Couinaud C (1957) Le foie. Etudes anatomiques et chirurgicales. Masson, Paris

Gillot C (1968) La phlébographie cave occlusive. Technique d'exploration des veines rénales, des veines sus-hépatiques et des anastomoses porto-caves. Arch Mal App Dig 57:25–37

Glickman MG, Handel SF (1972) Opacification of hepatic veins during celiac and hepatic angiography. Radiology 103:565–571

Hernandez C, Charleux H, Picard JM, Morin G (1961) Phlébographie sus-hépatique. Technique originale. Presse Med 69:1409–1410

Moreno AH, Ruzicka FF, Rousselot LM, Burchell AR, Buno RF, Slafsky SF, Burke JH (1963) Functional hepatography: A study of the hemodynamics of the outflow tracts of the human liver by intraparenchymal deposition of contrast medium, with attempts at fonctionnal evaluation of the outflow block concept of cirrhotic ascites and the accessory outflow role of the portal veins. Radiology 81:65–79

Paraf A, Chalut J (1958) L'exploration non opératoire du système porte chez les splénectomisés. L'hépatographie rétrograde transcutanée. Rev Med Chir Mal Foie 33:215–240

Rappaport AM (1951) Hepatic venography. Acta Radiol 36:165–171

Sabourin C (1900) Les communications porto-sus-hé-

patiques directes dans le foie humain. Rev Méd 20:74–83
Steinbach HL, Bierman HR, Miller ER, Wass WA (1953) Percutaneous transhepatic portal venography. A preliminary report. Radiology 60:363–373
Tori G (1953) Hepatic venography in man. Acta Radiol 39:89–96
Viamonte M, Martinez LO, Parks RE, Warren WD, Fomon JJ (1968) Liver shunts. AJR 102:773–775
Viamonte M, Warren WD, Fomon JJ (1970) Liver panangiography in the assessment of portal hypertension in liver cirrhosis. Radiol Clin North Am 8:147–167
Warren WD, Muller WH (1959) A classification of some hemodynamic changes in cirrhosis and their surgical significance. Ann Surg 150:413–427

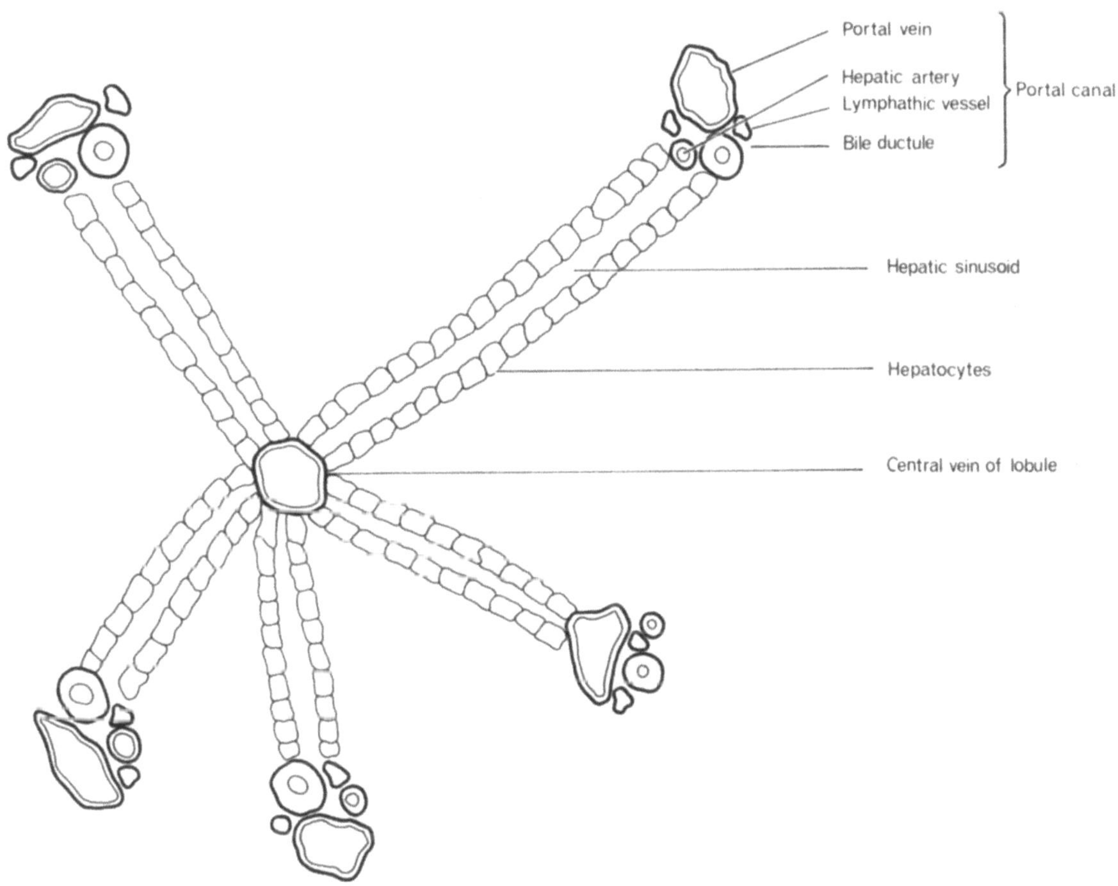

Fig. 12.1. Hepatic lobule

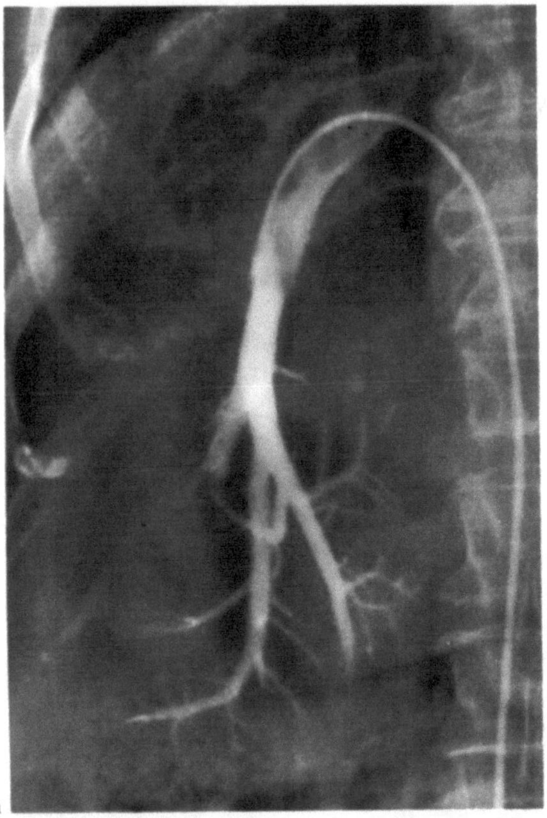
12.2a

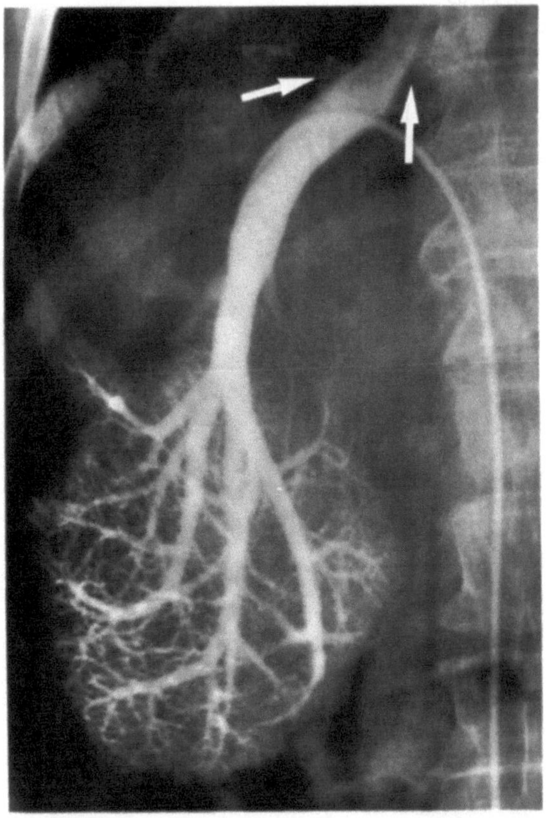
12.2b

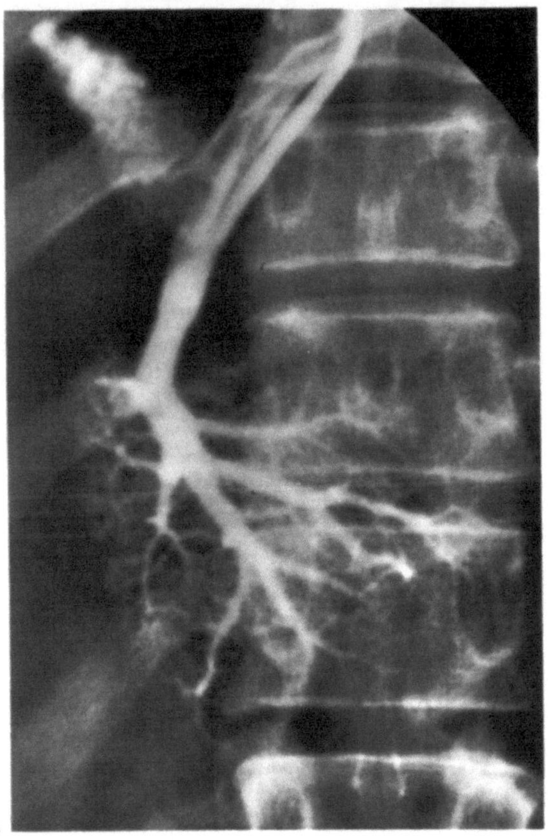
12.3a

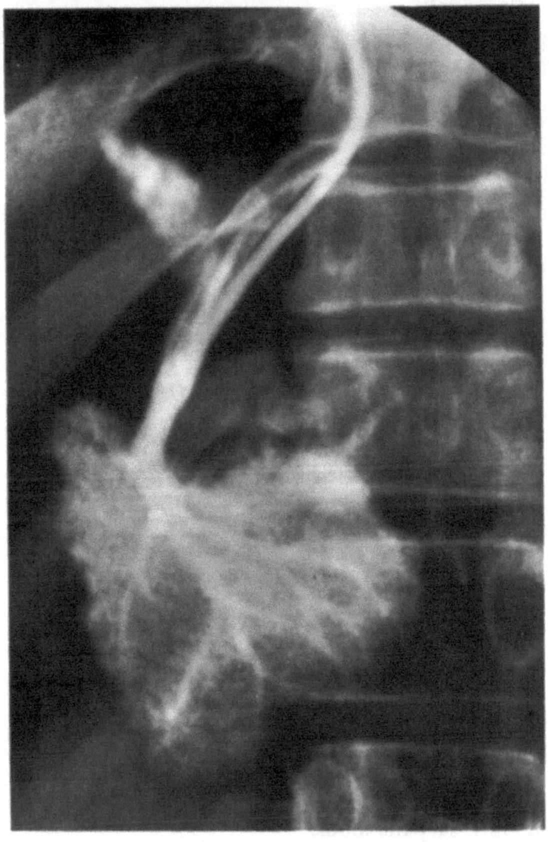
12.3b

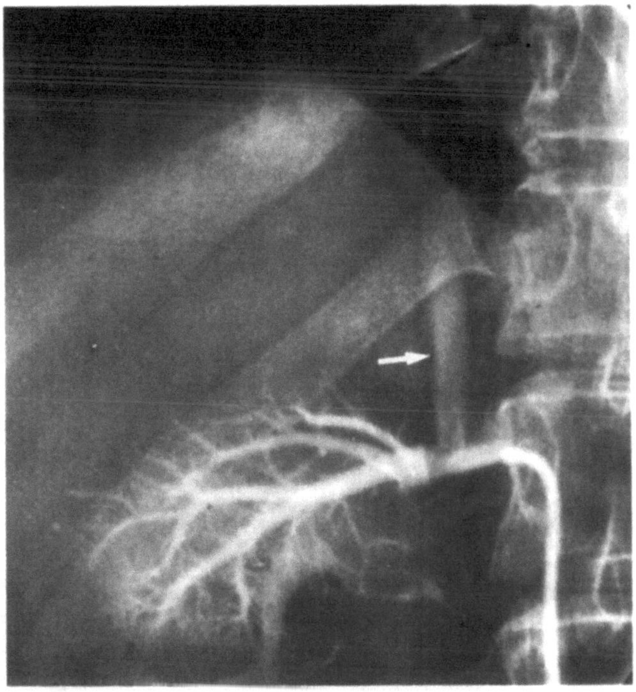

Fig. 12.4. Small hepatic veins. Free flow injection. Note the small caliber of the injected hepatic lobule. Slight reflux in the inferior vena cava (↗)

◁ Fig. 12.2a, b. Right hepatic vein. Free injection. Anatomical variations. a Onset of opacification. Only the trunk of the right hepatic vein and some of its origin branches are opacified. b At the 4th second, opacification of fine hepatic rami of segment IV. Dilution flow (↗) at the termination of the major hepatic vein

◁ Fig. 12.3. a Free injection showing a normal sagittal vein. a Harmonious and dense hepatic vascularization. The superior hepatic branches join to form the trunk of the sagittal vein. Its ostium is free. b Wedge injection. Good opacification of a hepatic lobule. It is homogeneous and has smooth contours

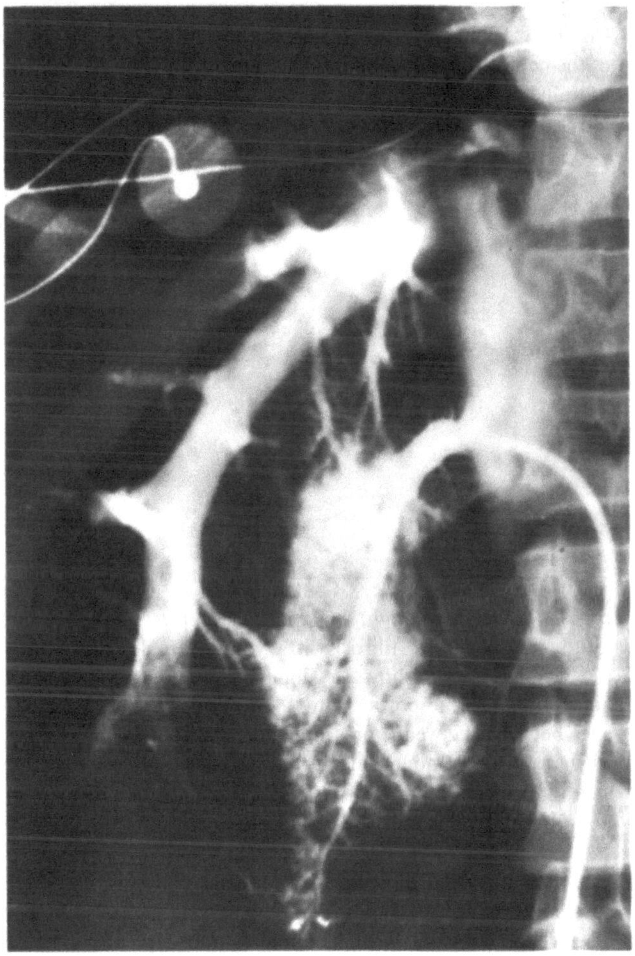

Fig. 12.5. Catheterization of a small hepatic vein. Via anastomoses between segment I and right liver lobe, opacification of the right hepatic vein is obtained; there occurs stagnation of the contrast due to right ventricular failure. Note also the moderate reflux in the inferior vena cava

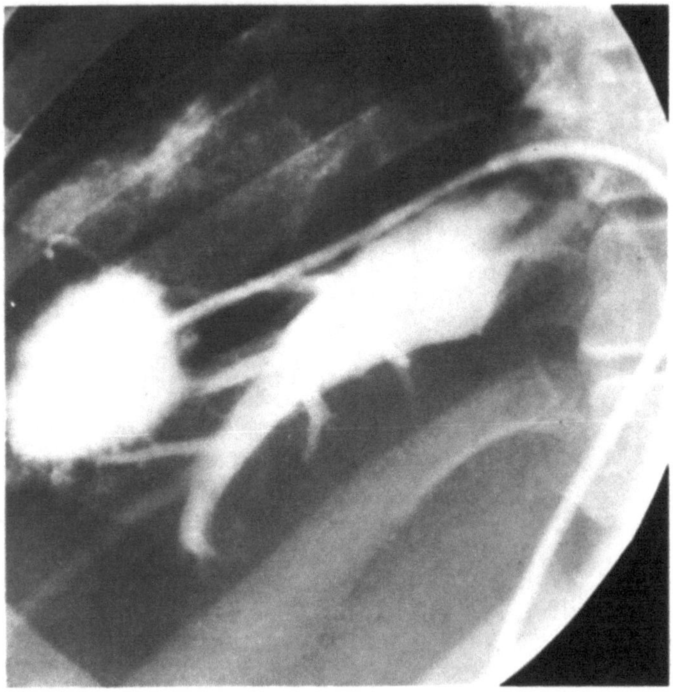

Fig. 12.6. Right hepatic vein. Wedge injection. Normal appearance of the hepatic lobule: dense and homogeneous. The contrast material is drained by all hepatic branches adjacent to the catheterized venule. No reflux into the portal vein

---

Fig. 12.7. Occlusive right hepatic venography (catheter with balloon). Cryptogenetic fibrosis in a young female. Opacification of the venous system shows a slightly inhomogeneous parenchyma and reflux into the portal vein (↗) secondary to cirrhosis. (Difference between the wedge pressure and the free pressure: 15 mm Hg). This occlusive venographic technique allows the visualization of small intrahepatic tumors, particularly metastases. But for that, all main hepatic veins must be catheterized ▷

Fig. 12.8. Diagram showing the difference between the wedge pressure and the free pressure in the hepatic vein in a case of cirrhosis. The wedge pressure is high, about 44 mm Hg; the free pressure is 12 mm Hg. Thus the gradient is 32 mm Hg, proof of severe portal hypertension

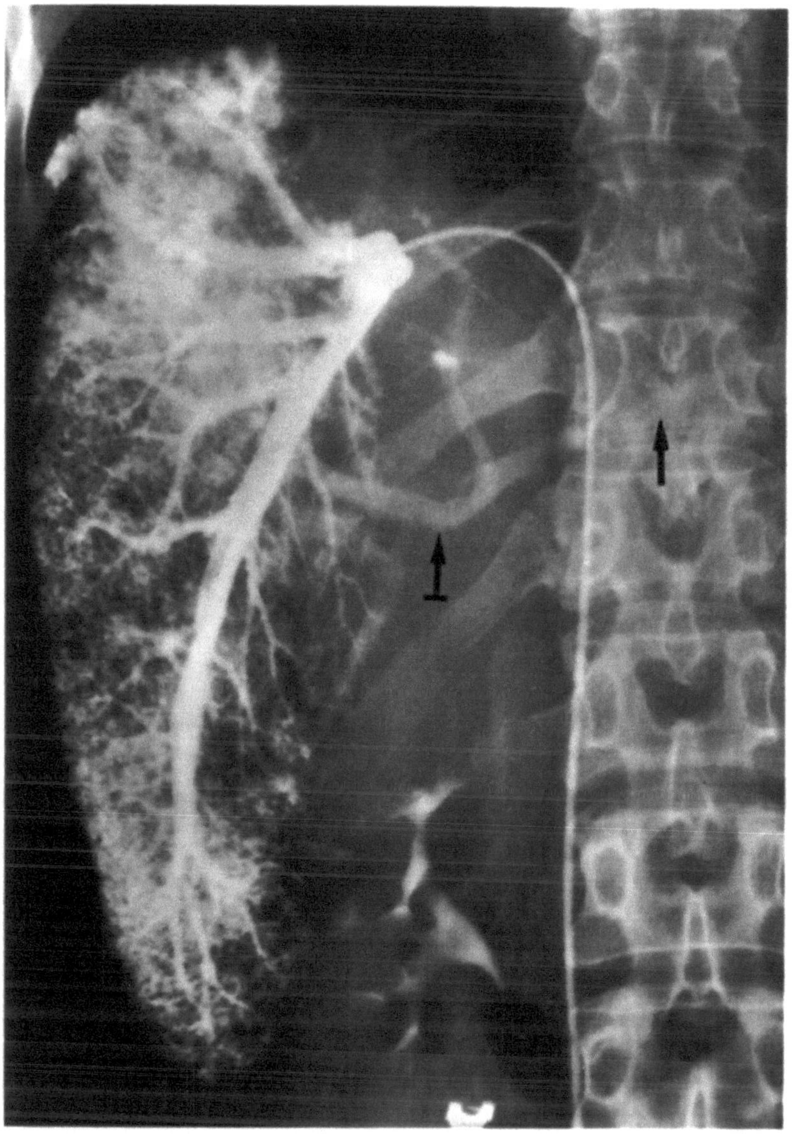

12.7

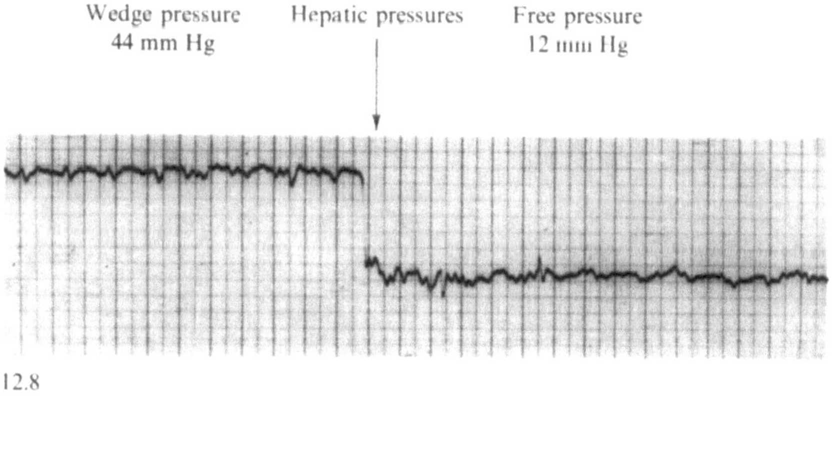
Wedge pressure
44 mm Hg
Hepatic pressures
Free pressure
12 mm Hg

12.8

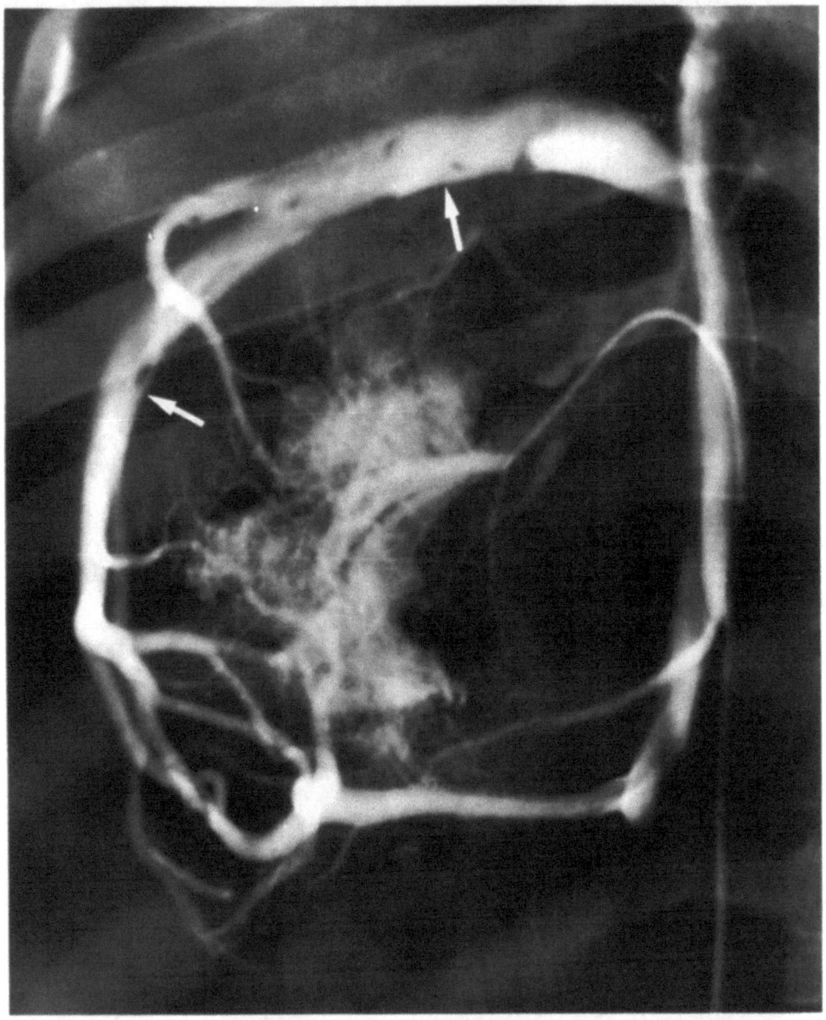

Fig. 12.9. Catheterization of an accessory hepatic vein. Bilharzian cirrhosis (presinusoidal obstacle). Via this accessory hepatic vein it was possible to opacify a right main hepatic vein (↗) and an accessory inferior hepatic vein entering directly the inferior vena cava. There is no pressure gradient in this case, since the sinusoidal pressure is normal. Note the small dilution flows on the trunk of the main hepatic vein (nonopaque hepatic branches)

Fig. 12.10. Cirrhosis. During wedge catheterization occurs very marked retrograde ▷ portal opacification which does, however, not reach the hilus (Stage II)

Fig. 12.11. Cirrhosis. Stage III with severe hyperpressure (45 mm Hg gradient). Wedge injection into the left hepatic vein showing massive hepatopetal portal reflux, with reflux into the right portal system. The hepatic lobule is heterogeneous

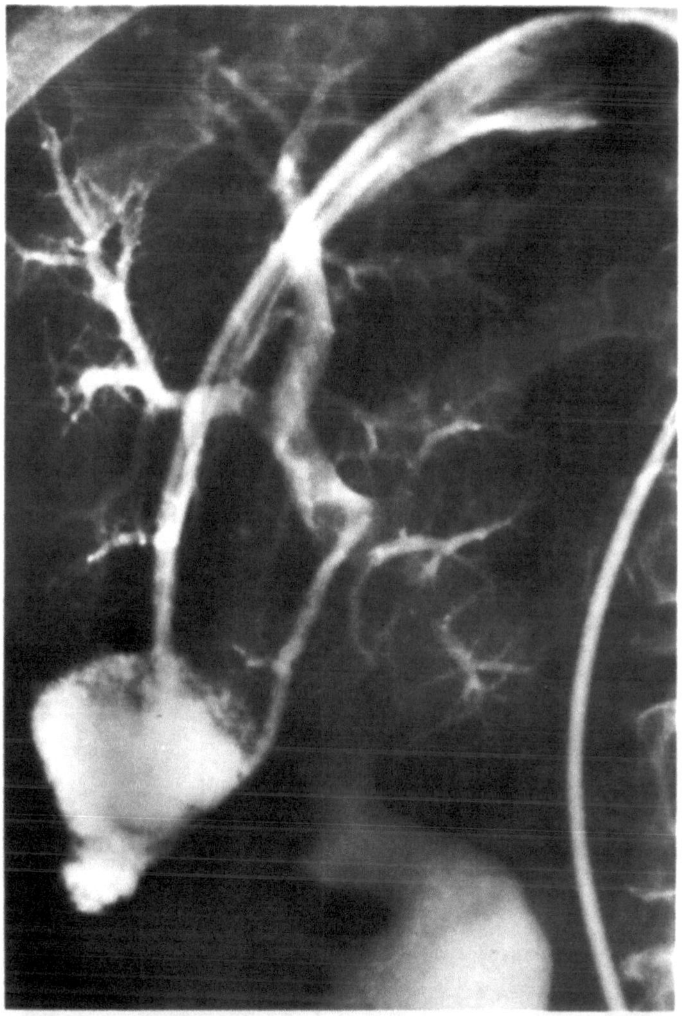

12.10

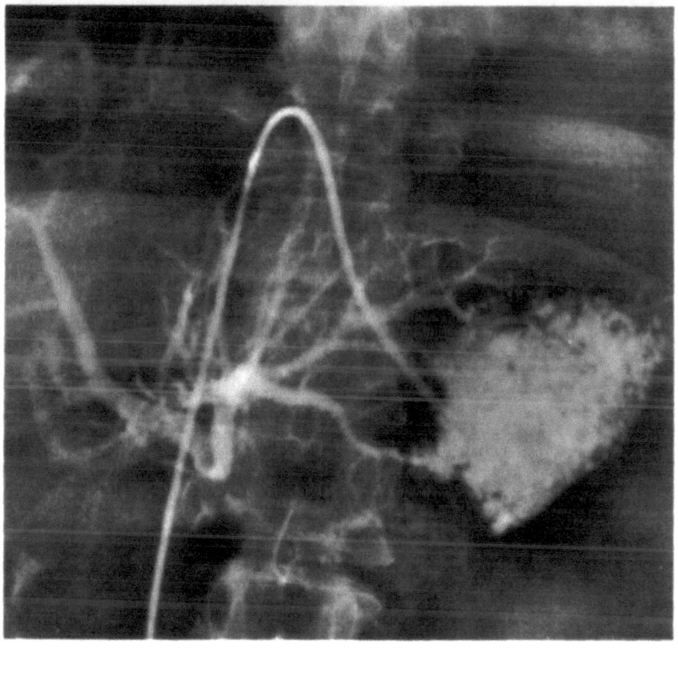

12.11

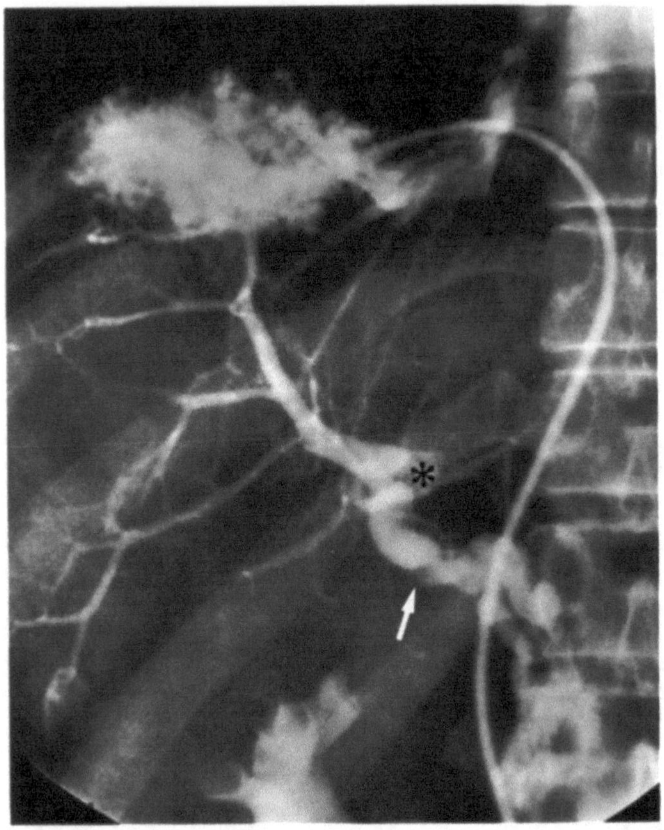
12.12

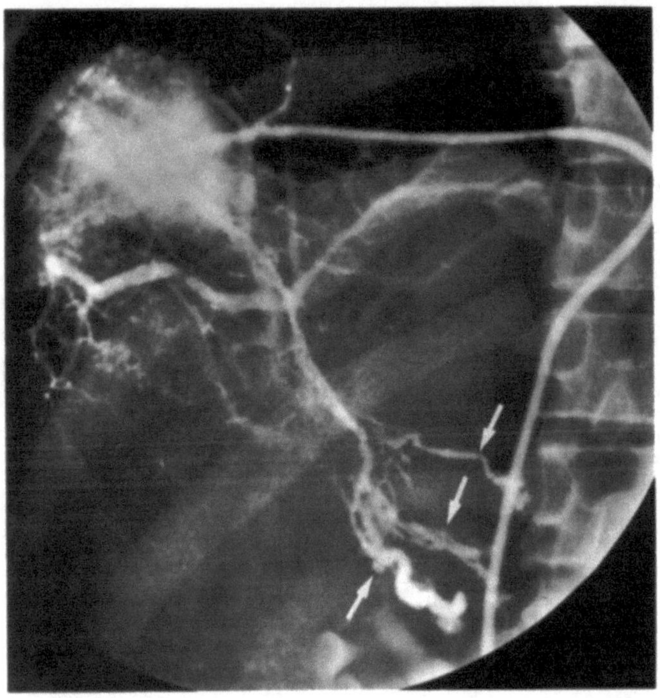
12.13

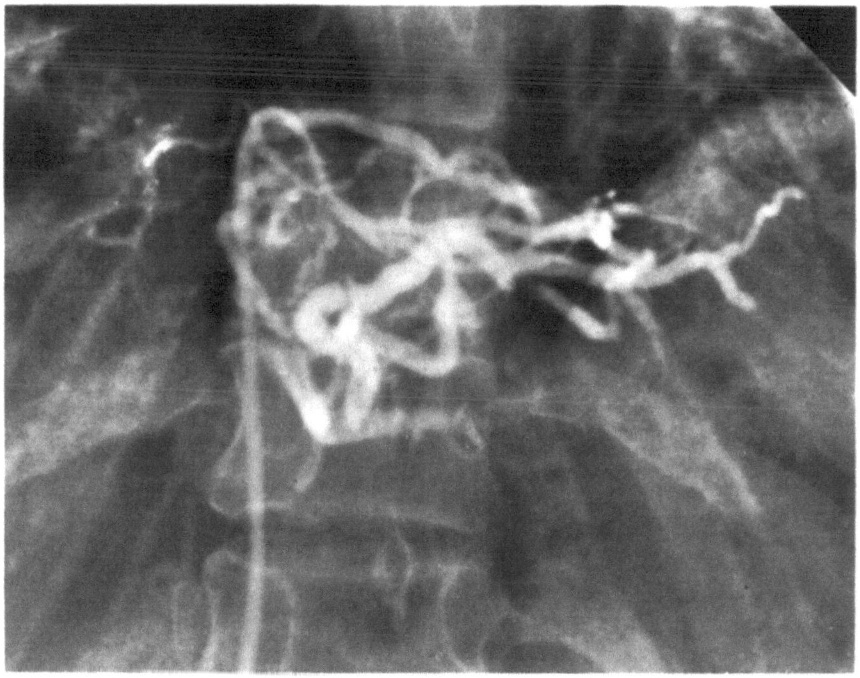

Fig. 12.14. Budd-Chiari syndrome. Retrograde catheterization of an accessory hepatic vein. The major hepatic veins are thrombotic. Small, nonsystematized veins arise in the left liver lobe

◁ Fig. 12.12. Stage IV cirrhosis. The opacification with wedge injection shows an inhomogeneous lobule and inversion of the portal flow toward the hilus. There is thrombosis (*) of the portal trunk and collateral circulation over Sappey's veins (↗). These disappear rapidly and are of large caliber which allows to differentiate them from the lymph vessels

Fig. 12.13. Cirrhosis with ascites. Opacification of lymph vessels. During wedge injection occurs marked portal reflux and also opacification of small tortuous canalicules coursing in the free edge of the lesser omentum, i.e. lymph vessels (↗). The contrast material remains there longer, which allows to differentiate them from the veins

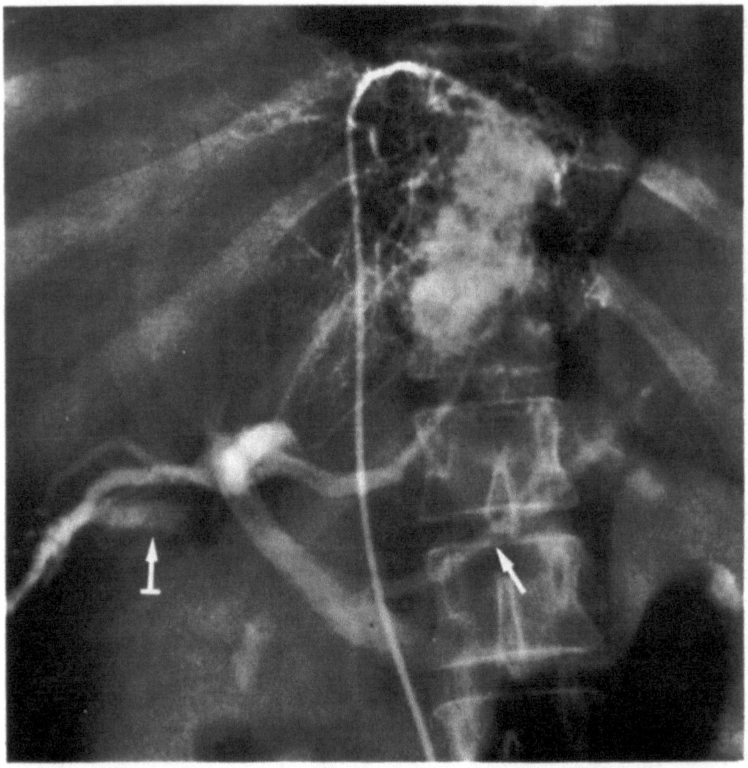

a

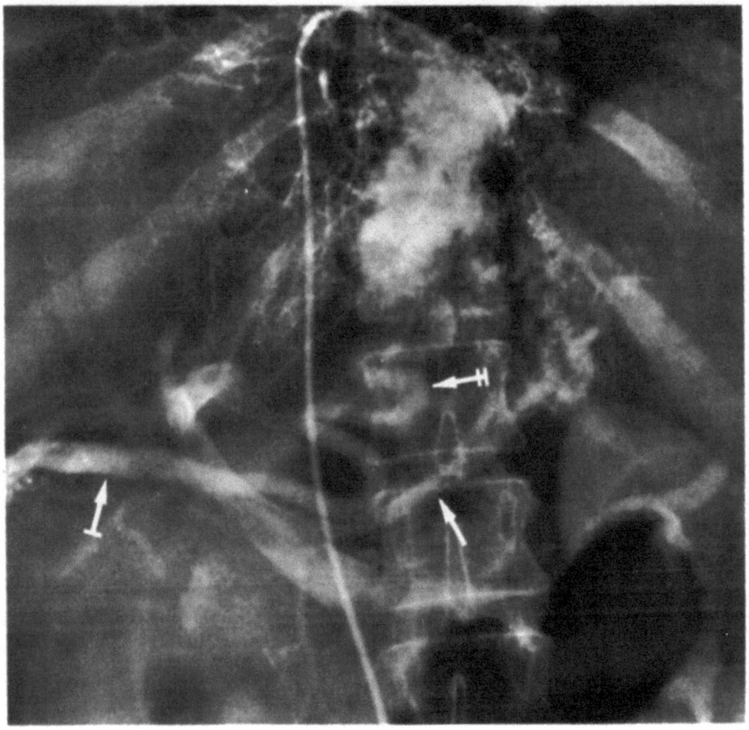

b

Fig. 12.15a, b. Budd-Chiari syndrome with ascites and severe portal hypertension. Catheterization of some accessory rami in the left liver lobe shows very thin and very irregular, collateral-type hepatic veins and massive portal reflux, since there is: – inversion of the flux in the portal trunk with retrograde opacification of the left gastric vein (↗) which allows the visualization of esophageal varices. – opacification of an umbilical vein (↗) which drains toward the internal mammary system (↗)

Fig. 12.16. Budd-Chiari syndrome. Catheterization of a small, dilated accessory venule permits partial opacification of some collateral, dilated and irregular intrahepatic veins. The major hepatic veins are thrombotic

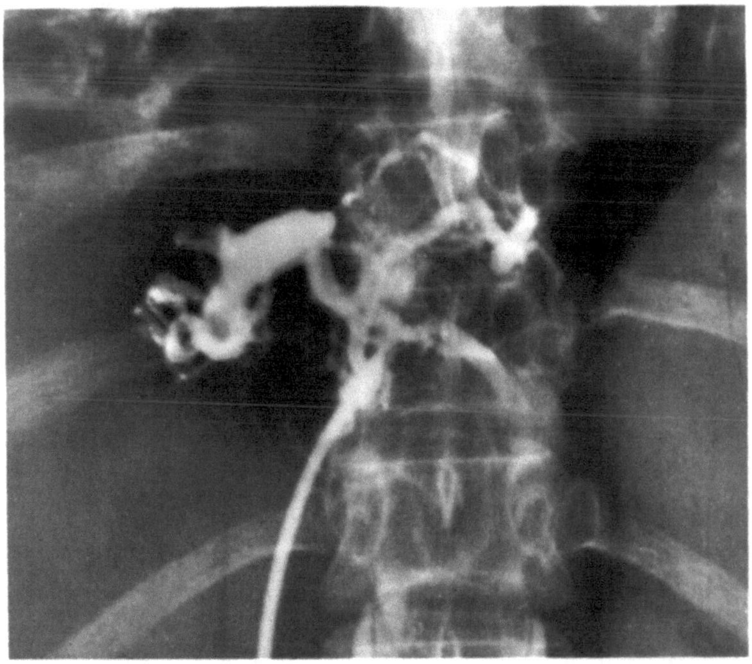

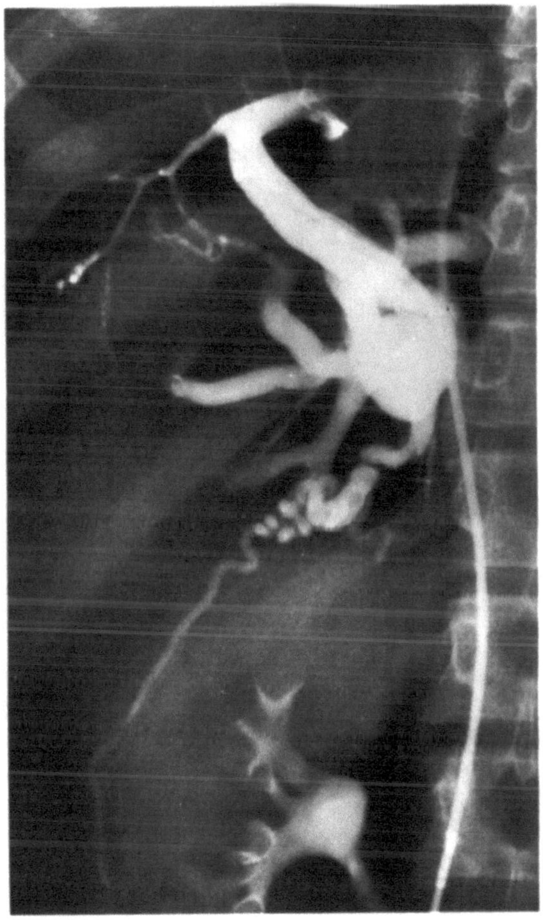

Fig. 12.17. Budd-Chiari syndrome. Distension of the hepatic veins of the caudate lobe. Thrombosis of the major hepatic veins. Compensating hypertrophy of the caudate lobe with dilated venules, visualized with echotomography and catheterized. Note the anastomosis of these hepatic veins with the exorenal venous ring

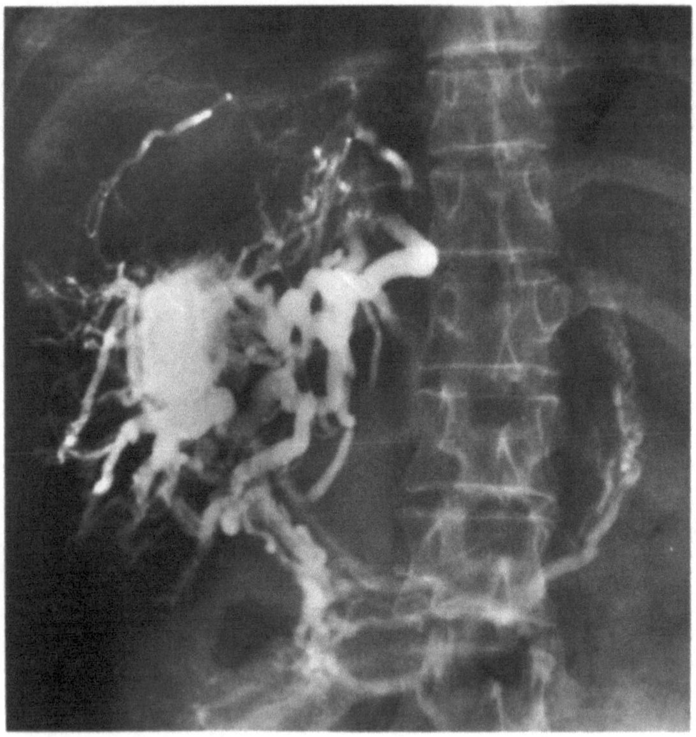

12.18

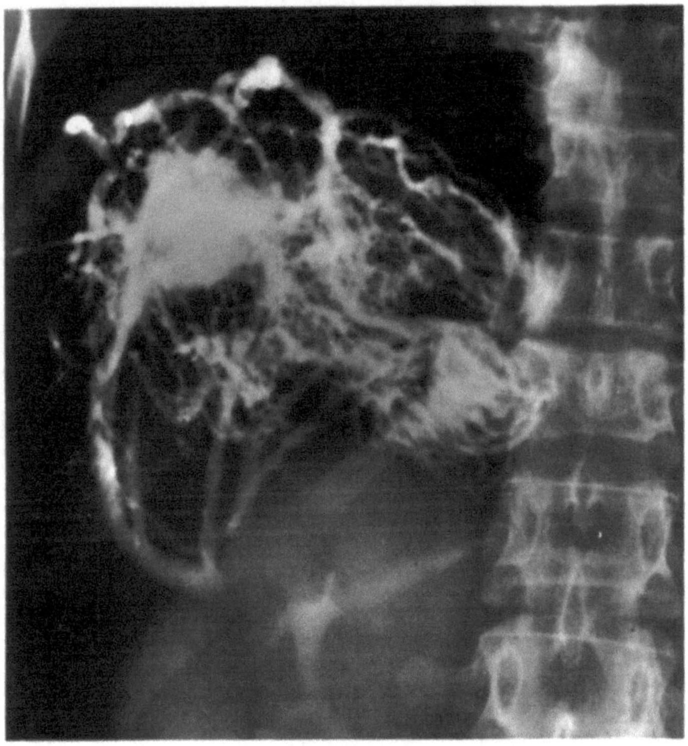

12.19

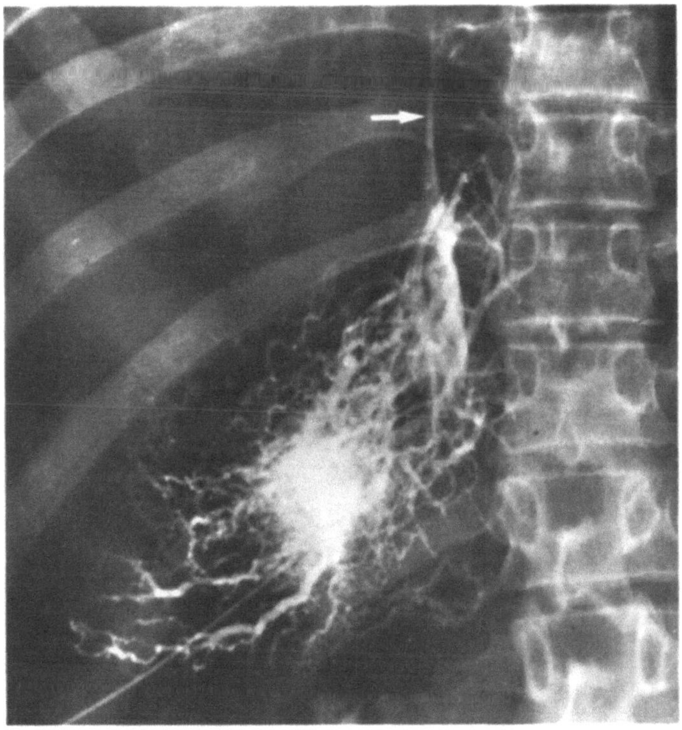

Fig. 12.20. Complete Budd-Chiari syndrome. Study by percutaneous puncture with posterior approach. Posterior hepatic puncture in the non-peritonized area is not indicated in a Budd-Chiari syndrome since the caudate lobe is often uninvolved and hypertrophic. In this case, there is also thrombosis of the drainage veins and opacification of small and very thin and irregular collateral channels with some drainage toward the inferior vena cava. Note the marked narrowing of the inferior vena cava (↗) on its retrohepatic segment

◁ Fig. 12.18. Budd-Chiari syndrome. Transhepatic puncture. Progressive, segmental opacification of some very irregular hepatic veins which drain via collateral venous channels (coursing in the lesser omentum and along the lesser gastric curvature). The right hepatic vein is not opacified

Fig. 12.19. Budd-Chiari syndrome. Transhepatic puncture. Stasis of contrast medium in the parenchyma with slow opacification of a collateral venous network, without drainage toward the inferior vena cava. Marked portal reflux accounts for insufficient collateral circulation

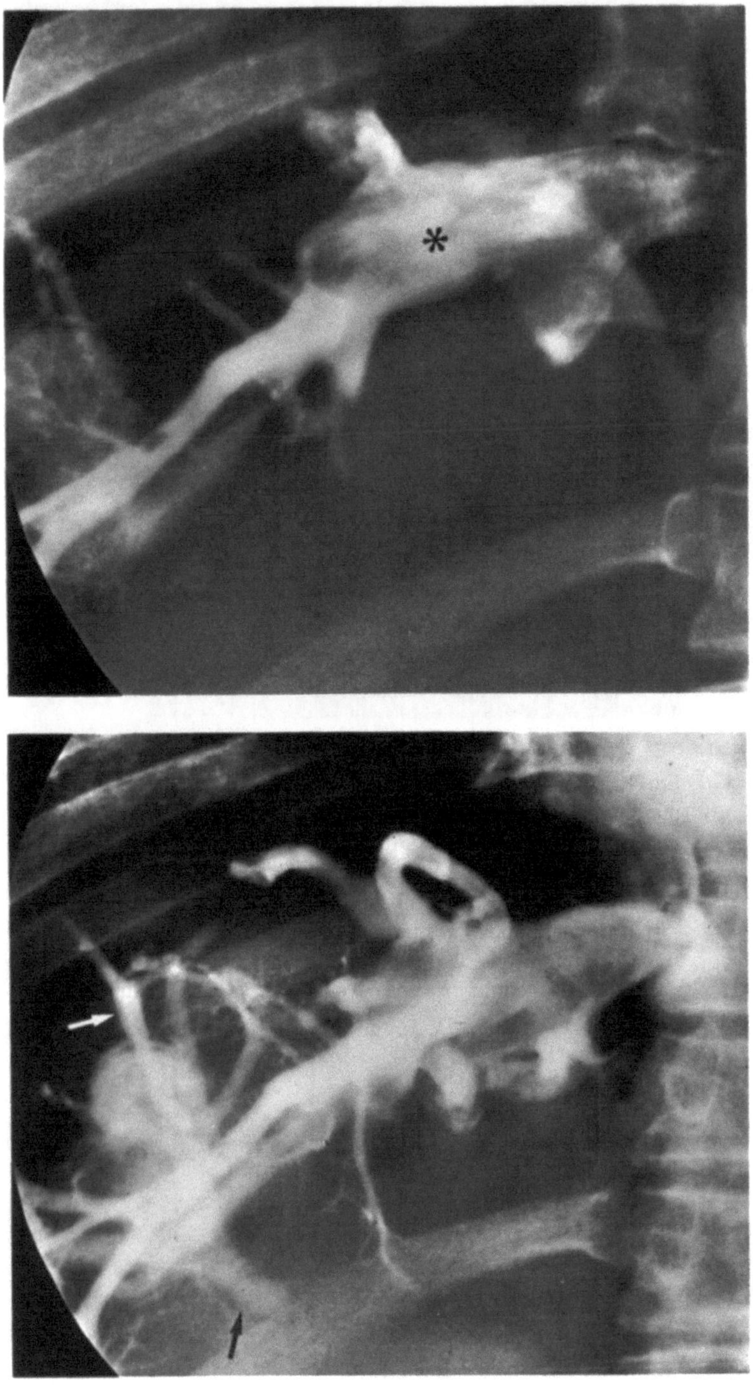

a

b

Fig. 12.21 a, b. Type III Budd-Chiari syndrome. a and b Transhepatic puncture. The hepatic veins are neither dilated nor anastomosed among each other. Filling defect in the ostium. These features correspond to ostial thrombosis (*) with partial recanalization. Secondary opacification of some portal rami (↗) is obtained as well as reflux in the adjacent hepatic branches, accounting for poor drainage

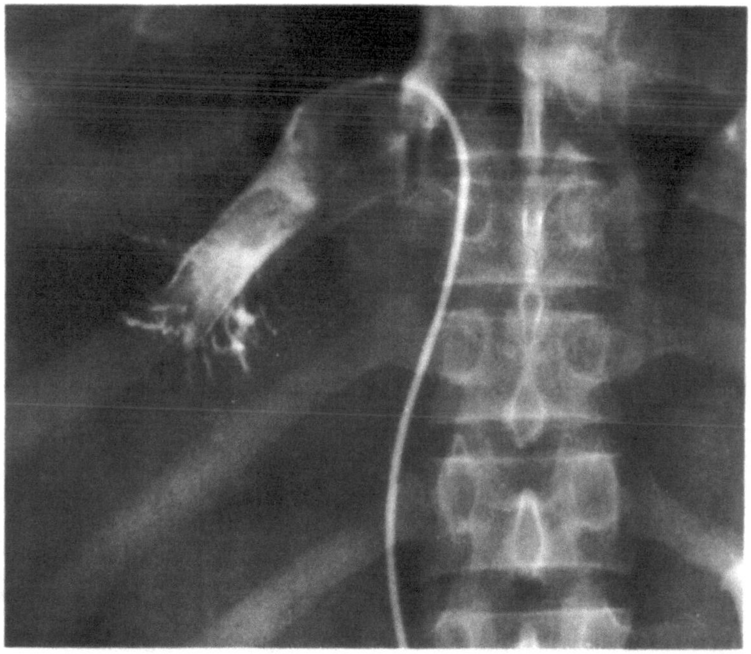

a

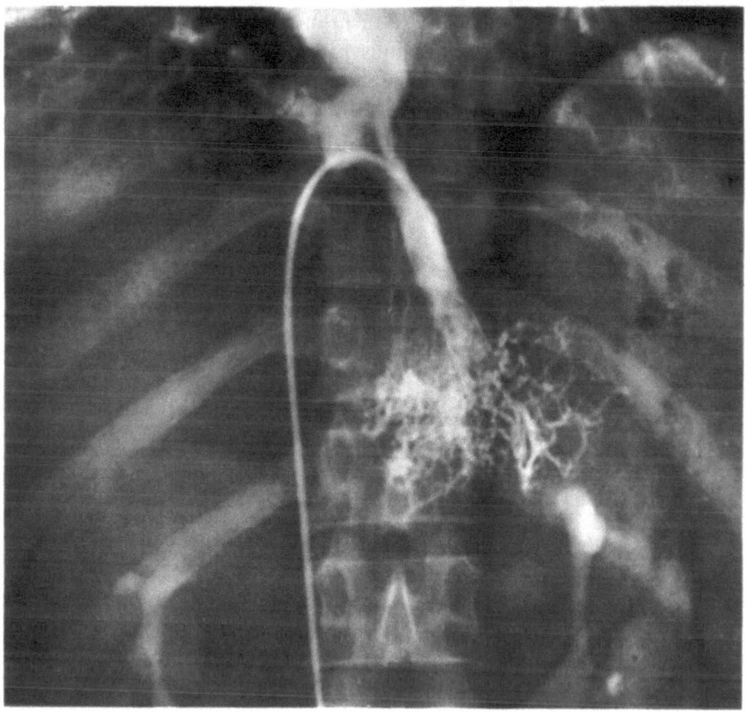

b

Fig. 12.22a, b. Budd-Chiari syndrome occurring in a Marchiafava-Michelli syndrome. a Right hepatic vein. This is patent over a distance of 2 cm commencing at its ostium, then there is a huge intraluminal thrombus. b Left hepatic vein. Similar appearance: intraluminal thrombus and beyond it, opacification of dilated venules which are not systematized

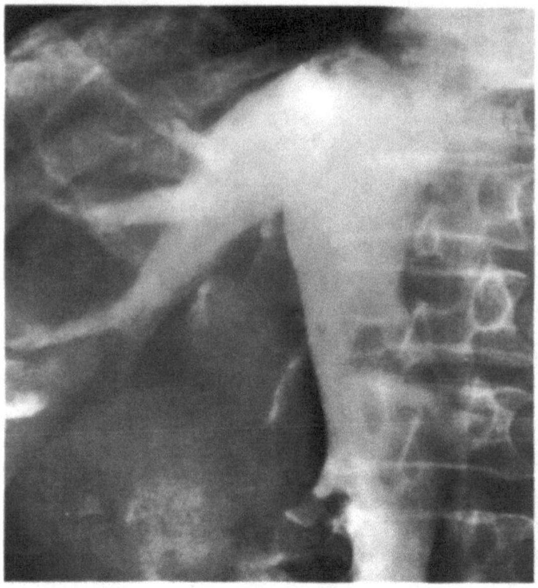

Fig. 12.23. Constrictive pericarditis. The investigation was carried out for suspicion of cirrhosis. Cavogram shows a stasis in the suprahepatic segment of the inferior vena cava with increased venous pressure. The vessels are markedly dilated, especially the main right hepatic vein

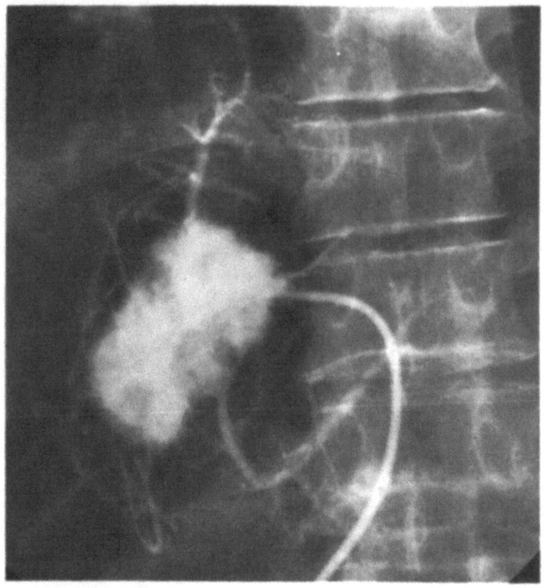

Fig. 12.24. Multinodular hepatoma. Venography of an accessory hepatic vein. The lobule is heterogeneous and irregular with some filling defects corresponding to the tumor nodules. Marked portal reflux

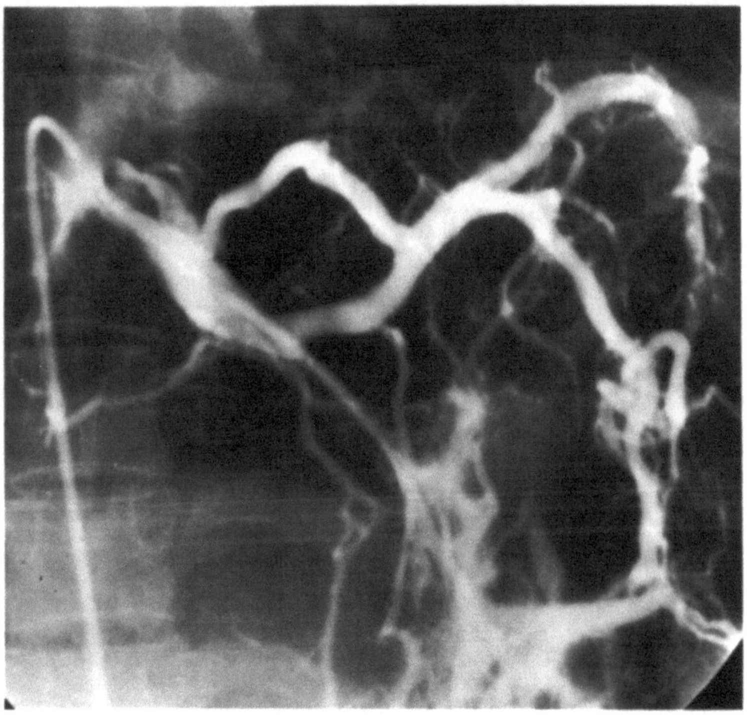

Fig. 12.25. Polycystic liver. Catheterization of the left main hepatic vein gives evidence of displaced and disorientated veins, winding around the numerous intrahepatic cysts

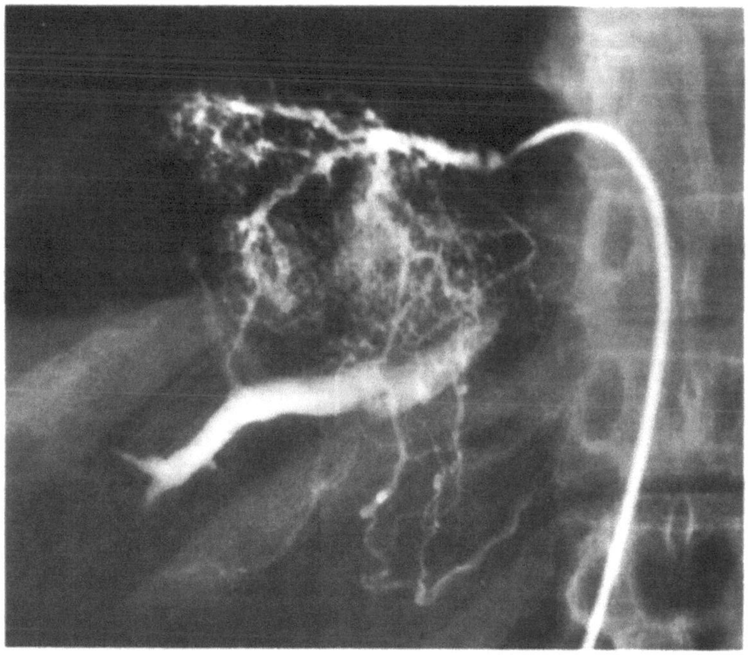

Fig. 12.26. Perihepatitis chronica hyperplastica with cirrhosis. Narrowed and very irregular appearance of a right hepatic vein which is probably subcapsular, with very marked and irregular collateral channels within the fibrous capsule

Chapter 13. Pelvic Venography in Females

13.1 Introduction

There are many different pelvic phlebography techniques. The diversity bears witness to their lack of perfection. The angiographic investigation of the veins of the lesser pelvis in females developed considerably between 1955 and 1960, since when interest has considerably decreased. At present, these techniques have only exceptional indications and provide no definite therapeutic clues.

13.2 Angiographic Exploration Techniques

13.2.1 Bifemoral Percutaneous Iliocavography

Opacification of the hypogastric venous system is insufficient or incomplete with this technique. Different means have been proposed to improve opacification, e.g., the Valsalva maneuver, and abdominal compression at the lower part of the vena cava. However, these only achieve incomplete opacification of the hypogastric venous system, which normally is valvulated. Opacification never reaches beyond the first or second valve, and is usually confined to the presacral venous plexuses, which are not very valvulated, if at all.

13.2.2 Selective Utero-ovarian Phlebography (Uni- or Bilateral)

This technique is performed with retrograde femoral venous catheterization and placement of a preshaped catheter, most often in the left ovarian vein (Fig. 13.1). It was described by Jacobs and is easy to perform in multiparous subjects, in whom the ovarian veins have a large caliber and incompetent valves. The technique is almost the same as with spermatic venography. Retrograde selective catheterization must reach quite far: Dopman and Chretien introduce the catheter as far as the iliac crest. These authors recommend bilateral injection which, according to them, is the only means of providing satisfactory data. The method achieves very good opacification of the venous plexus of the parametrium and of the uterine veins, and subsequently of the hypogastric veins.

Unilateral injection may produce contralateral opacification via the uterine veins. Bilateral injection is carried out with a Y-tube, with a delivery rate of 10 to 15 ml/s and 60 to 80 ml contrast medium. Serial filming is performed with the beam directed cranially, forming an angle of 30° with the coronal plane, so as to visualize the parauterine venous plexus.

13.2.3 Selective Hypogastric Venography

Selective catheterization of the hypogastric veins is usually performed by contralateral femoral approach; it is quite easy. Contrariwise, selective catheterization of the entire hypogastric venous system is rendered difficult by its very frequent anatomic variations: it often has double or even triple venous trunks.

13.2.4 Hypogastric Venography by Pertrochanteral Approach (Fig. 13.2)

Opacification of the iliac venous system by transosseous (transtrochanteral) approach is certainly one of the most effective techniques for the study of this system; unfortunately it entails the drawbacks and dangers of any intraosseous phlebographic injection. Lea Thomas has used it for a prospective study of the incidence of hypogastric venous thrombosis with regard to iliofemoral thromboses.

Opacification is obtained by introducing a trocar into both greater trochanters and injecting 50 ml contrast medium at a rate of 10 ml/s using a Y-tube. General anesthesia is essential.

Opacification of the entire internal iliac venous system with all its collaterals is better achieved with the patient supine than prone.

13.2.5 Injection into a Vulvar Varix or into the Dorsal Vein of the Clitoris

Injection of a vulvar varix can be done by percutaneous approach; 30 ml contrast at 3 ml/s will demonstrate, on an oblique projection, the drainage of the vulvar varices and the hypogastric venous system. Injection into the dorsal vein of the clitoris necessitates exposure of the vein by cutdown, and is hardly ever used.

13.2.6 Phlebohysteroangiography (Fig. 13.3)

This technique, advocated by Guilhem and Baux, involves the use of an instrument for puncturing the uterine muscle by endocavitary approach. Injection of 20 to 30 ml contrast at 3 ml/s produces opacification of the uterine and ovarian veins on both sides. The technique is hardly ever used.

13.2.7 Pelvic Phlebography by Transpubic or Transischiatic Approach

These techniques are no longer employed.

13.2.8 Conclusion

The techniques are highly diversified. Most of them have their place in the history of vascular radiology. Only selective utero-ovarian venography with retrograde catheterization is still in use.

13.3 Radioanatomy of the Pelvic Veins in Women

13.3.1 Hypogastric Venous System

Pertrochanteral venography provides the best opacification of the hypogastric venous system. The trunk of the internal iliac vein is very variable in length (from 3 to 7 cm), and has a width of about 1 cm. Its confluence with the external iliac vein is also variable and may be level with the sacroiliac articulation or be located much lower. Moreover, the left hypogastric vein may drain into the right external iliac vein, and vice versa.

The hypogastric venous trunk is formed by five groups of veins: medially, the lateral sacral veins; below them, a group of veins draining the inferior aspect of the lesser pelvis and the perineum, receiving thus the veins of the rectum, bladder, vagina, and uterus. On the lower part of the film, one can see the obturator veins, and more laterally, the ischiatic veins projected onto the femoral head. The gluteal veins are seen above and lateral to the ischiatic veins. For the radioanatomic appearance of the opacified veins, the reader is referred to the paper by Lea Thomas, (p. 664, Fig. II).

13.3.2 Uterine Venous Plexus

The veins of the uterus join the large uterine plexus, which is located laterally to the uterus and receives two anastomosed collecting trunks: one draining the anterior wall of the uterus, the other the posterior wall. These plexuses are anastomosed with the ovarian veins. The uterine veins also communicate with the veins of the bladder, pelvic floor, and external genital organs. They are also anastomosed with the veins of the round ligament and with the superior hemorrhoidal veins. All these veins have only rare valves. They are particularly well demonstrated with an endo-uterine injection.

13.3.3 Ovarian Veins

Left Ovarian Vein

The left ovarian vein empties into the left renal vein. In the event of a double left renal venous arch, it may empty into either portion of the arch. The mouth is located in the first 3 cm, to the left of the spine. The vein always joins the inferior surface of the left renal vein. There are two possible sources of error: on the one hand, there exists a short vein connecting the renal vein and the ascending lumbar vein, which has usually a larger caliber and a more medial course. On the other hand, there may exist a small vein connecting the left renal vein with the periureteral venous plexus. This vein is located more laterally on the renal vein, and communicates moreover with the left ovarian vein.

Right Ovarian Vein

Its termination is much less constant. It is usually located on the lateral or anterolateral aspect of the inferior vena cava, 3 to 5 cm below the right renal vein. It may also join the right renal vein itself or join at the angle between the inferior vena cava and the right renal vein. Besides, its termination may be double. There is frequently anastomosis of this vein (at the L3-L4 level, laterally) with the veins of the abdominal wall, which communicate caudally with the external iliac system. Connections of the ovarian veins with the retroperitoneal veins are frequent.

The Opacified Veins (Selective Ovarian Venography) the Valves and the Pelvic Anastomoses

The ovarian veins opacified by selective ovarian venography are seen to communicate extensively with the uterine and vaginal plexuses at the level of the broad ligament. In the case of unilateral injection, filling of the contralateral uterine plexuses often occurs. Uni- or bilateral opacification of the hypogastric venous system is also frequent with this technique. Filling of the anastomoses is better, the lower the selective injection has been made (at the level of the iliac crest). Classically, a valve is seen 1 cm beyond the ostium of the ovarian veins. Authors' experience is frequently contradictory on this point, since competence of the valves depends not only on the level of injection, but also on the delivery rate and on the frequent anatomic and physiologic variations. Multiparous subjects often have more or less valveless ovarian veins of large caliber (Fig. 13.4).

13.3.4 Veins of the Vulva

The venous drainage of the vulva is by four routes: (1) the internal pudendal vein and (2) the obturator vein, both branches of the internal saphenous vein; (3) the external pudendal veins, superficial and deep, which are branches of the internal iliac vein, and (4) the veins of the round ligament.

13.4 Pelvic Venography in Genital Tumors

Opacification of the veins of the parametrium at one time seemed a promising method for the early detection of invasion of the parametrium by tumors of the uterine cervix. Unfortunately, venous opacification seems too variable for nonfilling of a parauterine venous plexus to have diagnostic value. Moreover, it is not certain that involvement of the parametrial veins is an early sign of tumor of the uterine cervix; the cases reported concern more advanced stages. No statistics have been compiled in stages I and II from a large enough series of patients to show whether nonfilling of the parauterine and paravaginal venous plexuses has significant value. The most frequently used technique is retrograde selective utero-ovarian venography, which provides constant opacification of the parametrial plexuses.

13.5 Syndrome of Ureteral Compression by the Ovarian Vein

Several reports have pointed out the possibility of a left or right ureteral obstacle due to the ovarian vein. The retaining mechanism is dilatation of an ovarian vein secondary either to valvular incompetence or to extrinsic or intrinsic compression of the left renal vein (in the case of unilateral left syndromes). Bilateral syndromes have also been reported. In some cases selective venography has demonstrated dilatation of the ovarian vein associated with impression on the ureter. Association with pelvic varices is often encountered.

13.6 Pelvic Varices in Women

Pelvic varices (broad ligament) are sometimes considered to be the origin of some so-called pelvic congestive syndromes, in which they could be responsible for pain and menorrhagia. These varices are sometimes seen during celioscopy and may also

---

Fig. 13.1. Selective left utero-ovarian venography. Positioning of the catheter in the left ovarian vein. Normal left ovarian venogram. (By courtesy of Pr. J. Tavernier and Dr. J. Drouillard) ▷

Fig. 13.2. Right transtrochanteral venography. Drainage via the circumflex veins to the branches of the deep femoral vein, and drainage via the obturator vein and the hypogastric system. Opacification of the right common iliac vein. This transtrochanterian venography was performed for suspicion of ischemia necrosis of the right head of femur

Fig. 13.3. Phlebohysteroangiography. Bilateral varicose dilatation of the veins of the parametrium. (By courtesy of Pr. J. Tavernier and Dr. J. Drouillard)

Fig. 13.4. Selective left renal venography. The left ovarian vein has a very large caliber and is valveless with important downward reflux (↓)

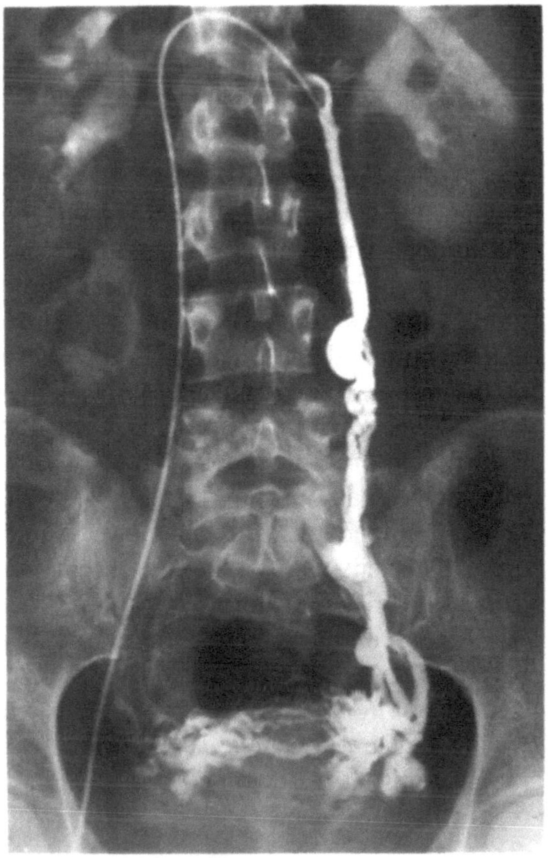

13.1

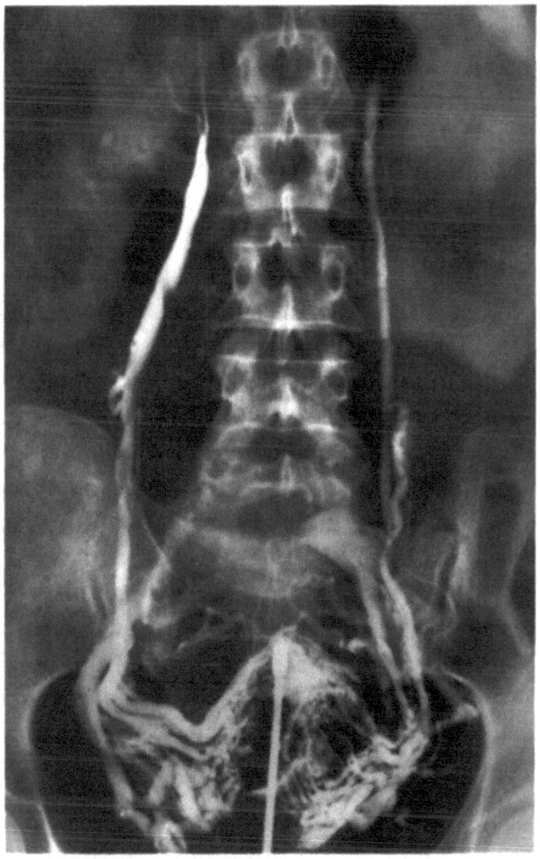

13.3

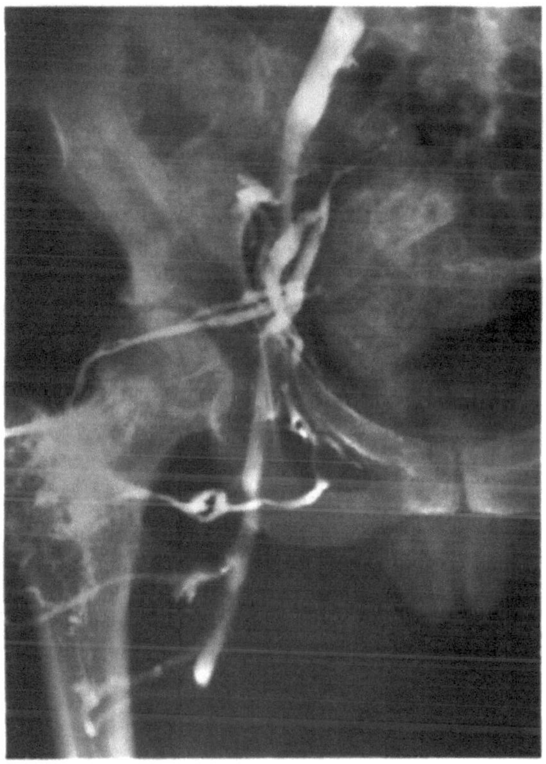

◁ 13.2

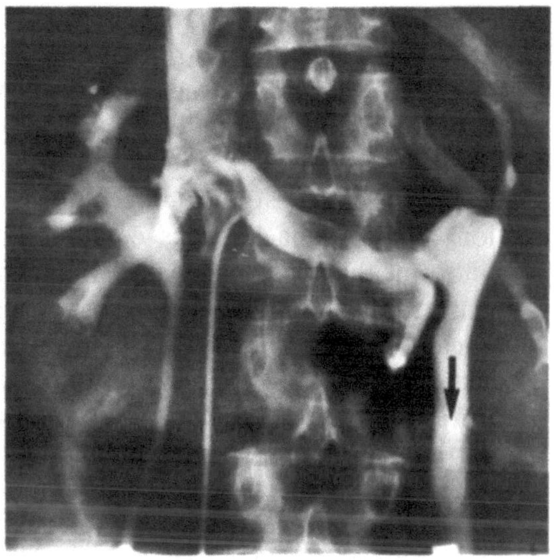

△ 13.4

be visualized by retrograde ovarian venography, which may, moreover, demonstrate incompetence of the valves, and distal retrograde opacification of the veins of the broad ligament and the hypogastric vein.

On the other hand, pelvic varices may also be related, according to Cockett, to an iliac venous compression syndrome (most often left). In some cases presenting this syndrome, Cockett has observed collateral circulation via the uterine, parametrial, and then ovarian veins. The uterus may in such cases become markedly vascularized and surrounded by large, congestive, tortuous veins. Drainage via the ovarian veins makes them dilated and sometimes tortuous. Consequently, in these patients, the greater part of venous return flow from the left lower limb may pass through the pelvic varices. This is of practical importance, since it results in three types of condition:

1) A pelvic algic syndrome with menorrhagia may be observed.
2) Left iliofemoral thrombosis secondary to hysterectomy: removal of the uterus and left ovarian vein may suppress most of the collateral venous return from the left lower limb and thus accelerate a latent stage of venous obstruction.
3) "White leg syndrome" after parturition: this consists of postpartum decompensation of a left iliac venous compression syndrome that was remarkably well compensated during pregnancy owing to significant development of the uterine circulation. Uterine compression after parturition may be responsible for a status of relative venous obstruction which had up to then been compensated by important endopelvic venous collateral channels. Some correlate this syndrome of left iliac venous compression with the higher incidence of recurrent varices on the left side.

13.7 Pelvic Veins and Pulmonary Embolism

Lea Thomas performed a prospective study (bilateral pertrochanteral venography) of the hypogastric venous system in patients who already had obstruction of the iliofemoral venous system. This study was aimed at determining the frequency of thromboses of the internal iliac vein and showed it to be 25% in a group of patients with high risk (iliofemoral thrombosis). It may, however, be pointed out that among all the patients examined, only three had patent common iliac veins. It would thus seem that isolated primary thrombosis of the internal iliac vein is extremely uncommon and that researching hypogastric thrombosis in a case of pulmonary embolism is not worthwile. Contrary to a classical notion, pulmonary embolism does not usually originate from the pelvic veins.

References

Chidekel N (1968) Female pelvic veins demonstrated by selective renal phlebography with particular reference to pelvic varicosities. Acta Radiol (Stockh) 7:193–209

Guilhem P, Baux R (1954) La phlébographie pelvienne par voie veineuse, osseuse, et utérine. Masson, Paris

Jacobs J (1969) Selective gonadal venography. Radiology 92:888–893

Revelli E, Baricalla A (1962) La phlebographie utérine au cours des syndromes douloureux pelviens. Presse Med 70:1634–1635

Tavernier J, Lange D (1965) La phlébographie utéro-ovarienne gauche. Presse Med 73:863–866

Thomas LM, Browse NL (1972) Internal iliac thrombosis. Acta Radiol (Stockh) 2:660–672

Vermeersch A, Claus D, Lecart C (1971) Technique séquentielle d'hystéro-phlébographie par voie endo-utérine. Gynecol Obstest (Paris) 70:589–607

Chapter 14. Lumbar Phlebography

Used for the study of vertebromedullary pathology, lumbar phlebography consists in the opacification of the intra- and extravertebral veins in order to appreciate changes determined by lesions situated in their neighborhood. It is an "indirect" investigation technique since the epidural veins themselves have no proven pathology.

14.1 Technique

The accuracy of the phlebographic diagnosis depends on the quality of opacification of the epidural veins. After having at one time been performed by injection into the spinous processes and subsequently by exclusive catheterization of the ascending lumbar veins, opacification of the lumbosacral veins is now achieved by injection into a lateral sacral vein – which depends on the hypogastric system – and/or into an ascending lumbar vein. In fact the angiographer adapts the technique to the pattern of the extravertebral venous system in each case. Bilateral injection of these veins is associated with abdominal compression, so as to compress the vena cava and force the contrast medium to enter the epidural veins.

The technique is almost painless when performed under local anesthesia. It is advisable systematically to inject 30–50 mg heparin during the examination, so as to prevent thromboembolic complications; these are very rare, but may be encountered in patients operated upon some days after phlebography. Moreover, anti-inflammatory drugs should be administered to the patient when surgery is considered. When all these precautions are taken, thromboembolic complications almost never occur.

14.2 Radioanatomy

Classical radioanatomic descriptions mention two pairs of intravertebral longitudinal epidural veins, an anterior and a posterior pair. In fact all epidural veins are located in the anterolateral angles of the spinal canal and there are no posterior longitudinal epidural veins. One may distinguish on each side a medial epidural vein and a lateral epidural vein. These veins course together all along the lumbar spine down to the L5-S1 vertebrae, where they spread apart and may thus be easily recognized on a frontal phlebographic projection (Fig. 14.1). On each side the epidural veins are connected to the corresponding ascending lumbar vein by the veins of the lateral foramina.

14.3 Indications

The epidural veins represent an important anatomic landmark, for two reasons:

1) They are situated in the anterolateral angles of the spinal canal, between the disk and the nerve roots: they are therefore affected by any disk herniation, even a very lateral one, which compresses the nerve root.
2) Their appearance reflects the state of the epidural space: localized or diffuse lumbar stenosis is always accompanied by nonopacification of the epidural space corresponding to the narrowed segment.

The indications are schematically divided into four groups: disk herniation, lumbar neuralgia, lumbar stenosis, and tumor.

14.3.1 Disk Herniation

Disk herniation is visualized in phlebography as a localized interruption (Fig. 14.2) which may involve either the lateral epidural vein (Fig. 14.3) or the medial epidural vein (Fig. 14.4), sometimes accompanied by dilatation of the adjacent veins secondary to stagnation and bypass of the obstacle by the venous blood flow. Extension into the lateral foramen causes interruption of the corresponding veins. In case of interruption of the epidural veins, it is necessary to visualize the upper and the lower limits of compression in order to rule out pseudointerruptions due to technical inadequacies.

The diagnostic accuracy of phlebography is superior to that of radiculography (Dimer X) as concerns very lateral disk herniations at any level. Moreover, at the L5-S1 level phlebography provides more precise data about median and paramedian disk lesions, because of the thickness of the epidural space and the particular disposition of the veins at this level. However, since phlebography is a more complex investigation than radiculography, it seems advisable to perform it only as second investigation in the following cases:

a) When radiculography is normal or insufficiently convincing to orientate surgery

b) When radiculography shows abnormal features at a level other than that of the clinical symptoms;

c) In cases of megadural sac (radiculography being particularly imprecise in this case)

d) When radiculography has demonstrated features of postoperative or postradiculographic arachnoiditis, but keeping in mind that interruption of the veins at a disk level already operated upon has no diagnostic value

14.3.2 Lumbar Neuralgia

In lumbar neuralgia without sciatica, phlebography sometimes shows interruption of the epidural veins secondary to a disk herniation which has no peculiarity beside the unusual clinical symptoms. In similar clinical conditions, radiculography would also show characteristic features of disk herniation. In fact, in most cases, radiculography is normal and phlebography only permits one to suspect the presence of disk lesions (Fig. 14.5), from the following features: dilatation of the venous anastomoses above and below a disk, tortuous appearance of the epidural veins at the level of this disk, and mild localized interruptions of the veins. These phlebographic features alone do not prove the degenerated disk responsible for lumbar neuralgia, but they do orientate a diskography. The latter investigation will confirm the degree of degenerescence of the disk and show whether pain is triggered by the injection.

This prevailing disk pathology should not lead one to forget the possibility of lesions of the articular facets as a factor in the etiology of lumbar neuralgia. Before any other investigation, an infiltration of xylocaine and steroids into the articular facets should be performed, which will serve as a diagnostic and therapeutic test: when the pain disappears, the "facet syndrome" may be affirmed, when it is unchanged or only diminished, radiologic investigation of the disk is undertaken, with phlebography and diskography.

14.3.3 Lumbar Canal Stenosis

Any localized or diffuse stenosis of the lumbar spinal canal is accompanied by compression of the corresponding epidural space. On the phlebogram the compression is seen as a nonopacification of the epidural veins. Two main schematic types of lumbar canal stenosis are recognized on a phlebogram:

a) Concentric stenosis involving all diameters of the canal, visualized on the phlebogram as a reduced distance between the epidural veins (Fig. 14.6a)

b) Anteroposterior stenosis, which affects the anteroposterior diameter of the lateral recessus of the canal,without abnormal position of the epidural veins with regard to the midline (Fig. 14.6b)

The major interest of phlebography consists in demonstrating localized areas of compression in the epidural space caused by an anterior lesion (disk, vertebral body arthrosis) or by a posterior lesion (articular facet arthrosis), which have given rise to earlier clinical symptoms, since they occur on a narrow canal (Fig. 14.7).

Whereas investigations with gas myelography have often led the surgeon to perform extensive laminectomy, these lesions, determined from the phlebogram, may often be treated by localized interventions. Computer tomography (CT) will certainly permit an even more precise diagnosis by analyzing the compression area that the phlebogram indicates.

Sometimes phlebography shows an extensive lack of opacification of the epidural veins (Fig. 14.8), which could schematically correspond either to very marked concentric stenosis in a young subject or to multiple disk lesions in an elderly subject. In these two types of lesion, phlebography makes it possible to determine the extent of compression and hence the extent of laminectomy necessary to relieve the contents of the lumbar spinal canal. When the phlebogram shows extensive nonopacification of the epidural veins, additional investigations with myelography should be performed, since the findings could also correspond to an intraspinal tumor (Fig. 14.9).

14.3.4 Tumor

On account of the location of the epidural veins in the anterolateral angle of the spinal canal, phlebography is not the method of choice for investigation of intraspinal tumor pathology. Indeed, a small tumor developing in the posterior part of the canal or a tumor hanging from the roots of the cauda equina does not compress the anterior epidural space, and thus does not change the phlebographic appearance. However, phlebography readily displays the extracanalar lateral extension of a larger tumor (Fig. 14.9) and shows very early venous changes in cases of metastatic epiduritis.

References

Babin E, Capesius P, Maitrot D (1977) Signes radiologiques osseux des variétés morphologiques des canaux lombaires étroits. Ann Radiol (Paris) 20:491–499

Bucheler E, Janson R (1975) Combined catheter venography of the lumbar venous system and the inferior vena cava. Br Radiol 46:655–661

Djindjian R, Pansini A, Dorland P (1963) Phlébographie vertébro-rachidienne par voie transépineuse. Acta Radiol 1:689–701

Fischgold H, Clement JC, Talairach J, Ecoiffier J (1952) Opacification des systèmes veineux rachidiens et crâniens par voie osseuse. Presse Med 60:599–601

Gargano FP, Meyer JD, Sheldon JJ (1974) Transfemoral ascending lumbar catheterization of the epidural veins in lumbar disc disease. Radiology 111:329–336

Ginestie JF, Fassio B, Connes H, Buscayret C, Castan PH, Vidal J (1976) L'apport des explorations modernes dans l'étude des colonnes postérieures du rachis lombaire. *Communication* GETROA

Larde D (1977) Les veines épidurales lombo-sacrées. Etude anatomique et radiologique. Intérêt de la phlébographie lombaire dans le diagnostic des discopathies. *These* Med Nancy

Lepage JR (1974) Transfemoral ascending lumbar catheterization of the epidural veins. Radiology 111:337–339

Maslow GS, Rothman R (1975) The facet joints: Another look. Bull N Y Acad Med 51:1294–1311

Massare C, Bard M, Benoist M, Cauchoix J, Bloch-Michel H (1974) Renseignements fournis par la discographie lombaire pour le diagnostic et le traitement chirurgical des discopathies douloureuses lombaires et lombo-sacrées. Rev Rhum 41:113–122

Moret J, Vignaud J, Doyon D (1976) Techniques d'opacification des plexus veineux intra-rachidiens lombaires. J Radiol Electrol Med Nucl 57:553–560

Pedersen HE, Blunck CFJ, Gardner E (1956) The anatomy of lumbosacral posterior rami and meningeal branches of the spinal nerves (sinu vertebral nerves): With an experimental study of their function. J Bone Joint Surg [Am] 38:377–391

Picard L, Roland J, Blanghot P, David R, Montaut J, Pourel J (1977) Scarring of the theca and the nerve roots as seen at radiculography. J Neuroradiol 4:29–48

Schobinger RA (1960) Intraosseous venography. Grune and Stratton, New York

Theron J, Houtteville JP, Ammerich H, Alves de Souza A, Adam H, Thurel C, Rey A, Houdart R (1976) Lumbar phlebography by catheterization of the lateral sacral and ascending lumbar veins with abdominal compression. Neuroradiology 11:175–182

Theron J, Moret J (1978) Spinal Phlebography. Springer, Berlin Heidelberg New York

Verbiest H (1976) Fallacies of the present definition, nomenclature and classification of the stenoses of the lumbar vertebral canal. Spine 1:217–225

Vogelsang H (1970) Intraosseous spinal venography. Excerpta Medica Amsterdam

Wackenheim A, Babin E (1977) Sténoses et etroitesses du canal rachidien lombaire. Journées nationales de radiologie. Cours de perfectionnement P. U., Paris

Fig. 14.1. a Schematic drawing of the intraspinal epidural veins on a frontal lumbar venogram.
1 Lateral longitudinal epidural vein
2 Medial longitudinal epidural vein. Down to the L5-S1 level it is often difficult to differentiate the medial from the lateral epidural vein. There, they spread apart and form four veins of four groups of veins.
2 Retrocorporeal anastomosis
4 Superior vein of the lateral foramen
5 Inferior vein of the lateral foramen. There are schematically two veins, but they may form a plexus.
6 Ascending lumbar vein. This vein is often more developed on the left side than on the right.
7 Lateral sacral vein, belonging to the hypogastric system

b Normal lumbar venography, performed by simultaneous catheterization of the left lateral sacral vein and of the left ascending lumbar vein, with compression of the inferior vena cava. Frontal view. The L5-S1 level is indicated by an open arrow.
1 Lateral longitudinal epidural vein
2 Medial longitudinal epidural vein. At the L5-S1 level the medial is clearly differentiated from the lateral epidural vein.
3 Medial epidural vein at the L3-L4 level. Above the L5-S1 level, the medial and the lateral epidural veins are coupled. The medial epidural vein is usually more tortuous than the lateral. It is sometimes impossible to differentiate the lateral from the medial. ▷
4 Right lateral sacral vein
5 Left ascending lumbar vein
6 Veins of the left L4-L5 lateral foramen. In this case they present as a plexus.
7 Catheter crossing from one iliac vein to the other to opacify more easily the left lateral sacral vein.

c Schematic drawing of the intra- and extravertebral venous system viewed from above on a section passing through an intervertebral disc (above L5-S1).
1 Lateral longitudinal epidural vein
2 Medial longitudinal epidural vein. At the L5-S1 level these two veins spread apart (see Fig. 14.1a)
3 Vein of the lateral foramen
4 Left ascending lumbar vein
5 Left lumbar vein
6 Inferior vena cava
7 Right lumbar vein
8 Right ascending lumbar vein

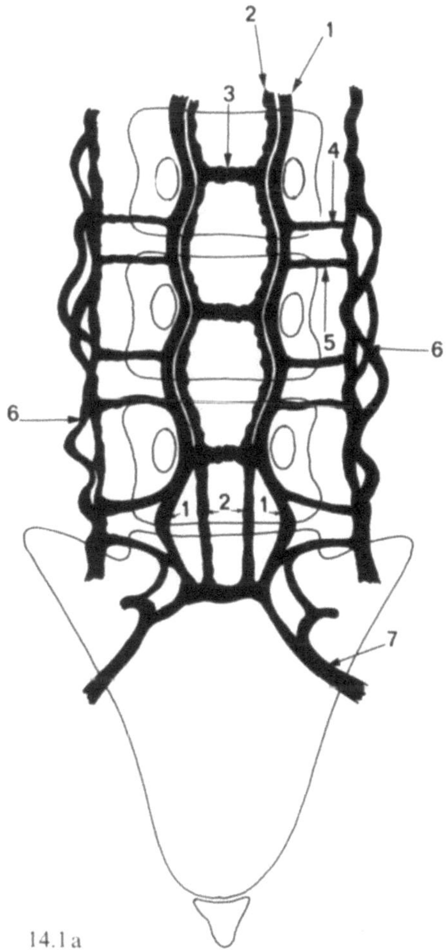

14.1a

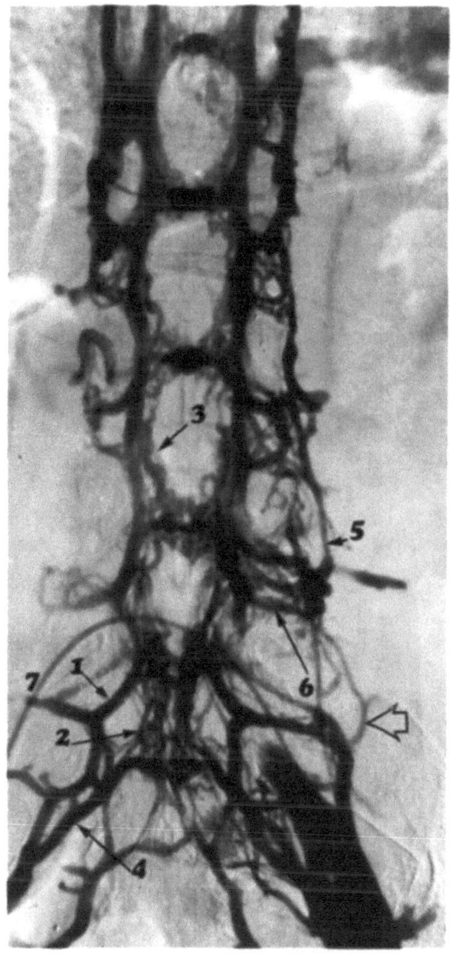

14.1b

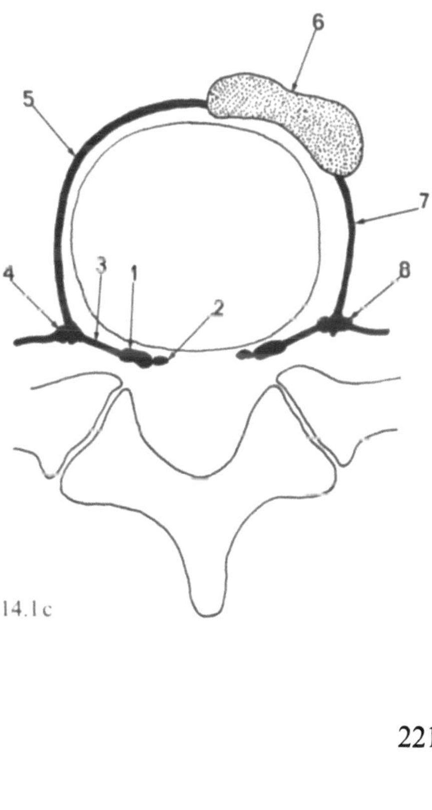

14.1c

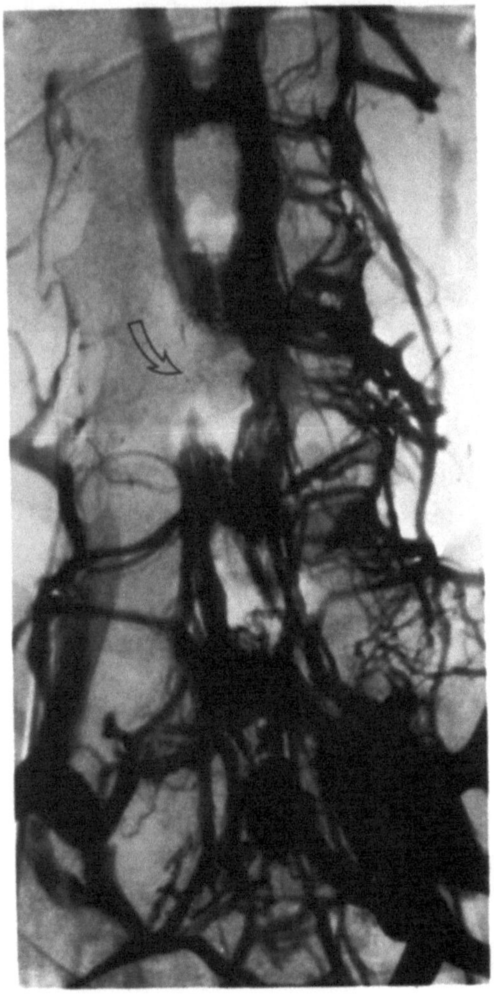

14.2

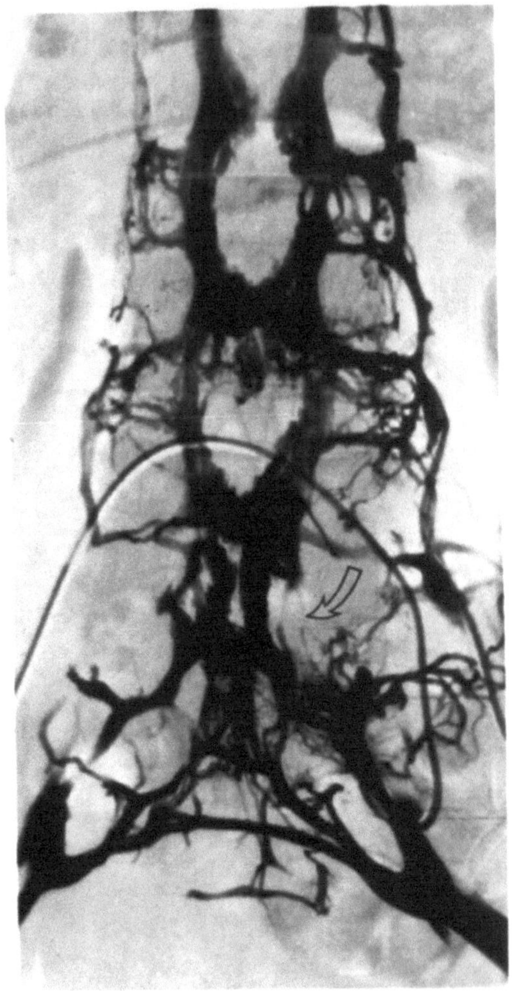

14.3

Fig. 14.2. Right L4–L5 disk herniation. The disk herniation interrupts the epidural venous strip formed by the medial and lateral epidural vein at the right side, in front of L4–L5 (⇘). It is necessary to visualize the upper and the lower limit of the venous interruption to affirm that this non-opacification is pathological

Fig. 14.3. Left L5-S1 disk herniation. The disk herniation interrupts the lateral epidural vein in front of the L5-S1 disk (⇙). The left medial epidural vein is dilated due to the bypass of the obstacle by the venous flow. Compare with the normal appearance of the same disk level (Fig. 14.1 b)

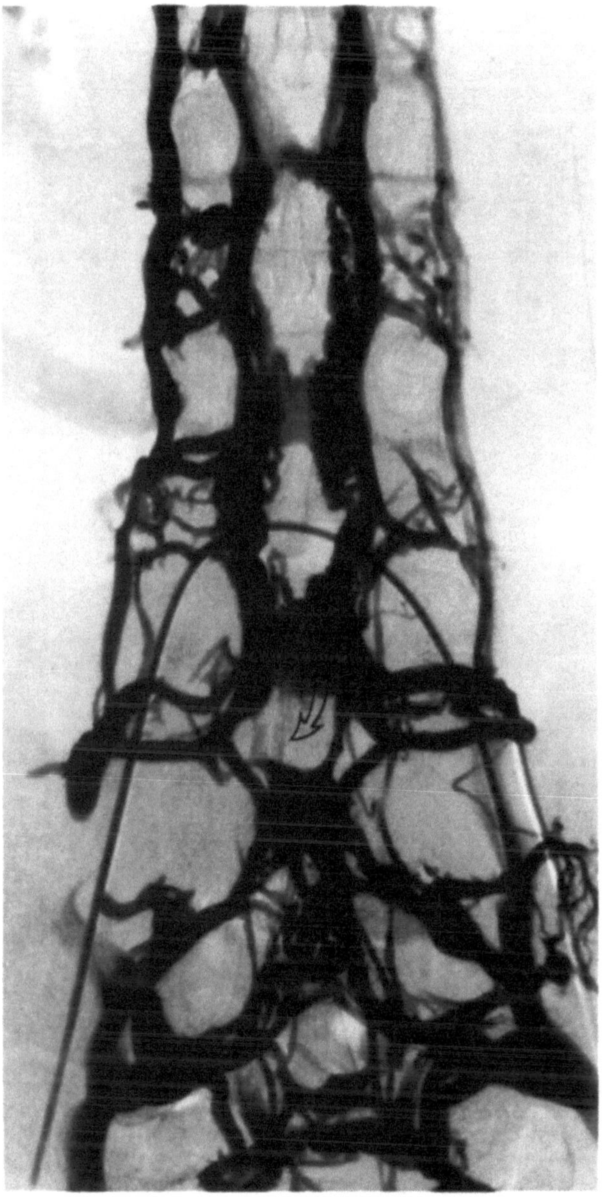

14.4

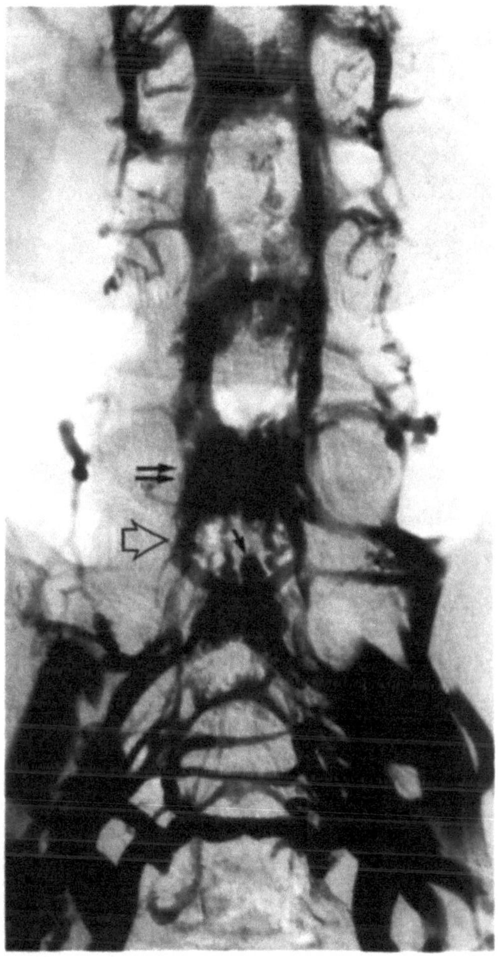

14.5

Fig. 14.4. Right paramedian L5-S1 disk herniation. Compression of the right median epidural vein by the disk herniation (⇨). The other veins are normal. Compare with the appearance of the four normal vein groups at the L5-S1 level in Fig. 14.1 b

Fig. 14.5. Low back pain without sciatic radiation. At the level of the L5-S1 disk (➧) the venogram shows slight changes in the epidural veins which are tortuous with a small partial interruption of the left medial epidural vein (↘), associated with dilatation of the retrocorporeal anastomoses in front of L5 (↗↗)

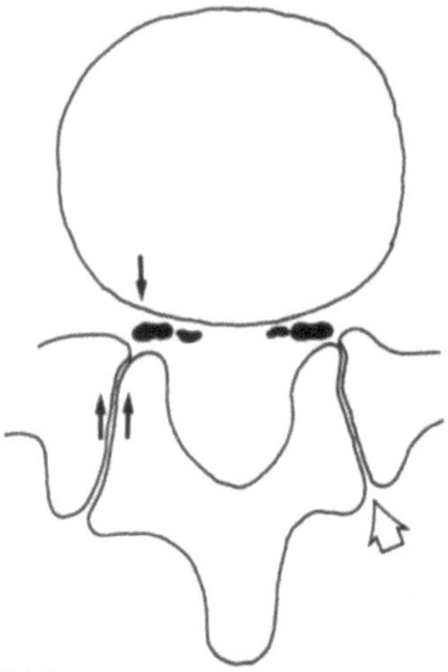

14.6a

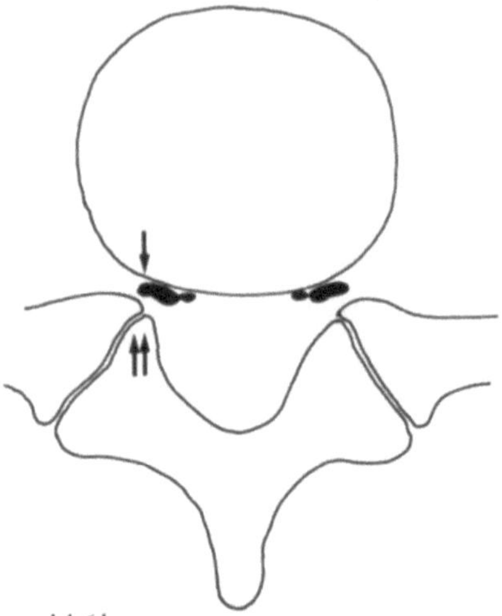

14.6b

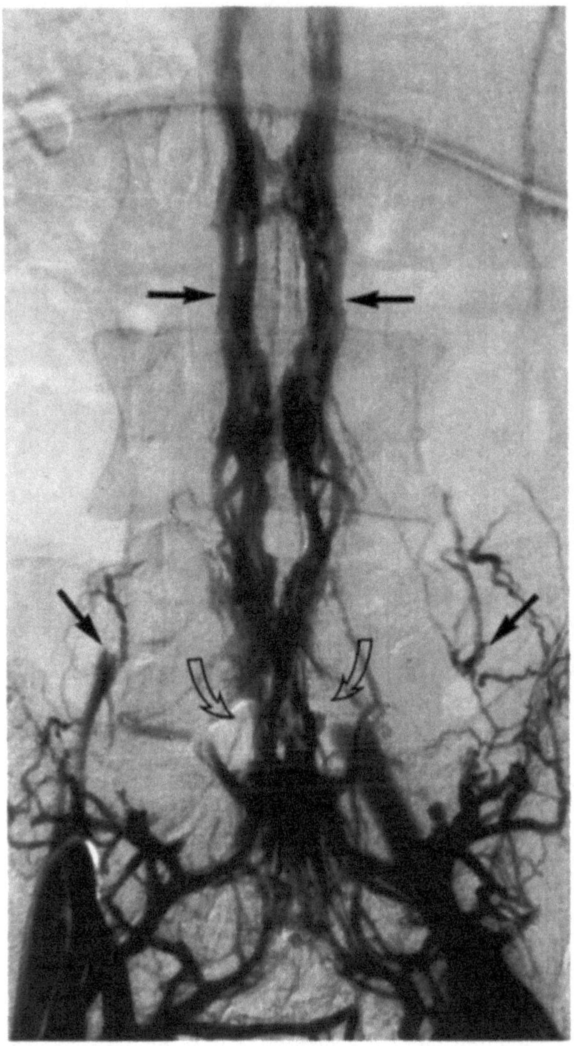

14.7

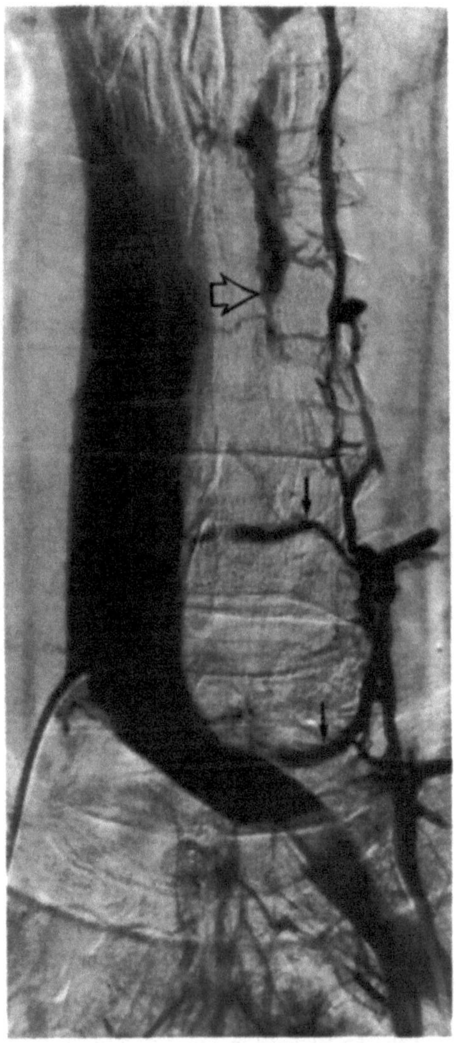

14.8

◁ Fig. 14.6a, b. Schematic drawing of the two types of narrow lumbar canal in a lumbar vertebra viewed from above. a Concentric stenosis characterized by hypertrophy of the posterior arch of the vertebra with sagittalization of the posterior articular facet interspace (✦). In this type of canal the epidural veins come closer to the midline (see Fig. 14.7). b AP stenosis of the lumbar canal. The reduction in diameter concerns mainly the lateral recesses. On the venogram the distance between the epidural veins and the midline seems normal. On account of this anomaly of the spine, any anterior (↗) (disk herniation, osteophytosis) or posterior (↗ ↗) (arthrosis of articular facets) lesion will determine more rapidly clinical symptoms than in a normal canal, and will interrupt the corresponding epidural veins. Other radiographic techniques (myelography, computerized tomography) will allow to differentiate anterior and posterior compressions since venography shows only venous interruption in both cases

◁ Fig. 14.7. Concentric narrow lumbar canal with bilateral L5-S1 disk herniation. The lumbar venogram shows abnormal epidural veins which are close to each other in the lateral recesses (distance between the two horizontal arrows). This feature suggests a concentric type narrow canal (see Fig. 14.6a). There is also a bilateral interruption of the lateral epidural vein (↘) at the L5-S1 level, corresponding to a bilateral disk herniation. Clinical symptoms have probably occurred more rapidly due to the congenital narrowness of the lumbar canal. The ascending lumbar veins are atrophic and replaced by an irregular venous network (*oblique closed arrows*). These features are due to the narrowness of the lateral recesses impeding the venous exchanges between the intra- and extraspinal venous systems

◁ Fig. 14.8. Narrow lumbar canal due to multiple disk protrusions. Lumbar venography shows absence of opacification of the intraspinal epidural veins at the level of the last three lumbar vertebrae. The venous flow is diverted from the ascending lumbar vein toward the inferior vena cava via the dilated lumbar veins (↗). The epidural veins are normally opacified from the upper aspect of L3 (↗). The extent of epidural space compression is thus precisely determined. Also, the area where decompression should be performed is determined, in case laminectomy were considered. These features are also encountered in severe concentric stenoses in young people. Venography has however no specific character and does not allow to rule out extensive compression of the epidural space by an intraspinal tumor (see Fig. 14.9). Additional myelography must be performed

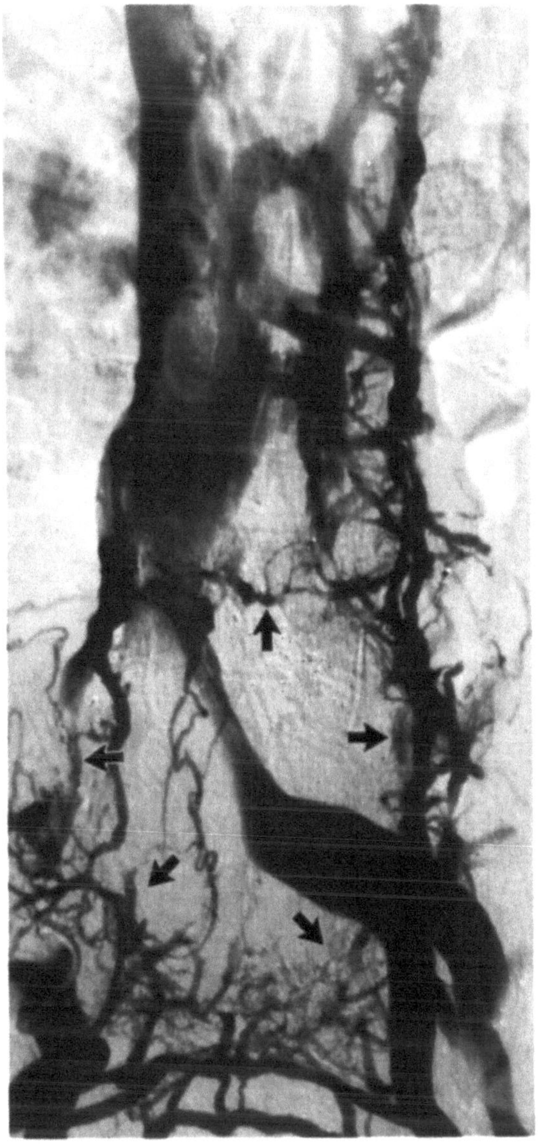

14.9

14.9

Fig. 14.9. Tumor of the sacral spinal canal. Venography shows interruption of the epidural and extraspinal veins, and delimits accurately (➘) the intra- and extra-spinal extension of the tumor

Subject Index

W. Wenz

Abdominal Angiography

In collaboration with G. van Kaick, D. Beduhn, F.-J. Roth

1974. 183 figures, some in color, comprising 351 radiographs and 34 drawings. VIII, 217 pages
ISBN 3-540-06508-3
Distribution rights for Japan: Igaku Shoin Ltd., Tokyo

G. B. Bradač, R. Oberson

Angiography in Cerebro-Arterial Occlusive Diseases

Including Computer Tomography and Radionuclide Methods
With a Foreword by A. Wackenheim

1979. 144 figures in 341 separate illustrations. IX, 228 pages
ISBN 3-540-08898-9
Distribution rights for Japan: Igaku Shoin Ltd., Tokyo

R. Djindjian, J.-J. Merland

Super-Selective Arteriography of the External Carotid Artery

With collaboration of J. Théron
Translated from the French by I. F. Moseley
Preface by R. Houdart

1978. 1068 figures, 5 plates, some in color. XVI, 550 pages
ISBN 3-540-08118-6

I. Yaghmai

Angiography of Bone and Soft Tissue Lesions

1979. 183 figures (689 separate illustrations). XI, 459 pages
ISBN 3-540-09147-5

J. Théron, J. Moret

Spinal Phlebography

Lumbar and Cervical Techniques
With a foreword by R. Djindjian
With the collaboration of D. Dilenge, J. P. Houtteville and H. Ammerich, P. Blanchot, D. Chevalier, A. Chevrot, J. F. Ginestic, D. Larde, L. Picard, J. Roland, J. Vignaud

1978. 113 figures in 182 separate illustrations, 1 table. XI, 165 pages
ISBN 3-540-08867-9

Springer-Verlag
Berlin
Heidelberg
New York

MIX
Papier aus verantwortungsvollen Quellen
Paper from responsible sources
FSC® C105338

If you have any concerns about our products,
you can contact us on
ProductSafety@springernature.com

In case Publisher is established outside the EU,
the EU authorized representative is:
Springer Nature Customer Service Center GmbH
Europaplatz 3, 69115 Heidelberg, Germany

Printed by Libri Plureos GmbH
in Hamburg, Germany